*…d or renewed on or before the*

*Recent.*

# Anaesthesia and in____Care

**22**

# *Recent Advances in*
# Anaesthesia and Intensive Care

*Edited by*

**A.P. Adams** MB BS, MRCS, LRCP, PhD, DA, FRCA, FANZCA
Emeritus Professor of Anaesthetics
University of London
Honorary Consultant Anaesthetist
Guy's, King's and St Thomas' Hospitals
London, UK
Emeritus Consultant to the Army

**J.N. Cashman** BSc, MB BS, BA, MD, FRCA
Consultant Anaesthetist, St George's Hospital, London
Honorary Senior Lecturer in Anaesthesia
University of London, UK

**R.M. Grounds** MB BS, MRCS, LRCP, MD, DA, FRCA
Consultant in Anaesthesia and Intensive Care Medicine
St George's Hospital, London
Honorary Reader in Intensive Care Medicine
University of London, UK

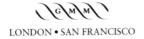

LONDON • SAN FRANCISCO

**\(G\M\M\)**

www.greenwich-medical.co.uk

© 2003
Greenwich Medical Media Limited
137 Euston Road
London
NW1 2AA

870 Market Street, Ste 720
San Francisco
CA 94102

ISBN 1 84110 1176

First Published 2003

Typeset by Mizpah Publishing Services, Chennai, India

Printed in the UK by the Alden Group Ltd, Oxford

Distributed by Plymbridge Distributors Ltd and in the USA by Jamco Distribution

# Contents

# Preface

*"An intellectual is a man
who takes more words than necessary
to tell more than he knows."*
Dwight D. Eisenhower (1890–1969)

In 1932 J & A Churchill Ltd published the first edition of *Recent Advances in Anaesthesia and Analgesia (Including Oxygen Therapy)*. Nearly 70 years later we commented in the Preface to the Millennium (21st) edition of *Recent Advances in Anaesthesia and Analgesia* that the pace of advances in anaesthesia showed no sign of abating. Although 2 years further on this statement remains true, change has now affected the title as well. Harcourt Publishers Ltd has transferred the title from Churchill Livingstone to Greenwich Medical Media Ltd. Coincident with the transfer it was decided to include more Intensive Care Medicine topics and consequently the title has been changed to *Recent Advances in Anaesthesia and Intensive Care*. In association with this change, we are pleased that Dr Michael Grounds has joined the editorial team.

The range of topics covered in this issue represent all aspects of anaesthesia from basic science to clinical practice, from training the anaesthetists of the future to relevant medical conditions, from optimization of patients to resuscitation of patients. As always, the editors are grateful to the many distinguished colleagues who have contributed to *Recent Advances in Anaesthesia and Intensive Care – 22*. The first three chapters present developments in pharmacology. It is now appreciated that there are two related, but unique isoforms, of the cyclo-oxygenase (COX) enzyme, which play important but different physiological and pathophysiological roles. An understanding of the differences between COX-1 and COX-2 is necessary for the logical development of new anti-inflammatory drugs. In their chapter on *The COX Enzyme System*, Dr Bishop-Bailey and Prof. Warner clearly elucidate these differences and their significance. Over recent years, drug stereochemistry has become a topic of considerable interest, with much discussion on the relative merits of using single isomer versus racemic mixtures of chiral drugs. Advances in chiral technology permit the commercial synthesis of single-isomer compounds. Dr Hutt considers the relevance of drug chirality to anaesthesia. With all of this interest in drug stereochemistry it is probably no surprise that chirality has been important in the development of new local anaesthetic agents. In his chapter on *New Local Anaesthetics*, Dr McLeod describes in detail recent advances in molecular biology with respect to nerve conduction as well as concepts of the method of action of local anaesthetics; he discusses both levobupivacaine and ropivacaine in detail.

The prevalence of asthma in society has increased dramatically over the past 30 years and at the same time the death rate has also been increasing alarmingly. Drs Cormican and Rees suggest that the reasons for the increase in the prevalence of atopy are still poorly understood, although a number of explanations have been proposed. They describe current understanding with regard to the epidemiology, genetics and immunopathology of asthma as well as discussing the implication of asthma for anaesthetists. In his chapter on reducing mortality and complications in high-risk surgical patients, Dr Grounds emphasizes that over the last quarter of a century the incidence of death following surgery, that is directly attributable to anaesthesia, has fallen. He suggests that deaths and complications after operation can nevertheless be reduced further in high-risk patients by the implementation of early aggressive goal-directed therapy aimed at temporarily improving the cardiovascular performance of these patients.

In the next chapter on an intensive care medicine topic, Prof. Gattinoni with Drs Chiumello and Pelosi argue the merits of prone position lung ventilation in patients with acute lung injury or the adult respiratory distress syndrome. They review the pathophysiology related to the prone position, the mechanisms for improving gas exchange and the existing clinical data on the use of prone position ventilation in patients with this spectrum of lung damage. Antibiotic resistance is a source of increasing concern, particularly among patients in the intensive care unit. In their chapter on *Antibiotics and Nosocomial Infection in the Intensive Care Unit*, Prof. Chastre and Dr Trouillet point out that the excess hospital costs due to antimicrobial resistance may reach tens of billions of dollars a year in the United States of America. They discuss the root cause of the problem and the core issues and suggest that apparently adequate control strategies are unlikely to succeed without clear strategic objectives.

*Neuropathic Pain*, as Drs Petrenko, Yamakura, Baba and Prof. Shimoji point out, is a formidable syndrome that complicates a variety of disease states. They describe the current understanding of the pathophysiology of neuropathic pain, in particular ectopic hyperexcitability and abnormal sodium channels, as well as central sensitization and NMDA receptor activation. Dr Petrenko and colleagues then consider in detail the clinical presentations and treatment of neuropathic pain states.

In *Managing Medical Mishaps: Learning lessons from industry*, Drs Parker and Lawton outline the factors that influence the likelihood of medical failure and how other safety-critical high-risk industries have tackled the problem of error. They stress the importance of moving from a person-centred approach towards a systems approach encompassing the basic premise that human beings are fallible and that errors will always be made. Nevertheless as Ms Hallinan and Dr Davies point out, anaesthesia today is remarkably safe, probably as a result of the high standards of training and of equipment. In their chapter on *Legal Issues in Anaesthesia and Intensive Care*, the principles behind legal actions for clinical negligence are reviewed together with a discussion of the issues of consent and criminal liability. Anaesthetists are involved in education and training both at an undergraduate and at a post-graduate level. As educational concepts continue to evolve, Drs Stanley and Cashman have reviewed the objectives and strategy for training anaesthetists for the future, and the objective of ensuring life-long learning within the profession. Finally, we make no apology for returning to the fast evolving subject of resuscitation. Not many years ago, the Royal College of Physicians of London stated that all persons involved in direct patient contact should be familiar with the latest resuscitation techniques. Drs Binns and Rowland have compiled a comprehensive review of the latest in resuscitation technology, including the most recent evidence on the beneficial effect of hypothermia in improving outcome after cardiac arrest.

*Recent Advances in Anaesthesia and Intensive Care* is committed to keeping anaesthetists abreast of the very latest developments in our specialty. The editors trust that the reader will find the chapters in this issue as stimulating and interesting as they themselves have done.

London                                                                                    A.P.A
September 2002                                                                          J.N.C
                                                                                        R.M.G

# Contributors

**Professor Hiroshi Baba**
Professor
Department of Anesthesiology
Niigata University School of Medicine
Niigata, Japan

**Dr Helen Binns**
Specialist Registrar in Cardiology
Department of Cardiology
St George's Hospital
London, UK

**Dr David Bishop-Bailey**
British Heart Foundation Basic Science Lecturer
Queen Mary University of London
London, UK

**Professor Jean Chastre**
Professor of Medicine
University of Paris
Assistant Director, MICU
Institut de Cardiologie
Groupe Hospitalier Pitié Salpêtrière
Paris, France

**Dr Davide Chiumello**
Ospedale Maggiore di Milano
Milan, Italy

**Dr Liam Cormican**
Specialist Registrar
Guy's, King's and St Thomas' School of Medicine
London, UK

**Dr Nicholas J.H. Davies**
Consultant Anaesthetist
Southampton University Hospitals NHS Trust
Southampton, UK

**Professor Luciano Gattinoni**
Universita di Milano
Ospedale Maggiore di Milano
Milan, Italy

**Miss Emma Hallinan**
Manager, Claims and Legal Services
Medical Protection Society
London, UK

**Dr Andrew J. Hutt**
Lecturer in Pharmaceutical Chemistry
Department of Pharmacy
King's College London
London, UK

**Dr Rebecca Lawton**
Lecturer
Department of Psychology
University of Leeds
Leeds, UK

**Dr Graeme A. McLeod**
Consultant and Senior Lecturer in Anaesthesia
Ninewells Hospital and Medical School
Dundee, UK

**Dr Dianne Parker**
Senior Lecturer
Department of Psychology
University of Manchester
Manchester, UK

**Professor Paolo Pelosi**
Universita dell'Insubria
Ospedale Circolo
Varese, Italy

**Dr Andrei B. Petrenko**
Research Fellow
Department of Anesthesiology
Niigata University School of Medicine
Niigata, Japan

**Dr John Rees**
Senior Lecturer and Consultant Physician
Guy's, King's and St Thomas' School of Medicine
London, UK

**Dr Edward Rowland**
Consultant Cardiologist
St George's Hospital
London, UK

**Professor Koki Shimoji**
Professor Emeritus
Department of Anesthesiology
Niigata University School of Medicine
Niigata, Japan

**Dr Glynne D. Stanley**
Assistant Professor and Director of Residency Education
Department of Anesthesiology
Boston University Medical Center
Boston, USA

**Dr Jean-Louis Trouillet**
Service de Réanimation Médicale
Institut de Cardiologie
Groupe Hospitalier Pitié Salpêtrière
Paris, France

**Professor Timothy D. Warner**
Head, Department of Vascular Inflammation Research
Queen Mary University of London
London, UK

**Dr Tomohiro Yamakura**
Lecturer
Department of Anesthesiology
Niigata University School of Medicine
Niigata, Japan

*D. Bishop-Bailey   T.D. Warner*

# The COX enzyme system

The cyclo-oxygenase (COX) enzymes are the target for inhibition by non-steroidal anti-inflammatory drugs (NSAIDs), such as aspirin, ibuprofen and indomethacin. By acting on COX enzymes, NSAIDs block the production of prostanoids, a large family of lipid mediators with diverse biological roles and activities. The inhibition of COX is known to account for both the majority of beneficial effects of NSAIDs, i.e. the anti-inflammatory and anti-pyretic actions, and their detrimental side-effects i.e. gastrointestinal toxicity. It is now established that COX exists in two distinct isoforms, a 'constitutive' COX-1 present in all tissues, and an 'inducible' COX-2, that is highly regulated upon cellular stress, and found at high levels within cells at inflammatory sites. For this reason, since its discovery, there has been a great impetus to discover groups of NSAIDs that selectively inhibit COX-2, thereby selectively blocking the inflammatory production of prostanoids without causing deleterious side-effects. This chapter aims to give an up to date review of the COX pathway, and its relevance to current NSAID therapies.

## COX Enzymes

### COX: the catalyst of prostaglandin and thromboxane production

COX catalyses the production of the unstable prostaglandin (PG) $H_2$, via initial production of $PGG_2$ (fig. 1). For this reason COX is also commonly termed PGH synthase, PGG/H synthase or prostaglandin endoperoxide synthase. $PGH_2$ is the precursor to all prostanoids, $PGD_2$, $PGE_2$, $PGF_{2\alpha}$, $PGI_2$ (prostacyclin), and thromboxane (TX) $A_2$, being the most commonly produced

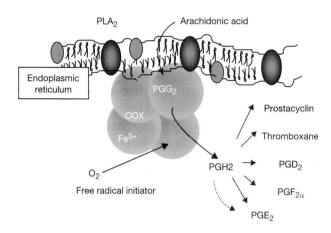

**Figure 1** COX catalyses the formation of $PGH_2$, the precursor of all prostanoids, from arachidonic acid.

in the body. COX is a particulate enzyme found in the microsomal fraction of all tissue types.[1] It is localised mainly in the endoplasmic reticulum, but is also found in the nuclear envelope and plasma membrane.[2,3] The catalytic site of COX is located in the cytosolic region of the protein.[4] Although COX can use the free fatty acids 8,11,14-eicosatrienoic acid and 5,8,11,14,17-eicosapenta-enoic acid as substrates, arachidonic acid (5,8,11,14-eicosatrienoic acid) is preferentially metabolised.[5] COX has two main catalytic components.[6,7] The first is a *bis*-oxygenase (a COX), which inserts two molecules of oxygen into the C20 carbon skeleton at C11 and C15 (forming a hydroperoxide group) of the arachidonic acid molecule. The resulting molecule, $PGG_2$, is a cyclopentane with an endoperoxide bridge. The second step, forming $PGH_2$, involves a hydroperoxidase, which reduces the C15-hydroperoxyl group to a hydroxyl. The *bis*-oxygenase and hydroperoxidase activities are distinct, but are catalysed by the same protein.[8] Both enzymic activities require the presence of a haem group ($Fe^{3+}$), and oxygen. Physiological inactivation of COX appears to be by two separate mechanisms:

a) the 'suicide' inactivation of the *bis*-oxygenase, and

b) inactivation of both enzymic activities by hydroperoxides.

Hydroperoxides, although required for COX activity, inactivate both catalytic centres, most likely through binding amino acids leading to conformational changes in the protein tertiary structure.[9]

## Formation of Arachidonic Acid

Arachidonic acid is an unsaturated 20 carbon chain (20 C: 4 double bonds) lipid usually found at the 2-acyl position of the membrane phospholipid.

Its liberation involves the activation of phospholipases,[10,11] mostly by direct action of phospholipase $A_2$ on phosphatidylcholine or phosphatidylethanolamine. However, arachidonic acid can also be formed through phospholipase D, or through phospholipase C and diacylglycerol lipase.[12] The free arachidonic acid can then either be utilised by a variety of metabolising enzymes, including COX, lipoxygenase or epoxygenase enzymes, or re-esterified back into the membrane lipids.[13] Phospholipase $A_2$ is considered the rate limiting enzyme for arachidonic acid and prostanoid production,[14] as well as another potent lipid mediator, platelet-activating factor.[15] Similar to COX, phospholipase $A_2$ exists in multiple isoforms (10 currently identified), which can be loosely classified into low molecular weight (14–18 kDa) secretory phospholipase $A_2$, high molecular weight (31–110 kDa) cytosolic phospholipase $A_2$ (cPLA$_2$)[16] and high molecular weight cytosolic calcium independent phospholipase $A_2$.[17] cPLA$_2$ isoenzymes are ubiquitously expressed, and preferentially cleave arachidonic acid containing phospholipids.[18] Moreover cPLA$_2$ have a lower requirement for $Ca^{2+}$ ($\mu$M) than phospholipase $A_2$ (mM).[19] Phospholipase $A_2$ are induced by cytokines such as interleukin-1 (IL-1),[20,21] and are mainly considered to act extracellularly.[22] cPLA$_2$ due to its low $Ca^{2+}$ requirements, its cytosolic location, and arachidonic acid substrate specificity has been considered the isoform that is most likely to link phospholipids to COX activity, under 'physiological' conditions.[18] Much less is known about the role of phospholipase $A_2$, though recent evidence suggests it may be involved in membrane phospholipid remodelling.[17]

Glucocorticoid steroids, such as dexamethasone, are potent anti-inflammatory agents that inhibit the actions of phospholipase $A_2$, and therefore inhibit eicosanoid/prostanoid production.[23] Glucocorticoids induce the synthesis of lipocortin-1, a $Ca^{2+}$/lipid binding protein that prevents the access of phospholipase $A_2$ to substrate phospholipids.[24]

## COX Exists in Constitutive and Inducible Isoforms

The hypothesis that multiple isoforms existed in the COX pathway was initially suggested by Flower and Vane.[25] In different organ homogenates they observed that the formation of prostanoids had different sensitivities to inhibition by NSAIDs, and acetaminophen (paracetamol). Further investigation into enzyme turnover rates also suggested the existence of different 'pools' of COX,[26] although not distinguished into structurally different isoforms.

COX-1 was first purified from sheep vesicular glands,[6] and was subsequently shown in the denatured state to have a molecular weight of approximately 70 kDa. The COX-1 protein from this tissue was not cloned and

**Table 1** Inducers of COX-2

| Cell Type | Reference | Inducers |
|---|---|---|
| Fibroblast (Chicken embryo) | 28 | rous sarcoma virus |
| Fibroblast (Swiss 3T3) | 29 | IL-1 |
| Human umbilical vein endothelial cells (HUVEC) | 27 | IL-1 |
| Monocyte (human) | 31 | IL-1 |
| Epithelial (lung human) | 32 | IL-1 |
| Smooth muscle (human vascular) | 33 | IL-1 |
| Smooth muscle (rat aorta) | 34 | PDGF, TGF-β, IL-1 |
| Mast cell (Mmmc-34) | 35 | IgG/antigen |

expressed until 12 years later.[1] The cDNA encoded a 2.8 kb mRNA which translated a protein with an approximate molecular weight of 66 kDa. Little is still known of how COX-1 is regulated, although small changes in mRNA levels (approximately three fold increase) was seen in phorbol 12-myrostrate 13-acetate-treated human umbilical vein endothelial cells (HUVEC).[27]

Soon after the cloning and expressing of COX-1, a novel lipopolysaccharide/cytokine-inducible isoform of COX (COX-2) was described,[28,29] which unlike its constitutive (constitutive COX: COX-1) counterpart, is regulated by glucocorticoids.[30] Table 1 gives an example of the cell types expressing COX-2 and agents that induce its activity.

Agents that have now been demonstrated to induce COX-2 also include tumour growth factor-β (TGF-β), forskolin, colony stimulating factor-1,[36] hormones such as progesterone, or luteinising hormone (rat granulosa cells[37]), bacterial lipopolysaccharide (macrophage[38]), phorbol ester (rat intestinal epithelial[39]), endothelin-1 (rat mesangial[40]), 5-HT (rat mesangial[41]), lysophosphatidylcholine (human umbilical vein endothelial cells[42]) and laminar shear stress (human umbilical vein endothelial cells[43]). In fact, almost without exception it is possible to induce COX-2 with at least one stimulus in any nucleated cell.

## Comparison of COX-2 vs. COX-1

The COX-2 gene is an immediate-early response gene,[44] a type of gene associated with control of the cell growth cycle. The COX-2 gene was identified in chicken embryo fibroblasts transformed by rous sarcoma virus (initially termed CEF-147[28]), and as an already discovered gene product (initially termed TIS10 early response gene) in phorbol ester treated Swiss 3T3 fibroblasts.[29] The cDNA for CEF-147 and TIS10 coded 4.1 kb and 3.9 kb mRNA products, respectively. The coding and expression of cDNA for a functional COX-2 has now been shown in mouse fibroblasts, human monocytes[31] and human umbilical vein endothelial cells.[27] COX-1 and COX-2 show about 60% homology at both the cDNA and amino acid level, the structural and enzymic components being the most highly conserved. The main difference in polypeptide structures is a longer N-terminal sequence of COX-1[37], and a 18 amino acid cassette in the C-terminus of COX-2.[27-29] However it is not clear, whether these differences serve any functional purpose.

The crystal structures of COX-1 and COX-2 indicate that they are virtually superimposable.[45] The genomic DNA and cDNA for COX-1 and COX-2 have now been isolated. COX-1 has 11 exons while COX-2 has only 10. The main differences occur in the 5′ flanking promoter region, which confer regulatory elements including binding sites for CAAT/enhancer binding protein, a TATA box, two activation protein-2 sites, three nuclear factor (NF)κB sites, cyclic adenosine monophosphate (cAMP) response element and Ets-1.[46] Furthermore, the gene encodes a large number of AU repeats in the 3′ untranslated region giving rise to the characteristic instability of the mRNA, seen with other early response genes.[46] Indeed, part of the mechanism of induction by IL-1α and IL-1β is considered to be stabilisation of the COX-2 mRNA,[47] while one of the actions of the glucocorticosteroids such as dexamethasone may be to reduce COX-2 protein expression by destabilising mRNA.[48]

Although the catalytic actions[45] and substrate use[49] of COX-1 and COX-2 are virtually identical, several differences have been demonstrated in substrate requirement and product formation. For example, COX-2 requires 10-fold less hydroperoxide activator for function.[50] In this respect, in a system where both COX-1 and COX-2 are present, it is possible that only COX-2 may be active.[50]

## Prostanoid Biosynthesis

$PGH_2$ is an unstable moiety, and is further converted enzymically and non-enzymically into the family of prostanoids. The main bioactive prostanoids produced are $PGI_2$, $PGE_2$, $PGF_{2\alpha}$, $PGD_2$ and $TXA_2$, the actions of which are summarised in table 2. The release of specific prostanoid metabolites from individual cell types depends on the relative abundance of their respective synthases; the actions of which are summarised in the following sections.

### PGI2 biosynthesis
$PGI_2$ was discovered in 1976, as a factor isolated from bovine aorta, with smooth muscle relaxant and anti-platelet properties.[51] Although produced in

**Table 2** Bioactivity of the prostanoids

| Metabolite | $PGI_2$ | $PGE_2$ | $PGF_{2\alpha}$ | $TXA_2$ | $PGD_2$ |
|---|---|---|---|---|---|
| Vascular | Vasodilation<br>Decrease blood pressure | Vasodilation<br>Decrease blood pressure | Vasoconstriction or vasodilation | Vasoconstriction<br>Increase BP | |
| Platelet | Anti-aggregation | Anti-aggregation | | Platelet aggregation | Anti-aggregation |
| Lung | Bronchodilation | Bronchodilation | Bronchoconstriction | | |
| Pain | Hyperalgesia | Hyperalgesia | | | Nociception<br>Hypothermia |
| Others | Decrease gastric secretion<br>Cytoprotection<br>Decrease cell proliferation<br>Anti-lipidaemic | Decrease gastric secretion<br>Cytoprotection<br>Decrease cell proliferation<br>Anti-lipidaemic | Constriction of gut and uterine smooth muscle<br>Luteolysis<br>ACh release | Lymphocyte proliferation<br>Increase cell profileration | Anti-convulsive<br>Sleep induction<br>Decrease LH release |

the smooth muscle, the majority of $PGI_2$ production is endothelium derived, due to the high levels of COX and $PGI_2$ synthase in this tissue. $PGI_2$ has a physiological half-life of 2–3 min[52] due to rapid hydrolysis to 6-keto $PGF_{1\alpha}$, a more stable product with very little biological activity, often used as an index for $PGI_2$ release.

### $PGE_2$ biosynthesis

$PGE_2$ can be synthesised via both enzymic and non-enzymic pathways,[12] both of which having degrees of glutathione dependency. Rat liver glutathione-S-transferases has PGE synthase activity,[53] while distinct PGH-PGE isomerases have also been isolated in bovine[54] and ovine vesicular glands.[55] However, high concentrations of glutathione alone can also cause the isomerisation from $PGH_2$ to $PGE_2$ non-enzymically. Recently a cytokine-inducible, glutathione-dependent, particulate PGE synthase has been identified, which may be functionally coupled to the induction of COX-2.[56]

### $PGF_{2\alpha}$ biosynthesis

PGF synthase[12] has two active sites, converting $PGH_2$ and $PGD_2$ to $PGF_{2\alpha}$ and 11-*epi*-$PGF_{2\alpha}$ respectively. The reaction is a reduction process requiring NADPH for the catalysis.

### $PGD_2$ biosynthesis

There appears to be atleast three different proteins capable of PGD synthase activity, which have been purified from the soluble fractions of rat spleen, liver and brain.[12] The enzymes purified from spleen[57] and liver[53] show glutathione-S-transferase activity, the catalysis of $PGD_2$ also being glutathione-dependent. The $PGD_2$ synthase purified from rat brain[58] (often also referred to as β-trace) is glutathione-independent, the cDNA codes for a 20 kDa protein with sequence homology to a set of transporter proteins, the lipocalin family.[59]

### $TXA_2$ biosynthesis

$TXA_2$ synthase has been purified[60] and cloned,[61] and like $PGI_2$ synthase is a cytochrome P-450 enzyme. $TXA_2$ is the major COX metabolite in platelets, where it was initially discovered.[62] It has a relatively short physiological half-life of approximately 30 s, and like $PGI_2$, is rapidly hydrolysed to a stable inactive metabolite, $TXB_2$.[63,64]

## Prostanoid receptors and second messenger systems

Molecular characterisation indicates that these receptors all belong to the family of seven transmembrane domain linked G-protein receptors. Table 3 is a brief summary of the classification of prostanoid receptors modified from the International Union of Pharmacology Classification of Prostanoid Receptors: Properties, Distribution, and Structure of the receptors and their subtypes.[65]

**Table 3** Characterisation of prostanoid receptors

| | Agonists | Distribution | 2nd messenger |
|---|---|---|---|
| $EP_1$ | $PGE_2$, iloprost, sulprostone | smooth muscle, myometrium | Increase in intracellular $Ca^{2+}$ via $G_{q/11}$, and phosphoinositol turnover |
| $EP_2$ | $PGE_2$, butaprost, misoprostol | Smooth muscle, epithelial cells (non acid secretions), mast cells, basophils, sensory afferent neurons | cAMP through stimulation of adenyl cyclase through $G_s$ |
| $EP_3$ | $PGE_2$, enprostil, sulprostone, misoprostol | Smooth muscle, autonomic nerves, adipocytes, gastric mucosa (acid secretion), renal medulla (water reabsorption) | At least six splice variants of $EP_3$ receptors have been identified linked to either inhibition ($G_{i/o}$) or activation ($G_s$) of adenyl cyclase, and increase in intracellular $Ca^{2+}$ via $G_{q/11}$, involving PI turnover |
| $EP_4$ | $PGE_2$ (other agonists weak), recently discovered and very little information available | Piglet saphenous vein smooth muscle (rabbit saphenous and jugular veins, rat trachea, and hamster uterus | cAMP through stimulation of adenyl cyclase through $G_s$ |
| IP | $PGI_2$, iloprost, cicaprost | platelets, vascular smooth muscle, sensory afferent neurones | cAMP through stimulation of adenyl cyclase through $G_s$ |
| $EP_2$ | $TXA_2$, $STA_2$, u46619 | platelets, arterial and venous vascular smooth muscle, airway smooth muscle, gastrointestinal epithelial cells, mesangial cells, myofibroblasts | Increase in intracellular $Ca^{2+}$ via $G_{q/11}$, involving activation of PLC and phosphoinositol turnover |
| FP receptors | $PGF_{2\alpha}$, fluprostenol | corpus luteum, iris, myometrium | increase in intracellular $Ca^{2+}$ via $G_{q/11}$, involving PLC activation and phosphoinositol turnover |
| DP receptors | $PGD_2$, 9-deoxy-$\Delta^9$-$PGD_2$ | Platelets, vascular smooth muscle, non-vascular smooth muscle, CNS | cAMP through stimulation of adenyl cyclase through $G_s$ |

## Peroxisome proliferator activated receptors (PPAR)

Peroxisome proliferator activated receptors are a family of three nuclear receptor/transcription factors termed PPARα, PPARδ(β), and PPARγ. Recently, the $PGD_2$ dehydration product 15-deoxy-$\Delta^{12,14}$-$PGJ_2$ was shown to activate the nuclear receptor PPARγ, promoting differentiation of fibroblasts into adipocytes,[66,67] indicating the possibility of a new intracellular receptor pathway on which COX- metabolites may exert their effects.[68] Subsequently, 15-deoxy-$\Delta^{12,14}$-$PGJ_2$ and $PGI_2$ have been shown to activate PPARα, and PPARδ.[68]

## Functional Studies

The roles of COX enzymes have been studied by a variety of methods. Outlined below are examples from animal studies using genetic knockout experiments, and animal and clinical studies using pharmacological inhibitors.

## Studies with Knockout Mice

In mice it is possible to selectively remove genes by a process called homologous recombination. This gene 'knockout' procedure can give extremely important information on the role of the particular gene studied. Both COX-1 and COX-2 have been successfully disrupted in mice. COX-1 knockout mice appear normal apart from their ability to produce viable offspring. The genetic disruption of COX-2 in mice appears to have more severe consequences, with effects being noted on the formation of nephrons, the heart, and female fertility (see table 4).

Table 4 Summary of the major findings in studies describing COX-1[69] and COX-2[70,71] knockout mice

| COX-1 knockout | COX-2 knockout |
|---|---|
| Good survival | Poor neonatal survival |
| No gastro-pathology | Chronic nephropathology |
| Reduced indomethacin induced gastric ulceration | Poorly developing nephrons Peritonitis |
| Reduced platelet aggregation | No reduction in TPA induced ear swelling |
| Decreased inflammatory response to AA | Responses to AA unchanged |
| No viable offspring | Females largely infertile |
| | Myocardial fibrosis |
| | Decreased TNF induced hepatocyte Necrosis |

## Inhibition of Prostanoid Biosynthesis: NSAIDs and COX-2 Inhibitors

The main therapeutic uses of the NSAID inhibitors of prostanoid biosynthesis are in inflammation and mild-to-moderate pain.[72] Elevated concentrations of prostanoids have been observed in almost all forms of human acute and chronic inflammatory conditions studied. $PGE_2$ and $PGI_2$ at physiological levels do not appear to directly cause oedema formation and pain, but strongly synergise with directly acting pro-inflammatory mediators, such as bradykinin and histamine to cause plasma exudation[73] and pain.[74] Furthermore, $PGE_2$ is also a potent pyrogenic factor.[75]

## NSAIDs – Non-selective COX Inhibitors

In 1971, Vane showed that aspirin, indomethacin and salicylate all inhibited COX activity.[76] Since then, three different mechanisms of inhibition have been described for the action of NSAIDs on COX:

1. aspirin is unique, as it irreversibly inhibits COX by acetylation of hydroxyl groups on serine residues, $Ser_{530}$ – acetylation results in inactivation of the *bis*-oxygenase activity.[77] Aspirin is also metabolised to the anti-inflammatory salicylate;

2. compounds including ibuprofen and salicylate act as reversible competitive inhibitors of the arachidonic acid binding site of COX;[78] while

3. compounds, including indomethacin-like drugs, non-competitively inhibit COX in a time-dependent manner, without covalent modification of the enzyme.[78]

It is also very important to note that the NSAIDs are of different chemical classes, and even within the same class can have different structures and properties; so in clinical usage one must also consider these physico-chemical properties (e.g. many NSAIDs are acidic), pharmacodynamic factors, which give rise to vastly different plasma half lives, binding to plasma proteins, plasma clearance and routes of excretion.

## The COX-2 Inhibitor Hypothesis

Most of the traditionally used NSAIDs are considered relatively safe drugs. The most common adverse reactions for NSAID users are gastrointestinal complications ranging from dyspepsia (at least 10–20%), to severe gastrointestinal complications (approximately 1%), of which there is a mortality rate of 4–10% per year.[79] However, due to the vast usage of these compounds throughout the world (the equivalent of 120 billion 300 mg doses of aspirin alone are consumed each year) this low incidence of severe events still equates to a very large amount of affected people.

Though the acidic chemical nature of many of the NSAIDs may account for some of the damaging effects seen[80] it is likely that most adverse events of NSAIDs occur through inhibition of COX activity. At best the traditional NSAIDs are equipotent inhibitors of COX-1 and COX-2 but many show selectivity towards the inhibition of COX-1.[81–83] Since COX-2 is thought to be responsible for prostanoid production associated with deleterious events in pathology, and COX-1 products for beneficial 'house-keeping' roles, most effort has centred on the development of COX-2 selective inhibitors for the treatment of musculoskeletal disorders such as osteoarthritis (OA) and rheumatoid arthritis (RA), as well as pain.

### Selective COX-2 inhibitors: experimental findings

A number of selective COX-2 inhibitors have been described over the last 10 years. It is important to note that the degree of selectivity for COX-2 vastly varies upon the assay system used,[83] making it difficult to state unequivocally what relative effects these drugs have on COX-1 and COX-2 *in vivo*. However what is generally common to all the assay systems tested, is that when comparing the relative selectivities of compounds between assays the rank orders of selectivities usually look very similar.

Mechanistically the actions of the inhibitors displaying selectivity towards COX-2 fall into two groups.

- The 'coxib' class which act in a manner similar to that of indomethacin, causing competitive, time-dependent inhibition of COX-2.[84–86] The mechanism by which these compounds work is by utilising their ability to access the hydrophobic arachidonic binding site of COX-2 due to the amino acid difference of isoleucine$_{509}$ (COX-1) to valine$_{509}$ (COX-2[87]).

- Meloxicam which is a competitive inhibitor of COX-2. Meloxicam modelled by crystal structure analysis within COX-2 fits within an additional flexible extra space created by the change at isoleucine$_{434}$ (COX-1) to valine$_{434}$ (COX-2), allowing it longer-term access. Other common NSAID/arachidonic acid binding sites such as Arg$_{120}$, near the mouth of the entrance into the active catalytic centre are not different between COX-1 and COX-2.[88]

Some of the earliest generated selective COX-2 inhibitors, such as NS-398,[89,90] L-745,337[91] and SC58125[92] were used for laboratory based studies and shown in various models to be anti-inflammatory without causing gastrointestinal lesions. This research led to the discovery of a number of compounds with COX-2 selectivity suitable for clinical use, e.g. celecoxib (Celebrex®), and rofecoxib (Vioxx®). Other compounds such as meloxicam (Mobic®), which also displays COX-2 selectivity, was discovered in earlier times through the pharmacological pursuit of compounds displaying anti-inflammatory activity but a reduced ability to promote gastrointestinal damage.

*Clinical use of NSAIDs*

Experience following the clinical use of NSAIDs and COX-2 inhibitors together with experimental animal and cell culture studies, has given us a great deal of information about the functional roles of COX-1 and COX-2 within the human body. Clinically traditional NSAIDs and COX-2-selective inhibitors are most widely used for the treatment of inflammation and pain. Use of NSAIDs, and to a lesser extent COX-2-selective inhibitors, is most commonly associated with gastrointestinal and cardiovascular side-effects, and less commonly with renal and reproductive complications. The functions of the COX-1 and COX-2 enzymes that may explain these drugs' beneficial and detrimental effects are discussed in detail below.

## Roles of COX Enzymes

### Inflammation and pain – experimental perspective

The classical signs of inflammation are heat (calor), redness (rubor), swelling (tumour) and pain (dolor) and loss of function. Prostaglandins can contribute to all these stages of the inflammatory response. Indeed, $PGE_2$ has been implicated as one of the major mediators in inflammation;[93] $PGE_2$ promotes local vasodilation within the microcirculation and so promotes oedema and erythema (calor, rubor, tumor), and although not directly pain-producing it also causes hyperalgesia (dolor). $PGE_2$ is also a potent pyrogenic mediator. Although NSAIDs have little effect on the allergic responses $PGD_2$ is also released peripherally by mast cells, and may therefore contribute to the inflammatory milieu of hypersensitivity type reactions.

Although COX-1 is likely to be involved in acute inflammatory responses, COX-2 is the major enzyme responsible for the production of chronic inflammatory prostanoids. Inflammatory mediators induce high levels of COX-2 protein, and prostanoid release, while COX-1 concentrations remain relatively stable. Furthermore, COX-2 is expressed in chronic inflammatory lesions in both animal models and human beings.[94]

### Inflammation and pain: clinical perspective

NSAIDs are clinically efficacious for the symptomatic treatment of osteoarthritis, rheumatoid arthritis and pain. The choice of NSAID is commonly a matter of patient preference due to tolerance, rather than any generalised comparative efficacy. Clinical trials have been performed to establish the efficacy of COX-2-selective inhibitors in osteoarthritis, rheumatoid arthritis and pain (tooth extraction).[95]

### Inflammation

Patients with osteoarthritis or rheumatoid arthritis are commonly recruited into these clinical trials after a flared response following withdrawal of their usual NSAID therapy. In osteoarthritis studies the patient or patient/physician assessment of global arthritis and/or level of pain shows that COX-2 inhibitors celecoxib (vs. naproxen[96]), rofecoxib (vs. ibuprofen[97]), or meloxicam (vs. diclofenac[98]) are as efficacious as compared with NSAIDs (in parentheses). Similar results have also been reported in trials of rheumatoid arthritis patients.

### Pain

A common clinical model to test the analgesic activity of these agents is their ability to reduce the pain following molar extraction. Analogous to the inflammation studies, celecoxib (vs. ibuprofen[99]), and rofecoxib (vs. ibuprofen[99–101]) are found to be at least as efficacious as traditional NSAIDs in time-to-effect, duration of effect, and overall analgesic effect.

### Fever

For fever studies, patients included were those with fever from a naturally occurring viral associated illness. Similar to previous discussed studies rofecoxib was as equi-active to ibuprofen when determining both time to effect or duration of reduction in the febrile response.[102]

Thus, many studies have now shown that COX-2 inhibitors are efficacious in the treatment of inflammation, pain and fever. The studies cited here were selected from this body of literature as they were all designed to allow comparisons between COX-2-selective inhibitors, and currently used non-selective NSAIDs, and a placebo. Currently in the USA rofecoxib is licensed for use in osteoarthritis and acute pain, celecoxib is licensed for osteoarthritis and rheumatoid arthritis, and meloxicam is licensed for osteoarthritis. It is clear that the new generation of COX-2-selective compounds are as efficacious as traditional NSAIDs on their therapeutic target areas.

### Gastrointestinal tract: experimental perspective

$PGE_2$ and $PGI_2$ released in the gastrointestinal tract reduce gastrointestinal gastric acid secretion, cause vasodilation of the gastric mucosa microcirculation, and stimulate protective mucus and bicarbonate secretion.[103] It is well established that traditional NSAIDs cause gastrointestinal damage, and this effect is often attributed to inhibition of PG production. COX-1 is found at high concentrations throughout the gastrointestinal tract, although there is now evidence for some expression of COX-2 in human gastric mucosa,[104] and so it is commonly held that it is inhibition of COX-1 that underlies the gastrointestinal toxicity of traditional NSAIDs. Indeed, there is generally a direct correlation between the selectivity of an NSAID for COX-1 and its ability to induce gastrointestinal damage.[83]

There are now several lines of evidence suggesting that although COX-1 is the most important isoform in gastrointestinal tract protection, it is a combination of inhibition of COX-1 and COX-2 that promotes damage. For example, in COX-1 deficient mice, in which gastric $PGE_2$ levels are decreased by 99%, no spontaneous ulcers were observed.[69] Moreover, if rats are treated with a selective COX-1 inhibitor no gastric damage is observed until the co-administration of a COX-2-selective inhibitor.[105] These observations suggest, in animal models at least, that in tissues such as the gastrointestinal tract where prostaglandins have protective effects it is not important which isoform of COX is responsible for their production. It may even be that inhibition of COX-1 promotes the expression of COX-2 to compensate for the lost prostanoids. Further evidence supports this idea of a protective role for COX-2 in the gastrointestinal tract, as COX-2 is also found at sites of gastric ulceration where it aids in the healing response. Similarly the administration of COX-2 inhibitors slows ulcer healing in animal models.[106–108]

*Gastrointestinal tract: clinical perspective*
The most common side-effects of NSAIDs are dyspepsia, and injury to the gastrointestinal mucosa. This injury in most patients is superficial, self-resolving, and goes mostly unnoticed. However, a number of serious adverse events can occur in a limited number of patients with NSAID use, these range from drug induced oesophagitis, small bowel ulceration, exacerbation of inflammatory bowel disease, and the formation or exacerbation of peptic ulcers, that may lead to perforation. Indeed, patients that have chronic arthritis, on long-term NSAIDs usage have 5–15 times the prevalence of gastric and duodenal ulcers compared to an age-matched healthy population.[79] The major risk factors associated with NSAID-induced gastropathy are increasing age, predisposition to ulcers, use of corticosteroids that also inhibit prostanoids production, dosage (i.e. the level of COX inhibition), concomitant use of anti-coagulants, and serious systemic disorders; possible other additive risks include, *H. pylori* infection, smoking, and alcohol consumption.[79,109] Additional therapies can be used concomitantly to prevent NSAID-induced gastropathy, including histamine $H_2$-receptor antagonists, proton-pump inhibitors, or the administration of a stable $PGE_2$ mimetic, misoprostol. The advantages of using a single COX-2-selective inhibitor rather than a traditional NSAID plus a gastrointestinal protective drug are

apparently clear. For example, as it is a single drug one should expect reduced side-effects compared to polypharmacy. Indeed, additional drugs though protecting the gastrointestinal tract can have their own adverse events associated.

As would be expected from the pre-clinical findings COX-2-selective inhibitors have appeared very promising in clinical use. All the COX-2 inhibitors tested at therapeutic dosing have been found not to affect gastric mucosal PG synthesis.[110,111] Similarly, very high dose of the COX-2 inhibitors rofecoxib or celecoxib do not cause a significant increase in acute mucosal injury compared to placebo.[112,113] Meloxicam caused slight mucosal injury, but was significantly lower than the comparator NSAID piroxicam.[111] In the majority of endoscopy and outcome trials rofecoxib and celecoxib have had significantly reduced occurrence of GI events including ulcers. The largest of these were the VIGOR (Vioxx Gastrointestinal Outcomes Research Study) and CLASS (Celecoxib Long-term Arthritis Safety Study) trials, the findings of which are summarised below.

## The VIGOR and CLASS Studies

The VIGOR trial[114] included 8,067 rheumatoid arthritis patients to study clinically significant or complicated GI events with rofecoxib compared to naproxen. Concomitant use of aspirin was not allowed. Rofecoxib and naproxen had similar efficacy against rheumatoid arthritis. During a median follow-up of 9.0 months, 2.1 confirmed gastrointestinal events per 100 patient-years occurred with rofecoxib, as compared with 4.5 per 100 patient-years with naproxen. The rates of complicated confirmed events (perforation, obstruction, and severe upper gastrointestinal bleeding) were 0.6 per 100 patient-years for rofecoxib compared to 1.4 per 100 patient-years for naproxen.

The CLASS trial[115] included 8,059 osteoarthritis or rheumatoid arthritis patients to study the incidence of symptomatic upper gastrointestinal ulcers and complications (bleeding, perforation, and obstruction) and other adverse effects. Aspirin was allowed for cardiovascular prophylaxis (325 mg/day), and diclofenac or ibuprofen used for comparison. For all patients, the annualised incidence rates of upper gastrointestinal ulcer complications alone and combined with symptomatic ulcers for celecoxib compared to diclofenac and ibuprofen were 0.76% (celecoxib), and 1.45% (diclofenac and ibuprofen). For patients not taking aspirin, the annualised incidence rates of upper gastrointestinal ulcer complications alone and combined with symptomatic ulcers for celecoxib compared to diclofenac and ibuprofen were 0.44% (celecoxib) and 1.27% (diclofenac and ibuprofen). For patients taking aspirin, the annualised incidence rates of upper gastrointestinal ulcer complications alone and combined with symptomatic ulcers for celecoxib to diclofenac and ibuprofen were 2.01% (celecoxib) and 2.12% (diclofenac and ibuprofen). Fewer celecoxib-treated patients than diclofenac and ibuprofen treated patients experienced chronic blood loss from the gastrointestinal tract, gastrointestinal intolerance, hepatotoxicity, or renal toxicity. No difference was noted in the incidence of cardiovascular events between celecoxib and NSAIDs, irrespective of aspirin use.

In these studies, rofecoxib and celecoxib use was associated with a lower incidence of ulcers and ulcer complications, compared with standard NSAIDs therapy. Interestingly in the CLASS trial where 'low-dose' aspirin use was allowed there was an increase in upper gastrointestinal toxicity. At least in terms of gastrointestinal toxicity, the concomitant prophylactic use of aspirin as an anti-platelet therapy may blunt the usefulness of COX-2 inhibitors as gastro-sparing NSAIDs. There were also problems to note from each of these trials. In the VIGOR trial a significant increase in severe cardiovascular events was observed with rofecoxib compared to naproxen. There has been a great deal of debate regarding this finding with rofecoxib and how this relates to findings with celecoxib, that showed no difference to its comparator NSAIDs. Currently this issue has not been resolved, and is likely that large-scale clinical trials are needed to address this issue. In the CLASS trial, although 6 month data on gastrointestinal events was strong, there was no difference between celecoxib and comparator NSAIDs at 12 months.[116] Whether this is a true effect again is uncertain, and may well be an artefact of the clinical trial design.

*Cardiovascular system*
Endothelial cell COX-1 is thought to be beneficial, contributing to the normal functioning of the cardiovascular system, via the release of $PGI_2$. $PGI_2$ is a vasodilator, with potent inhibitory actions on platelet function.[51,117] Indeed, $PGI_2$ analogues are one of the only clinical treatments for primary pulmonary hypertension. COX-2 becomes induced in animal arterial vessels after physical damage or exposure to pro-inflammatory cytokines.[34,118,119] Human vessels or vascular smooth muscle *in vitro*,[33] can be induced to express COX-2, and COX-2 can be found in human atherosclerotic lesions. The induction of COX-2 in human vascular smooth muscle cells and the subsequent release of $PGE_2$ and $PGI_2$ has protective functions. COX-2 expressed in the smooth muscle influences cell proliferation, cytokine release and adhesion receptor expression.[33] These observations strongly suggest that COX-2 can function as a protective pathway in human cardiovascular disease.[33]

In the VIGOR trial the incidence of myocardial infarction was lower among patients in the naproxen group than among those in the rofecoxib group

(0.1% vs. 0.4%; relative risk, 0.2). Recently, the group of Fitzgerald showed that, celecoxib[120] and rofecoxib[121] reduce circulating concentrations of prostacyclin in healthy human volunteers. This data suggests that COX-2 is a feature of the human cardiovascular system under physiological conditions, although it is not yet obvious where this COX-2 is expressed, as there appears little protein in the vessels of healthy individuals. One should also be cautious with these studies as the index for direct actions of COX-1 was platelet thromboxane production, and not the endothelial cell COX-1, originally considered responsible for the majority of circulating $PGI_2$.

$TXA_2$ synthesis by platelets is mediated by COX-1 and this is largely untouched by COX-2 inhibitors meaning that they have no anti-thrombotic effects. This can be contrasted with aspirin that irreversibly inhibits COX-1 in platelets via acetylation. As the platelets have no nuclei and cannot express replacement protein aspirin completely blocks $TXA_2$ production from platelets for their circulating lifetime. This explains the common use of aspirin as a prophylactic anti-thrombotic therapy for stroke.

### Kidney

$PGE_2$ is the major prostanoid product of kidney collecting tubule cells, regulating water absorption.[122] The formation of PGs generally only become important when the kidney is 'stressed', following for instance volume depletion, and $PGI_2$ in particular becomes essential to sustaining renal vasodilatation and blood flow. In animal kidneys COX-1 and COX-2 are co-localized in the macula densa,[123] while in man COX-2 appears most associated with podocytes. In addition, COX-2 has been identified in a subset of thick ascending limb cells, where it has been suggested to be involved in the handling of ions.[124] In rats, both selective and non-selective COX inhibitors decrease plasma renin activity.[125,126]

In human beings NSAIDs use leads to an increased risk of renal side-effects, though the incidence is much lower than gastrointestinal side-effects.[127] Interestingly, it appears that COX-2 is constitutively expressed in the kidney and influences salt and fluid resorption. This may well explain why clinical trials of COX-2-selective inhibitors have suggested at high dose a tendency to fluid retention and hypertension. Furthermore, in salt-depleted individuals celecoxib can cause sodium and potassium retention, leading to the conclusion that COX-2 selectivity does not spare the kidney under all circumstances.[128]

### Central nervous system

In the Central nervous system (CNS), $PGE_2$ promotes wakefulness, an effect apparently functionally antagonistic to $PGD_2$ in the sleep-wake regulation cycle.[129] $PGD_2$ seems to be the major COX metabolite in the brain, where in addition to the sleep-wake cycle it is known to be involved in homoeostatic temperature balance.[129] COX-1 and COX-2 are both localised in the brain and spinal cord. COX-2 is mainly expressed in the cortex, hypothalamus and hippocampus,[130,131] while COX-1 is expressed throughout the CNS, though it is particularly highly localised in the forebrain.[132] COX-2 appears also to be induced within the brain or the endothelium of brain blood vessels by pyrogens leading to a marked increase in $PGE_2$ production. This appears central to the fever response. For example, in experimental animals endotoxin-induced pyresis is strongly inhibited by COX-2-selective inhibitors or by COX-2 gene disruption.

There is now evidence that COX-2 in the CNS also plays a role in the generation of secondary hyperalgesia, i.e. sensitivity in the uninjured tissue surrounding an area of damage. Secondary hyperalgesia results from increased neuronal excitability in the spinal cord and is associated with widespread induction of COX-2 expression in spinal cord neurons and other regions of the CNS, and elevated prostaglandin $E_2$ levels in the cerebrospinal fluid. The intraspinal administration of COX-2 inhibitors decreased both the inflammation-induced central prostaglandin $E_2$ levels and mechanical,[133] or thermal[134] hyperalgesia. In contrast COX-1 inhibitors were only effective systemically and not when injected intraspinally.

*Alzheimer's disease*
Epidemiological evidence has suggested that patients taking NSAIDs have a reduced risk of developing Alzheimer's disease.[135] The protective effects of NSAIDs in this setting are most likely related to reduction of inflammation as acetaminophen (paracetamol) is without effect.[136] COX-2 expression is increased in the frontal cortex,[137] and COX-1 and COX-2 is increased in the temporal cortex[138] in Alzheimer's disease. The link between the prostaglandins and Alzheimer's disease is not completely understood, and it is possible that the epidemiological data showing that NSAIDs reduce Alzheimer's disease may have nothing to do with COX-2 inhibition. Indeed, the anti-platelet properties of NSAIDs may also relieve or prevent Alzheimer's disease.[139]

*Cancer*
The regular use of NSAIDs is associated with a reduction in the incidence of colon cancer. A retrospective study revealed that patients taking relatively low doses of aspirin, only 600–900 mg per week, over long periods of time had substantially reduced risks of developing colon cancer.[140] It is not entirely clear how this protective effect of NSAIDs is exerted. However, adenocarcinomas in human subjects display marked increases in COX-2 expression[141] and evidence from studies with isolated cells in culture[142] or

animal models[143] similarly points to COX-2 being the level at which the beneficial effects of NSAIDs are exerted. The process underlying these effects is thought to be the ability of prostaglandins produced by COX-2 to slow down the rate of apoptosis in cancerous cells. In addition, recent evidence suggests that both COX-1 and COX-2 may produce mediators that regulate the angiogenic process.[144] The effect of COX-2-selective inhibitors on the development of colon cancer in man is currently being investigated following the observation that celecoxib slows the development of polyp in familial polyposis. Since these earlier studies into colon cancer, COX-2 has now been identified in a number of other cancers including, oesophageal,[145] gastric,[146] and pancreatic[147] cancer. Whether or not COX-2 inhibitors can provide some level of protection in these forms of cancer remains to be established.

### Reproduction

Physiologically, $PGF_{2\alpha}$ is the main product of the uterine endometrium, and has been extensively studied in the utero-genital tract, being implicated in reproduction and induction of labour and parturition.[148,149] There is strong evidence from receptor knockout studies in the mouse that $PGE_2$ and $PGF_{2\alpha}$, and their respective E prostaglandin (EP) and F prostaglandin (FP) receptors mediated events during reproduction. EP2 receptor knockout mice have impaired ovulation and fertilisation, and impaired expansion of cumulus oophorus,[150] while in contrast EP4 receptor knockout mice have a patent ductus arteriosus that is not sensitive to closure by indomethacin insensitive unlike wild type animals.[151] FP receptor knockout mice have a normal early pregnancy and oestrous cycle. Interestingly, $PGF_{2\alpha}$ induces luteolysis in wild type animals, so again there seems to be mechanisms to compensate for the loss of this pathway. However in FP knockout mice there is no parturition, as there is no diminished progesterone at this stage.[152]

Therefore prostaglandins appear to be important throughout the stages of pregnancy.[153] Expression studies show a peak of COX-2 protein in pre-ovulatory follicles and endometrium prior to ovulation in the rat.[154] In COX-2 knockout mice there are severe ovulatory problems, with failure to induce follicle rupture prior to ovulation and a failure of fertilisation of ova.

During implantation there is up-regulation of COX-2 expression in the luminal epithelium and the subendothelial stromal cells in mice, rats, ewes and baboons. Blastocyte implantation is defective in COX-2 knockout mice but normal in COX-1 knockout mice. However, there is a complete failure of implantation when COX-1 deficient mice are treated with a selective COX-2 inhibitor.

COX-2-derived products may also influence development.[155] For instance, administration of a selective COX-2 inhibitor throughout and until weaning impaired renal cortex development and reduced glomerular volume in mice and rats, identical to that observed in COX-2 knockout mice. The period where these effects were most pronounced was the postnatal period when superficial nephrons begin developing and COX-2 expression peaks. This period of nephrogenesis in mice roughly corresponds to gestational weeks 24–32 in human beings, identified as critical time relating to NSAID-induced dysgenesis.

COX-2 activity is induced in foetal membranes prior to and during labour in rats, ewes, baboons as well as humans. Indomethacin delays delivery, but produces fetal side-effects, including closure of the ductus arteriosus, and impairment of renal development and function. However, in human beings it is still not clear whether ductus arteriosus patency is regulated by COX-1 or COX-2.

## Summary

COX enzymes play important roles in physiological and patho-physiological states in human beings. Prostanoid analogues can be used clinically in a limited number of clinical settings, such as to promote gastric ulcer, limit primary pulmonary hypertension, and induce labour. Importantly, however, for a number of years NSAID inhibitors of the COX pathway have been widely used clinically for the treatment of inflammation and pain, and aspirin as a prophylaxis for thrombosis. Recent findings suggest that NSAIDs may also be effective in limiting the development of Alzheimer's disease and various forms of cancer. However, a small proportion of the people taking NSAIDs can experience severe side-effects, and this is a major problem when one takes into account the extraordinarily large number of people world-wide who commonly take these drugs. The recent finding that COX exists in distinct isoforms generally associated with either a beneficial 'house-keeping' role (COX-1), or found at high levels in patho-physiological states (COX-2) provided the drive to find COX-2- selective inhibitors that could be anti-inflammatory without producing gastrointestinal side-effects. These COX-2-selective inhibitors are now in clinical use, and show much promise. The development of these selective COX-2 inhibitors has also highlighted beneficial roles of COX-2 in the body. In general we can say that where prostanoids are protective or detrimental it does not matter which isoform of COX underlies their production. However, in general apart from some particular tissues such as the reproductive and gastrointestinal tracts, COX-1 is present physiologically producing beneficial prostanoids, and COX-2 is present at high levels during patho-physiological processes.

## Acknowledgment

David Bishop-Bailey holds a British Heart Foundation Intermediate Fellowship (FS/99047).

## References

1. Smith WL, Marnett LJ. Prostaglandin endoperoxide synthase: structure and catalysis. Biochim Biophys Acta 1991; 1038: 1–17.
2. Rollins TE, Smith WL. Subcellular localization of the prostaglandin forming cyclooxygenase in Swiss 3T3 cells by electron microscopic immuno-cytochemistry. J Biol Chem 1980; 255: 4872–4876.
3. Smith WL, DeWitt DL, Allen ML. Bimodal distribution of the $PGI_2$ synthase antigen in smooth muscle cells. J Biol Chem 1983; 258: 4922–4926.
4. DeWitt DL, Rollins TE, Day JS, Gauger JA, Smith WL. Orientation of the active site and antigenic determinants of prostaglandin endoperoxide (PGH) synthase in the endoplasmic reticulum. J Biol Chem 1981; 256: 10375–10382.
5. Hamberg M, Samuelsson B. Oxygenation of unsaturated fatty acids by the vesicular gland of sheep. J Biol Chem 1967; 242: 5344–5354.
6. Miyamoto T, Ogmo N, Yamamoto S, Hayaishi O. Purification of prostaglandin endoperoxide synthetase from bovine vesicular gland microsomes. J Biol Chem 1976; 263: 3550–3553.
7. van der Ouderaa FJ, Buytenhek M, Nugteren DH, van Dorp DA. Acetylation of prostaglandin endoperoxide synthetase with acetylsalicylic acid. Eur J Biochem 1980; 109: 1–8.
8. Hamberg M, Svensson J, Samuelsson B. A new concept concerning the mode of action of release of prostaglandins. Proc Natl Acad Sci USA 1974; 71: 3824–3828.
9. Chen YNP, Bienkowski MJ, Marnett LJ. Controlled tryptic digestion of prostaglandin H synthase. J Biol Chem 1987; 262: 16892–16899.
10. Lands WEM, Samuelsson B. Phospholipid precursors of prostaglandins. Biochim Biophys Acta 1968; 164: 426–429.
11. Vonkeman H, Van Dorp DA. The action of prostaglandin synthetase on 2-arachidonyl lecithin. Biochim Biophys Acta 1968; 164: 430–432.
12. Smith WL, Marnett LJ, DeWitt DL. Prostaglandin and thromboxane biosynthesis. Pharmac Ther 1991; 49: 153–179.
13. Irvine RF. How is the level of free arachidonic acid controlled in mammalian cells? Biochem J 1982; 204: 3–16.
14. Flower RJ, Blackwell GJ. The importance of phospholipase $A_2$ in prostaglandin biosynthesis. Biochem Pharmacol 1976; 25: 285–291.
15. Venable ME, Zimmerman GA, McIntyre TM, Prescott SM. Platelet activating factor: a phospholipid autocoid with diverse actions. J Lipid Res 1993; 34: 691–702.
16. Glaser KB. Regulation of phospholipase $A_2$ enzymes: selective inhibitors and their pharmacological potential. Adv Pharmacol 1995; 32: 31–66.
17. Balsinde J, Dennis EA. Function of calcium-independent phospholipase A2 in arachidonic acid metabolism in P388D1 macrophages. Adv Exp Med Biol 1997; 407: 99–103.
18. Clark JD, Lin LL, Kriz RW *et al.* A novel arachidonic acid-selective cytosolic $PLA_2$ contains a $Ca^{2+}$-dependent translocation domain with homology to PKC and GAP. Cell 1991; 65: 1043–1051.

19. Leslie CC, Voelker DR, Channon JY, Wall MM, Zelarney PT. Properties and purification of arachidonoyl-hydrolyzing phospholipase $A_2$ from a macrophage cell line RAW 264.7. Biochim Biophys Acta 1988; 963: 476–492.
20. Kerr JS, Stevens TM, Davis GL, McLaughlin JA, Harris RR. Effects of recombinant interleukin-1β on phospholipase $A_2$ activity, phospholipase $A_2$ mRNA levels, and eicosinoid formation in rabbit chondrocytes. Biochem Biophys Res Commun 1989; 165: 1079–1084.
21. Gilman SC, Chang J. Characterisation of interleukin-1 induced rabbit coronary chondrocyte phospholipase $A_2$. J Rheumatol 1990; 17: 1392–1396.
22. VanDenBosch H, Aarsman AJ, Schaik RHNV, Schalkwijk CG, Neijs FW, Sturk A. Structural and enzymological properties of cellular phospholipase $A_2$. Biochem Soc Trans 1990; 18: 781–785.
23. Flower RJ, Blackwell GJ. Anti-inflammatory steroids induce biosynthesis of a phospholipase $A_2$ inhibitor which prevents prostaglandin generation. Nature 1979; 278: 456–459.
24. Davidson FF, Dennis EA, Powell M, Glenny JJR. Inhibition of phospholipase $A_2$ by "lipocortins" and calpactins: an effect of binding to substrate phospholipids. J Biol Chem 1987; 262: 1698–1705.
25. Flower RJ, Vane JR. Inhibition of prostaglandin synthetase in brain explains the anti-pyretic activity of paracetamol (4-acetamidophenol). Nature 1972; 240: 410–411.
26. Wu KK, Hatzakis H, Lo SS, Seong DC, Sanduja SK, Tai HH. Stimulation of de novo synthesis of prostaglandin G/H synthase in human endothelial cells by phorbol ester. J Biol Chem 1988; 263: 19043–19047.
27. Hla T, Nielson K. Human cyclooxygenase-2 cDNA. Proc Natl Acad Sci USA 1992; 89: 7384–7388.
28. Xie W, Chipman JG, Robertson DL, Erikson RL, Simmons DL. Expression of a mitogen-responsive gene encoding prostaglandin synthase is regulated by mRNA splicing. Proc Natl Acad Sci USA 1991; 88: 2692–2696.
29. Kujubu DA, Fletcher BS, Varnum BC, Lim RW, Herschman HR. TIS 10, a phorbol ester tumour promoter-inducible mRNA from Swiss 3T3 cells, encodes a novel prostaglandin synthase/cyclooxygenase homologue. J Biol Chem 1991; 266: 12866–12872.
30. Masferrer JL, Seibert K, Zweifel BS, Needleman P. Endogenous glucocorticoids regulate an inducible cyclooxygenase enzyme. Proc Natl Acad Sci USA 1992; 89: 3917–3921.
31. O'Banion MK, Winn VD, Young DA. cDNA cloning and functional activity of a glucocorticoid-regulated inflammatory cyclooxygenase. Proc Natl Acad Sci USA 1992; 89: 4888–4892.
32. Mitchell JA, Belvisi M, Akarasereenont P et al. Induction of cyclo-oxygenase-2 by cytokines in human pulmonary epithelial cells: regulation by dexamethasone. Br J Pharmacol 1994; 113: 1008–1014.
33. Bishop-Bailey D, Hla T, Mitchell JA. Cyclo-oxygenase-2 in vascular smooth muscle. Int J Mol Med 1999; 3: 41–48.
34. Rimarachin JA, Jacobson JA, Szabo P, Maclouf J, Creminon C, Weksler BB. Regulation of cyclooxygenase-2 expression in aortic smooth muscle cells. Arterioscle Thromb 1994; 14: 1021–1031.
35. Reddy ST, Herschman HR. Prostaglandin synthase-1 and prostaglandin synthase-2 are coupled to distinct phospholipases for the generation of prostaglandin D2 in activated mast cells. J Biol Chem 1997; 272: 3231–3237.

36. Thiemermann C. Biosynthesis and interactions of endothelium-derived vasoactive mediators. Eicosiniods 1991; 4: 187–202.

37. Sirois J, Levy LO, Simmons DL, Richards JS. Characterisation and hormonal regulation of the promoter of the rat prostaglandin endoperoxide synthase 2 gene in granulosa cells. J Biol Chem 1993; 268: 12199–12204.

38. Lee SH, Soyoola E, Chanmugam P *et al.* Selective expression of mitogen-inducible cyclo-oxygenase in macrophages stimulated with lipopolysaccharide. J Biol Chem 1992; 267: 25934–25938.

39. DuBois RN, Award J, Morrow J, Roberts LJ, Bishop PR. Regulation of eicosanoid production and mitogenesis in rat intestinal epithelial cells by transforming growth factor-$\alpha$ and phorbol ester. J Clin Invest 1994; 93: 493–498.

40. Kester M, Coroneous E, Thomas PJ, Dunn MJ. Endothelin stimulates prostaglandin endoperoxide synthase-2 mRNA expression and protein synthesis through a tyrosine kinase-signalling pathway in rat mesangial cells. J Biol Chem 1994; 269: 22574–22580.

41. Stroebel M, Goppelt-Struebe M. Signal transduction pathways responsible for serotonin-mediated prostaglandin G/H synthase expression in rat mesangial cells. J Biol Chem 1994; 269: 22952–22957.

42. Zembowicz A, Jones SL, Wu KK. Induction of cyclooxygenase-2 in human umbilical vein endothelial cells by lysophosphatidylcholine. J Clin Invest 1995; 96: 1688–1692.

43. Topper JN, Cai J, Falb D, Gimbrone MA. Identification of vascular endothelial genes differentially responsive to fluid mechanical stimuli: cyclooxygenase-2, manganese superoxide dismutase, and endothelial cell nitric oxide synthase are selectively up-regulated by steady laminar shear stress. Proc Natl Acad Sci USA 1996; 93: 10417–10422.

44. Herschman HR. Primary response genes induced by growth factors and tumor promoters. Annu Rev Biochem 1991; 60: 281–319.

45. Smith WL, Gravavito M, DeWitt D. Prostaglandin endoperoxide H synthases (cyclooxygenases)-1 and -2. J Biol Chem 1996; 271: 33157–33160.

46. Appleby S, Ristmaki A, Neilson K, Narko K, Hla T. Structure of the human cyclo-oxygenase-2 gene. Biochem J 1994; 302: 723–727.

47. Ristimaki A, Garfinkel S, Wessendorf J, Macaig T, Hla T. Induction of cyclo-oxygenase-2 by interleukin-1$\alpha$. J Biol Chem 1994; 269: 11769–11775.

48. Ristimaki A, Narko K, Hla T. Down regulation of cytokine-induced cyclo-oxygenase-2 transcript isoforms by dexamethasone: evidence for post-transcriptional regulation. Biochem J 1996; 318: 325–331.

49. Lanaeuville O, Breuer DK, Xu N, Huang ZH, Gage DA, Watson JT, Lagarde M, DeWitt D, Smith WL. Fatty acid substrate specificities of human prostaglandin-endoperoxide H synthase-1 and -2. J Biol Chem 1995; 270: 19330–19336.

50. Kulmacz RJ, Wang LH. Comparison of hydroperoxide initiator requirements for the cyclo-oxygenase activities of prostaglandin H synthase-1 and -2. J Biol Chem 1995; 270: 24019–24023.

51. Moncada S, Gryglewski R, Bunting S, Vane JR. An enzyme isolated from arteries transforms prostaglandin endoperoxides to an unstable substance that inhibits platelet aggregation. Nature 1976; 263: 663–665.

52. Dusting GJ, Moncada S, Vane JR. Disappearance of prostacyclin in the circulation of the dog. Br J Pharmacol 1977; 62: 414P–415P.

53. Ujihara M, Tsuchida S, Satoh K, Sato K, Urade Y. Biochemical and immunological demonstration of prostaglandin $D_2$, $E_2$, and $F_{2\alpha}$ formation from prostaglandin $H_2$

by various rat glutathione S-transferase isozymes. Archs Biochem Biophys 1988; 264: 428–437.

54. Ogino N, Yamamoto S, Hayaishi O, Tokuyama T. Isolation of an activator for prostaglandin hydroperoxidase from bovine vesicular gland cytosol and its identification as uric acid. Biochem Biophys Res Commun 1977; 87: 184–191.

55. Moonen P, Buytenhek M, Nugteren DH. Purification of PGH-PGE isomerase from sheep vesicular glands. Methods Enzymol 1982; 86: 84–91.

56. Jakobsson P-H, Thorén S, Morgenstern R, Samuelsson B. Identification of human prostaglandin E synthase: a microsomal, glutathione-dependent, inducible enzyme, constituting a potential novel drug target. Proc Natl Acad Sci USA 1999; 96: 7220–7225.

57. Christ-Hazelhof E, Nugteren DH. Isolation of PGH-PGD isomerase from rat spleens. Meth Enzym 1982; 86: 77–84.

58. Urade Y, Fujimoto N, Hayaishi O. Purification and characterisation of rat brain prostaglandin D synthetase. J Biol Chem 1985; 260: 12410–12415.

59. Toh H, Urade Y, Tanabe T. Molecular evolution of enzymes involved in the arachidonic acid cascade. Mediators of Inflammation 1992; 1: 223–233.

60. Haurand M, Ullrich V. Isolation and characterisation of thromboxane synthase from human platelets as a cytochrome P-450 enzyme. J Biol Chem 1985; 260: 15059–15067.

61. Yokoyama C, Miyata A, Ihara H, Ullrich V, Tanabe T. Molecular cloning of human platelet thromboxane A synthase. Biochem Biophys Res Commun 1991; 178: 1479–1484.

62. Hamberg M, Svensson J, Samuelsson B. Thromboxanes: a new group of biologically active compounds derived from prostaglandin endoperoxides. Proc Natl Acad Sci USA 1975; 72: 2994–2998.

63. Roberts LJ, Sweetman BJ, Oates JA. Metabolism of thromboxane B2 in man. Identification of twenty urinary metabolites. J Biol Chem 1981; 256: 8384–8393.

64. Fitzgerald GA, Pederson AK, Patrono C. Analysis of prostacyclin and thromboxane biosynthesis in cardiovascular disease. Circulation 1983; 67: 1174–1177.

65. Coleman RA, Smith WL, Narumiya S. International Union of Pharmacology classification of prostanoid receptors: properties, distribution of the receptors and their subtypes. Pharmacol Rev 1994; 46: 205–229.

66. Forman BM, Tontonoz P, Chen J, Brun RP, Spiegelman BM, Evans RM. 15-Deoxy-$\Delta^{12,14}$-prostaglandin $J_2$ is a ligand for the adipocyte determination factor PPARγ. Cell 1995; 83: 803–812.

67. Kliewer SA, Lenhard JM, Willson TM, Patel I, Morris DC, Lehmann JM. A prostaglandin $J_2$ metabolite binds peroxisome proliferator-activated receptor γ and promotes adipocyte differentiation. Cell 1995; 83: 813–819.

68. Bishop-Bailey D. Peroxisome proliferator-activated receptors in the cardiovascular system. Br J Pharmacol 2000; 129: 823–834.

69. Langenbach R, Morham SG, Tiano HF et al. Prostaglandin synthase 1 gene disruption in mice reduces arachidonic acid-induced inflammation and indomethacin-induced gastric ulceration. Cell 1995; 83: 483–492.

70. Morham SG, Langenbach R, Loftin CD et al. Prostaglandin synthase 2 gene disruption causes severe renal pathology in the mouse. Cell 1995; 83: 473–482.

71. Dinchuk JE, Car BD, Focht RJ et al. Renal abnormalities and an altered inflammatory response in mice lacking cyclooxygenase II. Nature 1995; 378: 406–409.

72. Mitchell JA, Warner TD. Cyclo-oxygenase-2: pharmacology, physiology, biochemistry and relevance to NSAID therapy. Br J Pharmacol 1999; 128: 1121–1132.

73. Williams TJ, Peck MJ. Role of prostaglandin mediated vasodilation in inflammation. Nature 1977; 289: 646–650.

74. Ferreira SH. Prostaglandin, aspirin-like drugs and analgesia. Nature 1972; 240: 200–203.

75. Saxena PN, Beg MM, Singhal KC, Ahmad M. Prostaglandin like activity in the cerebrospinal fluid of febrile patients. Indian J Med Res 1979; 70: 495–498.

76. Vane JR. Inhibition of prostaglandin synthesis as a mechanism of action for aspirin-like drugs. Nature 1971; 231: 232–235.

77. Roth GJ, Majerus PW. The mechanism of the effect of aspirin on human platelets. 1. Acetylation of a particulate fraction protein. J Clin Invest 1975; 56: 624–632.

78. Rome LH, Lands WEM. Structural requirements for time-dependent inhibition of prostaglandin biosynthesis by anti-inflammatory drugs. Proc Natl Acad Sci USA 1975; 72: 4863–4865.

79. Wolfe MM, Lichtenstein DR, Singh G. Gastrointestinal toxicity of nonsteroidal antiinflammatory drugs. N Engl J Med 1999; 340: 1888–1899.

80. Vane JR, Botting RM. The mode of action of anti-inflammatory drugs. Postgrad Med J 1990; 66 (Suppl.): S2–S17.

81. Meade EA, Smith WL, DeWitt DL. Differential inhibition of prostaglandin endoperoxide synthase (cyclooxygenase) isozymes by aspirin and other nonsteroidal antiinflammatory drugs. J Biol Chem 1993; 268: 6610–6614.

82. Mitchell JA, Akarasereenont P, Thiemermann C, Flower RJ, Vane JR. Selectivity of nonsteroidal antiinflammatory drugs as inhibitors of constitutive and inducible cyclooxygenase. Proc Natl Acad Sci USA 1993; 90:11693–11697.

83. Warner TD, Giuliano F, Vojnovic I, Bukasa A, Mitchell JA, Vane JR. Nonsteroid drug selectivities for cyclo-oxygenase-1 rather than cyclo-oxygenase-2 are associated with human gastrointestinal toxicity: a full in vitro analysis. Proc Natl Acad Sci USA 1999; 96: 7563–7568.

84. Copeland RA, Williams JM, Giannaras J et al. Mechanism of selective inhibition of the inducible isoform of prostaglandin G/H synthase. Proc Natl Acad Sci USA 1994; 91: 11202–11206.

85. Gierse JK, McDonald JJ, Hauser SD, Rangwala SH, Koboldt CM, Seibert K. A single amino acid difference between cyclooxygenase-1 (COX-1) and -2 (COX-2) reverses the selectivity of COX-2 specific inhibitors. J Biol Chem 1996; 271: 15810–15814.

86. Kargman S, Wong E, Greig GM et al. Mechanism of selective inhibition of human prostaglandin G/H synthase-1 and -2 in intact cells. Biochem Pharmacol 1996; 52: 1113–1125.

87. Guo Q, Wang LH, Ruan KH, Kulmacz RJ. Role of Val-509 in time dependent inhibition of human prostaglandin H synthase-2 cyclo-oxygenase activity by isoform selective agents. J Biol Chem 1996; 271: 19134–19139.

88. Kurumbail RG, Stevens AM, Gierse JK et al. Structural basis for selective inhibition of cyclo-oxygenase-2 by anti-inflammatory agents. Nature 1996; 384: 644–648.

89. Futaki N, Takahashi S, Yokoyama M, Arai I, Higuchi S, Otomo S. NS-398 a new anti-inflammatory agent, selectively inhibits prostaglandin synthase/cyclooxygenase (COX-2) activity in vitro. Prostaglandins 1994; 47: 55–59.

90. Masferrer JL, Zweifel BS, Manning PT et al. Selective inhibition of inducible cyclo-oxygenase-2 in vivo is antiinflammatory and nonulcerogenic. Proc Natl Acad Sci USA 1994; 91: 3228–3232.

91. Chan CC, Boyce S, Brideau C et al. Pharmacology of a selective cyclo-oxygenase-2 inhibitor, L-745,337: a novel nonsteroidal anti-inflammatory agent with an ulcerogenic sparing effect in rat and nonhuman primate stomach. J Pharmacol Exp Ther 1995; 274: 1531–1537.

92. Seibert K, Zhang Y, Leahy K *et al*. Pharmacological and biochemical demonstration of the role of cyclooxygenase 2 in inflammation and pain. Proc Natl Acad Sci USA 1994; 91: 12013–12017.

93. Williams TJ, Morley J. Prostaglandins as potentiators of increased vascular permeability in inflammation. Nature 1973; 246: 215–217.

94. Crofford LJ. COX-1 and COX-2 tissue expression: implications and predictions. J Rheumatol 1997; 24 (Suppl 49): 15–19.

95. Cannon GW, Breedveld FC. Efficacy of cyclooxygenase-2-specific inhibitors. Am J Med 2001; 110 (Suppl 3A): 6S–12S.

96. Bensen WG, Fiechtner JJ, McMillen JI *et al*. Treatment of osteoarthritis with celecoxib, a cyclooxygenase-2 inhibitor: a randomized controlled trial. Mayo Clin Proc 1999; 74: 1095–1105.

97. Day R, Morrison B, Luza A *et al*. A randomized trial of the efficacy and tolerability of the COX-2 inhibitor rofecoxib vs ibuprofen in patients with osteoarthritis. Rofecoxib/ibuprofen comparator study group. Arch Intern Med 2000; 160: 1781–1787.

98. Yocum D, Fleischmann R, Dalgin P, Caldwell J, Hall D, Roszko P. Safety and efficacy of meloxicam in the treatment of osteoarthritis: a 12-week, double-blind, multiple-dose, placebo-controlled trial. The meloxicam osteoarthritis investigators. Arch Intern Med 2000; 160: 2947–2954.

99. Malmstrom K, Daniels S, Kotey P, Seidenberg BC, Desjardins PJ. Comparison of rofecoxib and celecoxib, two cyclooxygenase-2 inhibitors, in postoperative dental pain: a randomized, placebo- and active-comparator-controlled clinical trial. Clin Ther 1999; 21: 1653–1663.

100. Ehrich EW, Dallob A, De Lepeleire I *et al*. Characterization of rofecoxib as a cyclooxygenase-2 isoform inhibitor and demonstration of analgesia in the dental pain model. Clin Pharmacol Ther 1999; 65: 336–347.

101. Morrison BW, Christensen S, Yuan W, Brown J, Amlani S, Seidenberg B. Analgesic efficacy of the cyclooxygenase-2-specific inhibitor rofecoxib in post-dental surgery pain: a randomized, controlled trial. Clin Ther 1999; 21: 943–953.

102. Schwartz JI, Chan CC, Mukhopadhyay S *et al*. Cyclooxygenase-2 inhibition by rofecoxib reverses naturally occurring fever in humans. Clin Pharmacol Ther 1999; 65: 653–660.

103. Whittle BJ, Lopez-Belmonte J. Actions and interactions of endothelins, prostacyclin and nitric oxide in the gastric mucosa. J Physiol Pharmacol 1993; 44: 91–107.

104. Zimmermann KC, Sarbia M, Schror K, Weber AA. Constitutive cyclooxygenase-2 expression in healthy human and rabbit gastric mucosa. Mol Pharmacol 1998; 54: 536–540.

105. Wallace JL, McKnight W, Reuter BK, Vergnolle N. NSAID-induced gastric damage in rats: requirement for inhibition of both cyclooxygenase 1 and 2. Gastroenterology 2000; 119: 706–714.

106. Reuter BK, Asfaha S, Buret A, Sharkey KA, Wallace JL. Exacerbation of inflammation-associated colonic injury in rat through inhibition of cyclooxygenase-2. J Clin Invest 1996; 98: 2076–2085.

107. Mizuno H, Sakamoto C, Matsuda K *et al*. Induction of cyclooxygenase 2 in gastric mucosal lesions and its inhibition by the specific antagonist delays healing in mice. Gastroenterology 1997; 112: 387–397.

108. Ukawa H, Yamakuni H, Kato S, Takeuchi K. Effects of cyclooxygenase-2 selective and nitric oxide-releasing nonsteroidal antiinflammatory drugs on mucosal ulcerogenic and healing responses of the stomach. Dig Dis Sci 1998; 43: 2003–2011.

109. Hernandez-Diaz S, Garcia-Rodriguez LA. Epidemiologic assessment of the safety of conventional nonsteroidal anti-inflammatory drugs. Am J Med 2001; 110 (Suppl 3A): 20S–27S.

110. Wight NJ, Gottesdiener K, Garlick NM et al. Rofecoxib, a COX-2 inhibitor, does not inhibit human gastric mucosal prostaglandin production. Gastroenterology 2001; 120: 867–873.

111. Lipscomb GR, Wallis N, Armstrong G, Rees WD. Gastrointestinal tolerability of meloxicam and piroxicam: a double-blind placebo-controlled study. Br J Clin Pharmacol 1998; 46: 133–137.

112. Lanza FL, Rack MF, Simon TJ et al. Specific inhibition of cyclooxygenase-2 with MK-0966 is associated with less gastroduodenal damage than either aspirin or ibuprofen. Aliment Pharmacol Ther 1999; 13: 761–767.

113. Smecuol E, Bai JC, Sugai E et al. Acute gastrointestinal permeability responses to different non-steroidal anti-inflammatory drugs. Gut 2001; 49: 650–655.

114. Bombardier C, Laine L, Reicin A et al. Comparison of upper gastrointestinal toxicity of rofecoxib and naproxen in patients with rheumatoid arthritis. VIGOR Study Group. N Engl J Med 2000; 343: 1520–1528.

115. Silverstein FE, Faich G, Goldstein JL et al. Gastrointestinal toxicity with celecoxib vs nonsteroidal anti-inflammatory drugs for osteoarthritis and rheumatoid arthritis: the CLASS study: A randomized controlled trial. Celecoxib Long-term Arthritis Safety Study. JAMA 2000; 284: 1247–1255.

116. Juni P, Rutjes AW, Dieppe PA. Are selective COX 2 inhibitors superior to traditional non steroidal anti-inflammatory drugs? BMJ 2002; 324: 1287–1288.

117. Radomski MW, Palmer RMJ, Moncada S. The anti-aggregating properties of vascular endothelium: interactions between prostacyclin and nitric oxide. Br J Pharmacol 1987; 92: 181–187.

118. Pritchard KA, O'Banion MK, Miano JM et al. Induction of cyclo-oxygenase-2 in rat vascular smooth muscle cells in vitro and in vivo. J Biol Chem 1994; 269: 8504–8509.

119. Belton O, Byrne D, Kearney D, Leahy A, Fitzgerald DJ. Cyclooxygenase-1 and -2-dependent prostacyclin formation in patients with atherosclerosis. Circulation 2000; 102: 840–845.

120. McAdam BF, Catella-Lawson F, Mardini IA, Kapoor S, Lawson JA, FitzGerald GA. Systemic biosynthesis of prostacyclin by cyclooxygenase (COX)-2: the human pharmacology of a selective inhibitor of COX-2. Proc Natl Acad Sci USA 1999; 96: 272–277.

121. Catella-Lawson F, McAdam B, Morrison BW et al. Effects of specific inhibition of cyclooxygenase-2 on sodium balance, hemodynamics, and vasoactive eicosanoids. J Pharmacol Exp Ther 1999; 289: 735–741.

122. Kirschenbaum AG, Lowe W, Trizna W, Fine LG. Regulation of vasopressin action by prostaglandins: evidence for prostaglandin synthesis in the rabbit cortical collecting tubule. J Clin Invest 1982; 70: 1193–1204.

123. Harris RC, McKanna JA, Akai Y, Jacobson HR, DuBois RN, Breyer MD. Cyclo-oxygenase-2 is associated with the macula densa of rat kidney and increase with salt restriction. J Clin Invest 1994; 94: 2504–2510.

124. Vio CP, Cespedes C, Gallardo P, Masferrer JL. Renal identification of cyclooxygenase-2 in a subset of thick ascending limb cells. Hypertension 1997; 30: 687–692.

125. Wang JL, Cheng HF, Harris RC. Cyclooxygenase-2 inhibition decreases renin content and lowers blood pressure in a model of renovascular hypertension. Hypertension 1999; 34: 96–101.

126. Harris RC, Cheng H, Wang J, Zhang M, McKanna JA. Interactions of the renin-angiotensin system and neuronal nitric oxide synthase in regulation of cyclooxygenase-2 in the macula densa. Acta Physiol Scand 2000; 168: 47–51.

127. Vane JR, Bakhle YS, Botting RM. Cyclooxygenases 1 and 2. Annu Rev Pharmacol Toxicol 1998; 38: 97–120.

128. Rossat J, Maillard M, Nussberger J, Brunner HR, Burnier M. Renal effects of selective cyclooxygenase-2 inhibition in normotensive salt-depleted subjects. Clin Pharmacol Ther 1999; 66: 76–84.

129. Hayaishi O. Molecular mechanisms of sleep-wake regulation: roles of prostaglandin $D_2$ and $E_2$. FASEB J 1991; 5: 2575–2581.

130. Breder CD, Dewitt D, Kraig RP. Characterization of inducible cyclooxygenase in rat brain. J Comp Neurol 1995; 355: 296–315.

131. Breder CD, Saper CB. Expression of inducible cyclooxygenase mRNA in the mouse brain after systemic administration of bacterial lipopolysaccharide. Brain Res 1996; 713: 64–69.

132. Breder CD, Smith WL, Raz A et al. Distribution and characterization of cyclooxygenase immunoreactivity in the ovine brain. J Comp Neurol 1992; 322: 409–438.

133 Samad TA, Moore KA, Sapirstein A, Billet S, Allchorne A, Poole S, Bonventre JV, Woolf CJ. Interleukin-1 beta-mediated induction of Cox-2 in the CNS contributes to inflammatory pain hypersensitivity. Nature 2001; 410: 471–475.

134. Yaksh TL, Dirig DM, Conway CM, Svensson C, Luo ZD, Isakson PC. The acute antihyperalgesic action of nonsteroidal, anti-inflammatory drugs and release of spinal prostaglandin E2 is mediated by the inhibition of constitutive spinal cyclooxygenase-2 (COX-2) but not COX-1. J Neurosci 2001; 21: 5847–5853.

135. Pasinetti GM. Cyclooxygenase and inflammation in Alzheimer's disease: experimental approaches and clinical interventions. J Neurosci Res 1998; 54: 1–6.

136. Stewart WF, Kawas C, Corrada M, Metter EJ. Risk of Alzheimer's disease and duration of NSAID use. Neurology 1997; 48: 626–632.

137. Pasinetti GM, Aisen PS. Cyclooxygenase-2 expression is increased in frontal cortex of Alzheimer's disease brain. Neuroscience 1998; 87: 319–324.

138. Kitamura Y, Shimohama S, Koike H et al. Increased expression of cyclooxygenases and peroxisome proliferator-activated receptor-gamma in Alzheimer's disease brains. Biochem Biophys Res Commun 1999; 254: 582–586.

139. de la Torre JC. Cerebromicrovascular pathology in Alzheimer's disease compared to normal aging. Gerontology 1997; 43: 26–43.

140. Giovannucci E, Egan KM, Hunter DJ et al. Aspirin and the risk of colorectal cancer in women. N Engl J Med 1995; 333: 609–614.

141. Smalley WE, DuBois RN. Colorectal cancer and nonsteroidal anti-inflammatory drugs. Adv Pharmacol 1997; 39: 1–20.

142. DuBois RN, Abramson SB, Crofford L et al. Cyclooxygenase in biology and disease. FASEB J 1998; 12: 1063–1073.

143. Williams CS, Smalley W, DuBois RN. Aspirin use and potential mechanisms for colorectal cancer prevention. J Clin Invest 1997; 100: 1325–1329.

144. Masferrer J. Approach to angiogenesis inhibition based on cyclooxygenase-2. Cancer J 2001; 7 (Suppl 3): S144–S150.

145. Zimmermann KC, Sarbia M, Weber AA, Borchard F, Gabbert HE, Schror K. Cyclooxygenase-2 expression in human esophageal carcinoma. Cancer Res 1999; 59: 198–204.

146. Murata H, Kawano S, Tsuji S *et al*. Cyclooxygenase-2 overexpression enhances lymphatic invasion and metastasis in human gastric carcinoma. Am J Gastroenterol 1999; 94: 451–455.

147. Tucker ON, Dannenberg AJ, Yang EK *et al*. Cyclooxygenase-2 expression is up-regulated in human pancreatic cancer. Cancer Res 1999; 59: 987–990.

148. Dennefors B, Hamberger L, Hillensjo T *et al*. Aspects concerning the role of prostaglandins for ovarian function. Acta Obstet Gynecol Scand 1983; 113: 31–41.

149. Senior J, Sangha R, Baxter GS, Marshall K, Clayton JK. In vitro characterisation of prostanoid FP-, DP-, IP-, and TP-receptors in the non-pregnant human myometrium. Br J Pharmacol 1992; 107: 215–221.

150. Hizaki H, Segi E, Sugimoto Y *et al*. Abortive expansion of the cumulus and impaired fertility in mice lacking the prostaglandin E receptor subtype EP(2). Proc Natl Acad Sci USA 1999; 96: 10501–10506.

151. Segi E, Sugimoto Y, Yamasaki A *et al*. Patent ductus arteriosus and neonatal death in prostaglandin receptor EP4-deficient mice. Biochem Biophys Res Commun 1998; 246: 7–12.

152. Sugimoto Y, Yamasaki A, Segi E *et al*. Failure of parturition in mice lacking the prostaglandin F receptor. Science 1997; 277: 681–683.

153. Chakraborty I, Das SK, Wang J, Dey SK. Developmental expression of the cyclo-oxygenase-1 and cyclo-oxygenase-2 genes in the peri-implantation mouse uterus and their differential regulation by the blastocyst and ovarian steroids. J Mol Endocrinol 1996; 16: 107–122.

154. Dong YL, Gangula PR, Fang L, Yallampalli C. Differential expression of cyclooxygenase-1 and -2 proteins in rat uterus and cervix during the estrous cycle, pregnancy, labor and in myometrial cells. Prostaglandins 1996; 52: 13–34.

155. Komhoff M, Jeck ND, Seyberth HW, Grone HJ, Nusing RM, Breyer MD. Cyclooxygenase-2 expression is associated with the renal macula densa of patients with Bartter-like syndrome. Kidney Int 2000; 58: 2420–2424.

*A.J. Hutt*

# Drug chirality: stereoselectivity in the action and disposition of anaesthetic agents

Drug stereochemistry, particularly drug chirality, has become a topical subject being discussed not only in the popular medical[1,2] and scientific literature[3-5] but also within the 'quality' lay press.[6,7] This interest in stereochemistry has arisen as a result of advances in chemical technology associated with the synthesis, separation and analysis of stereoisomers, together with an increasing realisation of the potential significance of the differential biological properties of the enantiomers of chiral drugs administered as racemic mixtures. Such mixtures, a racemate being an equal parts mixture of a pair of enantiomers, account for approximately 25% of all prescribed drugs[8] including many agents used in anaesthetic practice. The use of such mixtures may present problems particularly if the adverse effects of the drug mixture are associated with the less active enantiomer or do not show stereoselectivity.

To the physician the complexities of stereochemistry and the intricacies of the associated terminology are of little interest. A not unreasonable attitude as they could expect the pharmaceutical industry and the regulatory agencies to provide them with the most appropriate material irrespective of stereochemical considerations. However, it is important that physicians are aware of the nature of the material they are prescribing, mixture or single chemical entity, particularly with the advent of the Chiral Switch[9] (see below) and the possibility that both racemate and single stereoisomer products of some agents either are, or will be, available at the same time.

The aims of this chapter are to provide the reader with a brief background to stereochemistry with respect to the terminology and nomenclature employed, to illustrate the significance of stereochemical considerations in pharmacology with a particular emphasis on anaesthetic agents, and the current regulatory position with respect to chiral pharmaceuticals.

## Stereochemical Terminology and Nomenclature

Stereoisomers are compounds which differ in the three-dimensional spatial arrangement of their constituent atoms and may be divided into two groups, namely enantiomers and diastereoisomers. Enantiomers are stereoisomers which are non-superimposable mirror images of one another and are pairs of compounds related as an object to its mirror image, in the same way that an individual's left and right hands (or feet, or ears) are related. Such molecules are said to be chiral, from the Greek *chiros* meaning handed. Stereoisomers of this type are also referred to as optical isomers due to their ability to rotate the plane of plane polarized light, which is equal in magnitude but opposite in direction. In terms of the majority of drug molecules the most frequent, but not the only, cause of chirality arises due to the presence of a tetrahedral atom in a molecule to which four different atoms or groups are bonded (fig. 1). Such atoms are referred to as centres of chirality or asymmetry. The presence of one such centre in a molecule gives rise to a pair of enantiomers, the presence of $n$ such different centres yields $2^n$ stereoisomers and half that number of pairs of enantiomers. Those stereoisomers which are not enantiomeric, i.e. are not mirror image related, are diastereomeric (fig. 2).

The fundamental distinction between enantiomers and diastereoisomers is that in a pair of enantiomers the intramolecular distances between non-bonded

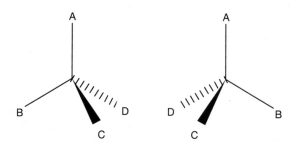

**Figure 1** Structural representation of a pair of enantiomers. This diagram depicts a tetrahedral atom to which four different groups are bonded, the structure on the right being a non-superimposable mirror image of that on the left. The chemical bonds represented by the wedge project above the plane of the paper (towards the reader), those drawn as dashed lines project below the plane (away from the reader), whereas the solid lines represent bonds in the plane of the paper.

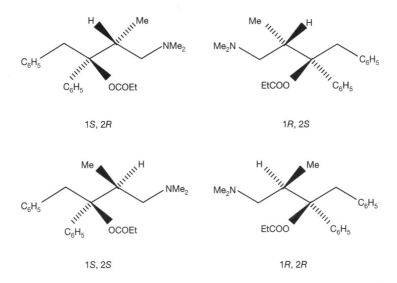

**Figure 2** Stereoisomers of propoxyphene. Propoxyphene contains two centres of chirality in its structure and four stereoisomers, i.e. two pairs of enantiomers are possible. In this diagram those compounds related horizontally (the upper and lower pairs) are enantiomeric, whereas those related vertically are diastereomeric. In the case of propoxyphene the upper enantiomeric pair are used therapeutically. The compound on the left, the 1S, 2R-stereoisomer is dextrorotatory and is the analgesic dextropropoxyphene, that on the right is laevorotatory (1R, 2S-stereoisomer) and is the antitussive levopropoxyphene. In this case the biological activity of the two enantiomers is such that both are marketed with different therapeutic indications. The trade names of the two agents Darvon and Novrad for the analgesic and antitussive respectively are also mirror-image related.

atoms are identical, whereas in a pair of diastereoisomers they are not. Thus the physicochemical properties, other than the direction of rotation of the plane of plane polarized light, e.g. solubility, melting/boiling point, ionization constant, partition coefficient etc., of a pair of enantiomers are identical. As a result the separation, or resolution, of enantiomers was, until relatively recently, fairly difficult. In contrast diastereoisomers differ in their physico-chemical properties and, in principle at least, may be separated relatively easily.

As enantiomers differ in the direction of rotation of the plane of plane polar-ized light this property is frequently used in their designation and nomenclat-ure. Those enantiomers which rotate light to the right are said to be dextrorotatory, indicated by either a (+)-sign or lower case italized *d-* before their name, or alternatively the prefix 'dex' or 'dextro' to the drug name. Enantiomers which rotate light to the left are termed laevorotatory indicated by a (−)-sign or lower case italized *l-* before the name, or the prefix 'lev' or 'levo'. A racemic mixture, an equal parts mixture of enantiomers being indicated by (±)- or *d,l-* before the name or, in some instances, the prefix 'rac'.

It is important to appreciate that this form of nomenclature provides information concerning a physical property and indicates the stereochemical composition, i.e. single enantiomer or racemic mixture, of the material. Considerable care is required when using the direction of rotation as a stereochemical descriptor as both the magnitude and direction of rotation may vary with experimental conditions.[10–13] This approach to nomenclature does not provide information with respect to the three-dimensional structure, or absolute configuration, of the stereoisomer which is the important feature with respect to the pharmacological activity of the compound. Once the three-dimensional structure of a stereoisomer has been determined, by for example, X-ray crystallography, then the spatial arrangement, or absolute configuration may be indicated by the use of a prefix letter to the name of the compound. Two systems are currently in use, the Cahn-Ingold-Prelog[14] Sequence Rule or R/S (Rectus/Sinister) designation and the older D/L notation.

The D/L notation relates the stereochemistry of a molecule to that of a standard reference compound either the carbohydrate D-glyceraldehyde or the amino acid L-serine. A particular stereoisomer being designated as a member of either the D- or L-series and the racemate as D,L-. The use of this system has lead to ambiguities, particularly in molecules with two, or more, centres of chirality in their structures where the configuration at one centre can be related to the D-series and that at the other to the L-series. Additional confusion also occurs as the upper case letters are used to indicate the configuration and the lower case the direction of rotation of light. Problems also arise in the literature as journal editors frequently alter the lower case letters to upper case in the titles of articles and thus a defined, correct physicochemical property is transformed into a configurational designation which may be incorrect. This system should now be restricted in use for the designation of the stereoisomers of the carbohydrates and amino acids.

The alternative Sequence Rule system uses a 'ranking' approach for the designation of configuration.[14] The substituent atoms bonded to the centre of chirality are placed in an order of priority based upon their atomic number, the higher the atomic number the greater the priority. The molecule is then 'viewed' from the side opposite the group of lowest priority and if the three remaining highest to lowest priorities are in a clockwise direction (to the right) the stereoisomer is assigned the Rectus configuration and if anticlockwise (to the left) the Sinister configuration. The designatory prefix letters being R- and S-, or R,S- for the individual enantiomers and racemate, respectively. In cases where two, or more, centres of chirality are present in a molecule each centre is defined and indicated by an appropriate number based on standard chemical nomenclature (fig. 2).

As pointed out above, the prefix terms 'dex', or 'dextro', and 'lev' or 'levo' have been used for a number of years to indicate the stereochemical nature of some agents, e.g. dextropropoxyphene, levodopa, and a number of agents are listed in the most recent British National Formulary (BNF 43; March 2002). This approach has also been used where both single enantiomer and racemic mixture preparations are, or were, available at the same time, e.g. dexfenfluramine/fenfluramine, dexketoprofen/ketoprofen, levobupivacaine/bupivacaine. More recently the configurational designation of the single enantiomer has been incorporated into the nomenclature of the agent, e.g. the S-enantiomers of the proton pump inhibitor omeprazole and the selective serotonin reuptake inhibitor citalopram have been named esomeprazole and escitalopram respectively.

## Discrimination of Stereoisomers in Biological Systems

That the individual enantiomers of a chiral drug could exhibit different pharmacological properties has been known since the early years of the last century[15] when the British pharmacologist Cushny[16] demonstrated differences in the activity of atropine (racemic hyoscyamine) and (−)-hyoscyamine and naturally occurring (−)-epinephrine and its (+)-enantiomer. Such differences in biological activity should not be surprising as many of the endogenous substrates or ligands of drug targets, i.e. receptors and enzyme active sites, are chiral single stereoisomer molecules, e.g. endogenous opioids, hormones, neurotransmitters, etc.

Differences between enantiomers are under normal circumstances difficult to detect, however when placed in a chiral environment such differences become more marked. Biological systems at a molecular level are intensely chiral environments being composed of 'handed' biopolymers (proteins, glycolipids, polynucleotides) from the chiral building blocks of D-series carbohydrates and L-series amino acids. Additionally the macromolecular helical structures of some of these biopolymers exhibit chirality, e.g. the protein α-helix and DNA double-helix, in the same way that a spiral staircase, or corkscrew, may be left handed or right handed. In the case of the above examples both have a right handed turn.

The interaction between a drug and its target is associated with bonding interactions between the functionalities of the drug and complementary sites on the biological macromolecule, enzyme or receptor. The relative orientation, spatial arrangement, of the functionalities in the drug structure being of considerable significance. This situation, with respect to a pair of enantiomers, is illustrated in figure 3. This model was originally proposed by Easson and Stedman[17] in the 1930s in order to rationalize the differential

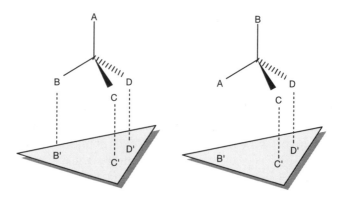

**Figure 3** Stereochemical discrimination on interaction of a pair of enantiomers with a biological macromolecule. The stereoisomer on the left is involved with three bonding interactions with complementary sites on the macromolecular surface whereas its enantiomer (on the right) can interact at two sites only. Alternative orientations of the enantiomer on right to the target are possible but only two interactions may take place at any time.

biological activity of drug enantiomers. In this model the 'more' active enantiomer is involved in a minimum of three simultaneous bonding interactions with the receptor, whereas the 'less' active, or 'inactive' enantiomer may take part in two such interactions. Thus, the 'fit' of the enantiomers to the target surface differs as does their energy of interaction. This model is a useful, if relatively simplistic, representation of the drug-target interaction since it is assumed that the drug adopts a particular orientation in relation to the biological target. In addition, conformational changes in both the drug and target macromolecule may take place during the interaction such that the final 'model' may be fairly complex. The chiral recognition process continues to be a topic of considerable interest and alternative models and refinements to existing models have been proposed.[18,19]

The differential biological activity of drug enantiomers has also resulted in additional terminology, the stereoisomer with the greater affinity, or activity, being termed the Eutomer and that with the lower affinity, or activity, the Distomer. The ratio of activities, essentially a measure of the stereoselectivity of the system under examination, is known as the Eudismic Ratio.[20,21] The magnitude of the eudismic ratio varies with the compound and biological system under examination, but values of 100 to 1000 are not uncommon and eudismic ratios of greater than one million have been reported, i.e. stereospecificity rather than stereoselectivity.

The above terminology refers to a single activity of a drug and for a dual action compound the eutomer for one activity may be the distomer for the other, or the stereoisomers may be of equal potency. For example in the case of the anaesthetic ketamine the anaesthetic-analgesic activity resides predominantly in the *S*-enantiomer, whereas (*R*)-ketamine is associated with central stimulation[22] and their action on nicotinic acetylcholine receptors shows no stereoselectivity.[23]

Differentiation between stereoisomers may also occur during drug disposition and is of significance for those processes which depend upon a direct interaction with a chiral biological macromolecule, e.g. enzyme systems involved in drug metabolism,[24,25] transporter systems during absorption, distribution and/or renal excretion, and binding to plasma or tissue proteins.[26,27]

The magnitude of the differences between enantiomers observed in their pharmacokinetic parameters, generally 1–3 fold, tend to be much smaller than those observed in their pharmacodynamic effects.[26] This is particularly the case for parameters such as systemic clearance, volume of distribution and half-life, which represent the whole body level of organization.[27] Differences between enantiomers tend to increase as the organizational level that the parameters represent decreases from the whole body to organ and macromolecular, e.g. hepatic and renal clearance at the organ level and intrinsic metabolite formation clearance at the macromolecular level. Pharmacokinetic parameters representing the whole body level of organization being determined by multiple organ parameters, which in turn are determined by multiple macromolecular interactions, which may show opposite stereoselectivities. Thus, stereoselectivity may be either amplified or attenuated with each organizational level.[27]

As a result of stereoselectivity in the processes of drug disposition the plasma profiles of the enantiomers of a drug administered as a racemate frequently differ and an evaluation of plasma-concentration-effect relationships or calculation of pharmacokinetic parameters based on 'total' drug present in biological samples is of limited value and potentially misleading.[28,29]

## Pharmacological Complexity

That a pair of enantiomers are different compounds rather than different forms of the same compound, and that in some instances a racemate may be regarded as a third 'compound', is emphasized on examination of their biological properties. There are relatively few examples of drugs in which the pharmacodynamic activity is restricted to a single enantiomer, the other being totally devoid of activity. In the majority of instances a pair of enantiomers will differ either quantitatively or qualitatively in terms of their biological activity and the idealized examples where the beneficial, or required, activity resides in one enantiomer with the adverse effects, or toxicity, residing in the other are rare. In the case of drugs administered as racemates, interactions between enantiomers may occur such that the observed pharmacodynamic profile is not simply the product of the activities of the individual enantiomers.

Evaluation of the biological properties of a pair of enantiomers may give rise to a number of different situations with respect to their activity as follows:

- The required activity resides in a single enantiomer, e.g. the antihypertensive agent (S)-α-methyldopa.

- The individual enantiomers have similar pharmacodynamic activity, e.g. the antihistamine promethazine.

- The activity of the enantiomers differs such that they are both marketed with different therapeutic indications, e.g. the analgesics dextropropoxyphene and levomethorphan and their enantiomers the antitussives levopropoxyphene (fig. 2) and dextromethorphan.

- The enantiomers have opposite effects at the same biological target, e.g. picenadol, the (+)- and (−)-enantiomers being an agonist and antagonist respectively at the μ-receptor, the racemate being a partial agonist due to the greater potency of the (+)-enantiomer.

- The activity of one enantiomer may antagonize the side effects of the other, e.g. the loop diuretic indacrinone, the diuretic and natriuretic activity residing predominantly in the R-enantiomer with the uricosuric activity in (S)-indacrinone.

- The required activity is predominantly associated with one enantiomer the adverse effects being predominantly associated with the other, e.g. the intravenous anaesthetic-analgesic ketamine (see later).

- The activity of the individual enantiomers is such that the use of the racemate has advantages over either of the individual enantiomers, e.g. the inotropic sympathomimetic agent dobutamine.

In addition to the examples cited above relatively little is known regarding the influence of route of administration, formulation, drug interactions, disease state, age, gender and pharmacogenetics on the action and disposition of a number of agents currently administered as racemates. Further discussion of the possibilities which may arise, together with their consequences may be found in references 30–35.

## Drug Chirality and Anaesthesia

A number of agents used in anaesthetic practice are either natural products, or are derived from natural sources, e.g. (−)-morphine, (+)-tubocurarine,

(−)-cocaine etc., and as nature frequently produces a particular isomer these agents have always been used as single stereoisomer products. The significance of molecular geometry in the action of opioid analgesics has been appreciated for 50 years and the application of stereochemical probes both agonists and antagonists, of the opioid receptors, to our ideas and concepts of analgesic action cannot be over emphasized, particularly as many of these investigations were carried out before the isolation and identification of the natural receptor ligands.[36] More recently stereochemical considerations have focused towards the differentiation of the anti-inflammatory and analgesic actions of the nonsteroidal anti-inflammatory drugs (NSAIDs). Examination of the differential pharmacological activity of some of these agents is complicated as the less active, or inactive, enantiomers undergo metabolic inversion of chirality in a number of species, including man.[37–40] However, pharmacological evaluation has indicated that in the case of the 2-arylpropionic acid NSAIDs the anti-inflammatory activity, inhibition of cyclo-oxygenase (COX) mediated prostaglandin synthesis, resides in the enantiomers of the S-configuration,[38,40] whereas the antinociceptive activity of some agents, e.g. flurbiprofen, resides in both enantiomers.[41–45] While the analgesic potency of the S-enantiomer may be greater, the adverse effect profile, particularly with respect to gastrointestinal effects[46,47] could be used as an argument for the use of the single R-enantiomer for its analgesic properties.

Although the stereochemical nature, and in some instances the differential pharmacological properties, of many chiral anaesthetic agents has been appreciated for a number of years only relatively recently have such considerations become significant in practice, due to the marketing of single enantiomer versions of ketamine and bupivacaine in some countries. Additionally, the availability of highly purified enantiomers of the volatile liquid agents and their biological evaluation will provide insight into their mechanisms of action and molecular theories of anaesthesia. The biological properties of the enantiomers of these agents will be addressed in the following sections.

## Intravenous Anaesthetics

### Etomidate

Etomidate (fig. 4) is the only intravenous agent currently listed in the BNF which is used as a single stereoisomer, the R-enantiomer, (S)-etomidate being reported to be 'devoid of hypnotic activity'.[48] The site of action of etomidate is thought to be the gamma-aminobutyric acid$_A$ (GABA$_A$) receptor[49] and both enantiomers potentiate GABA-induced PA3 cells expressing the GABA$_A$ receptor. However, the potentiation was stereoselective with the R-enantiomer being considerably more potent than (S)-etomidate and the eudismic ratio

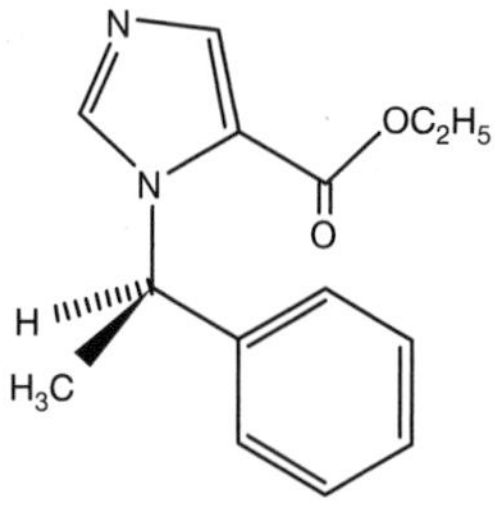


(R)-Etomidate

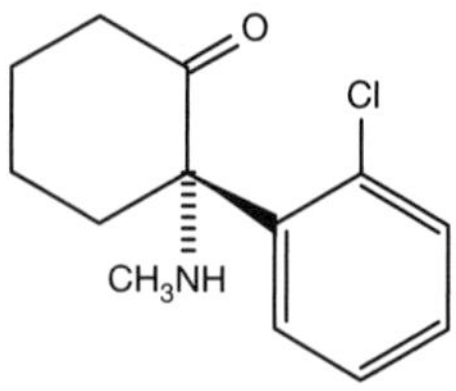


(S)-Ketamine

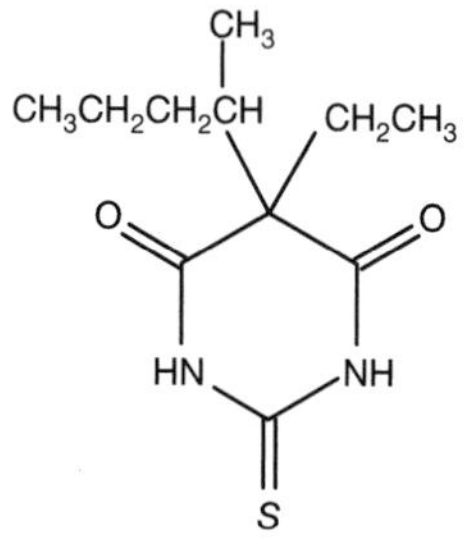


Thiopental

**Figure 4** Structures of the intravenous anaesthetic agents (*R*)-etomidate, (*S*)-ketamine and thiopental.

increased with drug concentration from a value of ca. 5 to 10 at concentrations of 1 and 10 μM respectively.[50] Such increases in eudismic ratio with concentration are unusual, but may be rationalized as being due to a modification of the binding site via drug induced allosteric conformational changes. Using loss-of-righting reflex in tadpoles as an indicator of anaesthetic potency the *R*-enantiomer was found to be 15 fold more potent than (*S*)-etomidate.[50]

## Ketamine

Ketamine (fig. 4) is an anaesthetic-analgesic agent the action of which is associated with non-competitive inhibition of N-methyl-D-aspartate (NMDA) receptors.[51] The drug is used, with the exception of Germany, as the racemate even though the *S*-enantiomer is 3–4 fold more potent than (*R*)-ketamine.[22] The use of the drug is complicated by postanaesthesia emergence reactions, including hallucinations, vivid dreams and agitation, it is also the subject of abuse.[52,53] The emergence reactions are reported to be more common following the administration of the *R*-enantiomer.[22,52]

Stereoselectivity in the pharmacological activity of the enantiomers of ketamine has been known since the 1970s when the greater analgesic (ca. 3 fold) and hypnotic (ca. 1.5 fold) activity and reduced locomotor activity of the S-enantiomer was shown following administration of the individual enantiomers to rats and mice.[54-56] In addition the therapeutic index, ratio of $LD_{50}$ to $ED_{50}$ (hypnosis) determined in the rat, yielded values of 10, 6.25 and 4 for (S)-, (R,S)- and (R)-ketamine respectively.[54] Similarly, studies in dogs have indicated a eudismic ratio (S/R) in anaesthetic potency of ca. 3.[57,58]

Ketamine interacts with multiple binding sites including NMDA and non-NMDA glutamate receptors, nicotinic and muscarinic cholinergic, monoaminergic and opioid receptors.[53] The NMDA receptor, considered to be the main site of action, shows stereoselectivity with (S)-ketamine having a 3 fold greater affinity for the phencyclidine binding site than the R-enantiomer.[53] In vitro studies have also shown that the S-enantiomer is twice as potent as (R)-ketamine in the blockade of NMDA receptor currents in cultured neurons.[59] Similarly the enantiomeric binding to the $\mu$- and $\kappa$-opioid receptors shows a 2–4 fold selectivity for (S)-ketamine, but with a 10–20 fold reduction in affinity compared to the NMDA receptor.[60] However, not all the actions of the drug exhibit stereoselectivity, e.g. inhibition of calcium channels,[61] and inhibition of neuronal nicotinic[23] and muscarinic cholinergic receptors.[62] In the latter case the enantiomers exhibited synergy in action, the inhibitory concentration ($IC_{50}$) of the racemate being significantly lower than that of the individual enantiomers.[63]

Initial studies in surgical patients, following administration of equianaesthetic doses of the enantiomers of ketamine indicated a reduced dose requirement (2.4 mg/kg) of the S-enantiomer compared to 8.5 mg/kg of (R)-ketamine) and lower plasma concentrations at the termination of anaesthesia for the S- compared (0.5 µg/ml) to the R-enantiomer (1.7 µg/ml) associated with a potency ratio (S/R) of 3.4.[22] The S-enantiomer was judged to produce more effective anaesthesia, less emergence reactions and agitated behaviour than either racemic or (R)-ketamine.[22] Pharmacodynamic modelling, monitoring electroencephalographic (EEG) median frequency, following infusion of the racemic drug and individual enantiomers to healthy volunteers has also shown differences between the enantiomers.[64] The maximal decrease ($E_{max}$) resulting from the central nervous system (CNS) depressant effects attained was significantly greater following administration of the S-enantiomer and the racemate compared to (R)-ketamine. The inhibitory concentration ($IC_{50}$) values obtained for (S)-ketamine (0.8 ± 0.4 µg/ml) were significantly lower than that of the R-enantiomer (1.8 ± 0.5 µg/ml) or the racemate (2.0 ± 0.5 µg/ml). These data were interpreted as indicating partial agonist activity of (R)-ketamine in comparison to the S-enantiomer, and partial antagonism following administration of the racemate.[64]

The principle metabolite of ketamine, the N-demethylated product norketamine, is also pharmacologically active. Studies in mice indicate a longer duration of action and reduced spontaneous locomotor activity following administration of (S)- compared to (R)-norketamine.[65] Enantioselectivity in the tissue distribution of both ketamine and norketamine has been reported following drug administration to rats, the plasma and tissue concentrations of (R)-ketamine and (R)-norketamine exceeding those of the S-enantiomers in the majority of tissues examined. The metabolite also binds stereoselectively to the NMDA receptor the Ki values being 1.7 and 13 $\mu$M for (S)- and (R)-norketamine respectively.[67]

Ketamine has recently undergone the Chiral Switch process (see below) and has been marketed in Germany as the single S-enantiomer[9] with the potential advantages of a reduction in dose and more rapid recovery with fewer psychotomimetic emergence reactions as compared with racemate. The greater clinical use of the single enantiomer will allow evaluation of the relative therapeutic merits of the drug compared to the racemate in man.

## Thiopental

Stereoselectivity in the action and toxicity of the barbiturates has been known for a number of years,[68] the (+)-enantiomers of some of these agents being excitatory whereas the (−)-enantiomers are depressant.[69] For example in the case of N-methyl-5-propyl-5-phenylbarbiturate[70] and 5-(1,3-dimethylbutyl)-5-ethylbarbituric acid (DMBB) the (+)-enantiomers are convulsants whereas the anaesthetic properties reside in the (−)-enantiomers. In addition (−)-DMBB is an antagonist of the convulsant effects of (+)- DMBB[71] which is ca. 24 fold more toxic, as measured by the $LD_{50}$ in mice, compared to the (−)-enantiomer. Similarly differences in the pharmacokinetic properties of the enantiomers of some of these agents have been reported in man, the extent of which appears to depend on age,[72,73] sex[73] and interactions with other drugs.[74]

Thiopental (fig. 4) exhibits a biphasic activation/depression concentration effect relationship following administration to both animals [75,76] and man.[77,78] Although differences in the potency and toxicity of the enantiomers of thiopental have been known since the 1970s only recently have EEG studies in rats indicated that both enantiomers, and the racemate, cause an initial EEG activation followed by depression, the extent of the latter response being significantly less for the R-enantiomer and the racemate compared to (S)-thiopental.[79] Such investigations are obviously of significance because as a result of potential stereoselectivity in action the two effects may have been associated with the individual enantiomers.

Barbiturates exert their sedative and anaesthetic effects primarily by potentiation of the GABA response at $GABA_A$ receptors via an increase in the duration of the chloride ion channel open-time. They are also able to directly
activate $GABA_A$ receptors and at high concentrations the chloride channel
may be blocked. The enantioselectivity of action of thiopental on the potentiation of the GABA response has been investigated[80] using *Xenopus laevis*
oocytes expressing human $GABA_A$ receptor subtype $\alpha_1 \beta_2 \gamma_2$, thought to be
the major human receptor subunit combination *in vivo*. The *S*-enantiomer
was found to be approximately 2 fold more potent than (*R*)-thiopental, the
mean effective concentration 50% ($EC_{50}$) being 26.0, 52.5 and 35.9 µM for
(*S*)-, (*R*)- and (*R*,*S*)-thiopental respectively,[80] a potency ratio in good agreement with that observed for anaesthetic doses in laboratory animals.[68]

Studies combining pharmacodynamic activity and drug distribution
following administration of the three stereoisomeric forms of thiopental
to rats confirmed the greater potency and lower therapeutic index of the
*S*-enantiomer ($S > R,S > R$) in terms of both administered dose or arterial
plasma concentration (table 1). Examination of tissue to plasma distribution
coefficients of the individual enantiomers following administration of the
racemate indicated a modest, ca. 10%, excess of the *R*-enantiomer in the
majority of CNS and peripheral tissues. However, following administration
of the individual enantiomers significantly greater ratios were observed for
the *R*-enantiomer in the CNS but not in peripheral tissues, possibly indicating an enantiomeric interaction following administration of the racemate.
Comparison of heart to brain ratios yielded a rank order of $S > R,S > R$.
Based on these data Mather *et al.*[81] presented arguments for the possible use
of (*R*)-thiopental as a single enantiomer drug as a result of the greater safety
margin, higher distribution coefficient for CNS penetration, lower heart to
brain ratio and minimal pharmacokinetic differences in man (see below).

There is also evidence that the enantiomeric distribution of thiopental in the
rat is influenced by the chiral volatile anaesthetic halothane.[82] Following
infusion of racemic thiopental to either conscious or halothane anaesthetized
rats the plasma concentrations and tissue distribution coefficients were found
to be lower in the halothane treated group, the effect being slightly greater
on (*R*)-thiopental. It was concluded that halothane reduces the relative
uptake of the drug into the brain but the mechanism of the reduction is by
no means clear.[82]

The systemic and cerebral pharmacokinetics of the enantiomers of thiopental
have been reported following administration of the racemate to sheep.[83] The
cerebral parameters were determined by comparison of the concentration
differences between arterial and superior sagittal sinus plasma. No significant

**Table 1** Anaesthetic and lethal doses, corresponding arterial plasma concentrations and therapeutic index of thiopental enantiomers following intravenous infusion to rats

| Stereoisomeric form | Dose (mg/kg) | | Plasma concentration (μg/ml) | | Therapeutic index | |
|---|---|---|---|---|---|---|
| | Anaesthesia | Lethality | Anaesthesia | Lethality | Dose | Concentration |
| R | 55.8 ± 2.4 | 176.2 ± 11.2 | 66.3 ± 4.5 | 89.8 ± 5.2 | 3.16 | 1.37 |
| S | 35.6 ± 1.9 | 74.2 ± 5.2 | 55.0 ± 1.9 | 64.1 ± 2.8 | 2.10 | 1.17 |
| R,S | 39.3 ± 2.1 | 97.5 ± 3.9 | 56.7 ± 2.0 | 77.8 ± 2.8 | 2.52 | 1.32 |

Data expressed as mean ± SEM, n = 7.[81]

differences were observed in the cerebral pharmacokinetic properties of the enantiomers of thiopental and no evidence was found for the faster brain uptake of either enantiomer. In contrast, the systemic clearance of the R-enantiomer was found to be significantly greater (17%) than that of (S)-thiopental.[83]

Differences in the pharmacokinetic properties of the enantiomers of thiopental following their individual administration to man were initially investigated in 1976 by Mark et al.[84] who reported a shorter half-life of the R-enantiomer. In spite of subsequent studies with related agents, e.g. pentobarbital,[85] hexobarbital[72,74] and mephobarbital,[73] indicating stereoselective pharmacokinetics in man the enantiomeric disposition of thiopental was not examined again until the mid-1990s, when Nguyen et al.[86] investigated the stereoselective disposition of the drug following intravenous bolus and infusion administration of the racemate to patients. These authors reported small, but statistically significant differences in the clearance, volume of distribution at steady state and fraction unbound between the enantiomers, the values for (R)-thiopental being greater than those of the S-enantiomer. When the pharmacokinetic parameters were based on unbound plasma concentrations no differences were observed between the enantiomers (table 2). Following intravenous infusion no differences in plasma concentrations, either total or free, for either the enantiomers of thiopental, or the metabolic oxidation product, pentobarbital were observed.[86]

Similar observations were reported following intravenous bolus administration of the racemate by Cordato et al.,[87] clearance and volume of distribution at steady state showing a trend towards higher values for (R)- compared to (S)-thiopental, which disappeared when unbound concentrations were taken into account (table 2). The free fraction of (R)-thiopental, was found to be significantly greater than that of the S-enantiomer and the 24 h urinary recovery of unchanged drug was also significantly greater for the R-enantiomer, but at less than 1% of the dose this is unlikely to be of significance. In one patient drug enantiomer concentrations were determined in cerebrospinal fluid (CSF): the values were ca. 20% of the corresponding plasma concentrations, with the R-enantiomer in excess. Taking protein binding into account these data are indicative of passive diffusion into the CSF.

Thiopental is also used in high doses for prolonged periods for treatment of intracranial hypertension and neuroprotection in head-injured patients. Under such conditions the drug shows nonlinear pharmacokinetics at total plasma concentrations of approximately 30 mg/L. Cordalo et al.[88] have examined the enantiomeric disposition of the drug under these conditions. Small, but statistically significant differences (10–20%) in the steady-state clearance and

**Table 2** Pharmacokinetic parameters of the enantiomers of thiopental following intravenous administration of the racemic drug to patients

| Method of administration | Bolus | Bolus | Infusion | Infusion | Infusion** |
|---|---|---|---|---|---|
| Number (sex) | 7 (M6, F1) | 12 (M7, F5) | 7 (M5, F2) | 5 (M4, F1) | 20 (M13, F7) |
| Age (years) | 43–72 | 38–82 | 37–73 | 20–47 | 15–69 |
| Dose (g) | 0.25–0.50 | 0.125–0.50 | 0.750–1.125 | 26.1–54.5 | 12.5–86.9 |
| Duration (h) | – | – | 1.75–3 | 31–92 | 31–285 |
| *Pharmacokinetic parameters* | | | | | |
| Clearance (L/min) | $R$ 0.295 ± 0.132* <br> $S$ 0.230 ± 0.104 | $R$ 0.59 ± 0.23 <br> $S$ 0.56 ± 0.20 | – | $R$ 0.022–0.160 <br> $S$ 0.021–0.156 | $R$ 0.10 ± 0.05* <br> $S$ 0.08 ± 0.04 |
| Volume of central compartment (L) | $R$ 2.0 ± 1.1 <br> $S$ 1.8 ± 1.1 | $R$ 20.2 ± 9.7 <br> $S$ 18.8 ± 7.9 | – | – | – |
| Volume of distribution at steady-state (L) | $R$ 139 ± 38* <br> $S$ 114 ± 47 | $R$ 91 ± 53 <br> $S$ 80 ± 37 | – | – | $R$ 313 ± 145* <br> $S$ 273 ± 115 |
| Half-life (h) | $R$ 9.6 ± 5.4 <br> $S$ 9.0 ± 4.5 | – | – | – | $R$ 14.6 ± 7.0 <br> $S$ 14.7 ± 7.2 |
| Fraction unbound | $R$ 0.124 ± 0.006[+] <br> $S$ 0.100 ± 0.010 | $R$ 0.165 (n = 6) <br> $S$ 0.156 | – | – | $R$ 0.20 ± 0.05* (n = 7) <br> $S$ 0.18 ± 0.04 |
| Unbound clearance (L/min) | $R$ 2.39 ± 1.07 <br> $S$ 2.31 ± 1.04 | $R$ 4.8 ± 2.3 <br> $S$ 5.3 ± 1.6 | – | – | – |
| Unbound volume of distribution at steady-state (L) | $R$ 1126 ± 311 <br> $S$ 1145 ± 476 | $R$ 680 ± 585 <br> $S$ 684 ± 464 | – | – | – |
| Steady-state concentration (mg/L) | – | – | $R$ 2.29 ± 0.99 <br> $S$ 2.76 ± 0.81 | – | – |
| Pentobarbital steady-state concentration (mg/L) | – | – | $R$ 0.28 ± 0.13 [‡] <br> $S$ 0.27 ± 0.16 | – | – |
| Reference | 86 | 87 | 86 | 87 | 88 |

*Significant difference between enantiomers. [+]Protein binding determined using plasma samples obtained from six healthy volunteers. **Protein binding determined in samples obtained from four patients. **Following administration of high doses of thiopental nonlinearity in the pharmacokinetics of the drug is observed and the following parameters were calculated in the study by Cordato et al.[88] $K_m$ (mg/L): $R$ 20 ± 19, $S$ 24 ± 23; $V_{max}$ (mg/L/h): $R$ 0.86 ± 0.54, $S$ 1.01 ± 0.69*; clearance (L/min) at pseudo steady state: $R$ 0.108 ± 0.05, $S$ 0.096 ± 0.04*; unbound clearance (L/min) at pseudo steady state: $R$ 0.582 ± 0.26, $S$ 0.588 ± 0.25.
[‡]Pentobarbital detected in samples obtained from four patients.

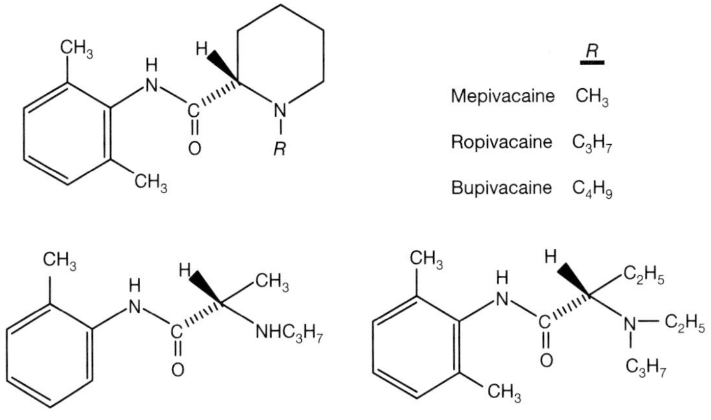

Figure 5 S-Enantiomers of chiral amide derivative local anaesthetic agents.

volume of distribution between enantiomers were observed $(R > S)$ and in $V_{max}$ but not $K_m$ (table 2), both enantiomers showing saturation.

In summary, only modest differences in the pharmacokinetic parameters of the enantiomers of thiopental are observed following either bolus or prolonged intravenous infusion of the racemate which are unlikely to be of clinical significance as compared with the pharmacodynamic differences.

## Local Anaesthetics

A number of commercially available local anaesthetics, e.g. prilocaine, mepi-vacaine, ropivacaine, bupivacaine, etidocaine (fig. 5) are chiral[89,90] and while the majority are marketed as racemates single enantiomers, e.g. ropivacaine,[91] or in the case of bupivacaine both the racemate and single $(-)$-S-enantiomer, levobupivacaine,[92,93] are available.

That the enantiomers of these agents may differ in their duration of action, disposition and acute toxicity following intravenous infusion or subcutaneous injection to experimental animals has been known since the late 1960s.[94–97] As the individual enantiomers differ in their effects on local blood flow these differences in duration of action may be accounted for by differences in rates of systemic absorption.[94–98] For example, following intradermal injection of the enantiomers of bupivacaine to healthy volunteers both enantiomers caused vasodilation at the highest concentrations examined but only the S-enantiomer showed a vasoconstrictor effect and consequently a longer dur-ation of action.[98] Thus the pharmacodynamic activity of the drug indirectly influences the stereoselectivity of absorption. A more recent investigation, concerned with an evaluation of the cutaneous analgesia following subcutaneous injection of the enantiomers of bupivacaine to rats, indicated that the addition of low concentrations of epinephrine results in vasoconstriction such that the duration of action of (R)-bupivacaine is similar to that of the S-enantiomer.[99] In addition the permeability of the individual enantiomers of bupivacaine through meningeal tissue *in vitro* has been shown to be equivalent confirming that the differences arise as a result of pharmacodynamic properties rather than differences in absorption.[100]

Local anaesthetics block voltage-gated sodium channels and their potency is modulated by channel state, open and inactivated states being favoured over resting states. The enantiomers of bupivacaine show modest stereoselectivity (eudismic ratio R/S of 1.5) for sodium channel blockade using a sciatic nerve preparation isolated from *Xenopus laevis*. The activity being determined by the decrease in sodium ion current at low-depolarization frequencies, which is associated with drug binding to the channel resting state and inactivated states at rest.[101] Blockade of inactivated sodium channels in guinea pig ventricular myocytes shows a similar stereoselectivity with a eudismic ratio of 1.7.[102] In contrast to the above bupivacaine shows marked stereoselectivity on the flicker potassium ion channel with a eudismic ratio (R/S) of 73 which appears to be predominantly associated with drug dissociation from the binding site, the enantiomeric ratio of the dissociation rate constants being R/S 64.[101]

Bupivacaine cardiotoxicity is associated with the R-enantiomer which presumably relates to its greater potency in blocking cardiac sodium and potassium channels. Stereoselectivity of blockade has been shown in hKv 1.5 channels, with the R-enantiomer being 7 fold more potent than (S)-bupivacaine as measured by the ratio of the apparent affinity constants,[103] but not Kv 2.1 or Kv 4.3 channels.[104,105] Bupivacaine has also been shown to inhibit L-type calcium ion channels in isolated cardiac myocytes but not stereoselectively.[106]

A number of studies have compared the clinical efficacy and dose response of (S)-bupivacaine and the racemate. The majority of which have indicated that sensory block and the clinical profile resulting from administration of the single enantiomer is essentially the same as that following the racemate.[90,92,107,108] For example following comparison of the two forms of the drug for epidural analgesia in labour the minimum ratio of local analgesic concentration was S/R,S 0.98.[109,110] As the clinical profile of the single enantiomer and racemate are similar the relative merits of the different forms of the drug are essentially associated with toxicity. Serious CNS and cardiovascular adverse reactions, including deaths, following accidental intravenous injection of local anaesthetics have been reported.[111-114] The cardiovascular effects of (S)- and (R,S)-bupivacaine have been investigated following intravenous infusion to healthy volunteers.[114] The negative inotropic effect, as measured by stroke index, acceleration index and ejection fraction, was found to be significantly less, approximately half, following the single enantiomer compared to racemic bupivacaine.[114] Both agents caused small increases in PR and QTc intervals which were greater following the racemate, but the differences did not achieve statistical significance.

*In vitro* studies using heart muscle preparations have reported smaller conduction changes with levobupivacaine as compared with the R-enantiomer or the racemate,[115-117] and a study comparing the S-enantiomer with the racemic drug *in vivo* in sheep has indicated the greater margin of safety following the single enantiomer.[118] Taken together these data indicate that the single enantiomer is a potentially safer agent in comparison to the racemate.

Evidence associated with the greater risk of cardiotoxicity occurring following administration of bupivacaine compared to shorter acting drugs, together with the stereoselectivity of the adverse effect, resulted in the development of ropivacaine, the N-propyl analogue of bupivacaine (fig. 5) as a single enantiomer.[89,91]

Bupivacaine also undergoes stereoselective disposition following administration to man.[119,120] Following intravenous administration of the racemate the systemic clearance, volume of distribution at steady-state and half-life of (R)-bupivacaine are greater than that of the S-enantiomer (table 3). However, stereoselectivity was also observed in plasma protein binding, the free fraction of the R-enantiomer being greater than that of (S)-bupivacaine, and

**Table 3** Pharmacokinetic parameters of the enantiomers of bupivacaine following intravenous administration to man

| Parameter (units) | Enantiomer | |
|---|---|---|
| | R | S |
| Clearance (L/min) | 0.395 | 0.317* |
| Volume of distribution at steady-state (L) | 84 | 54* |
| Half-life (h) | 3.5 | 2.6* |
| Fraction unbound | 0.066 | 0.045* |
| Unbound clearance (L/min) | 7.26 | 8.71 |
| Unbound volume of distribution at steady-state (L) | 1576 | 1498 |

*Significant difference between enantiomers; mean data following drug administration to 10 male volunteers. Data from Burm *et al.*[119]

when binding is taken into account there were no differences between the enantiomers in unbound volume of distribution but the unbound clearance of the S-enantiomer was greater than that of (R)-bupivacaine.[119] Stereoselectivity in the metabolism of bupivacaine has been reported following epidural infusion of the racemate to five patients. The urinary recovery of the R-enantiomer was, in the majority of cases, greater than that of (S)-bupivacaine with R/S ratios varying between 1.0 and 4.3. Examination of the stereochemical composition of the urinary metabolites, 4-hydroxy-, 3-hydroxy- and desbutylbupivacaine indicated considerable stereo- and regioselectivity with the excretion of (R)-4-hydroxybupivacaine exceeding that of the S-enantiomer in all subjects, whereas in the case of the other two products considerable variability in stereoselectivity was observed.[120] Such studies are of significance as investigations in animals[97,120] have indicated that the desbutyl metabolite may contribute to the toxicity of the drug, which may also show stereoselectivity.

Prilocaine (fig. 5), as a result of its high metabolic clearance, has a relatively low potential for CNS toxicity, but its use is limited due to a metabolic association with methaemoglobinaemia. Following the report of Åkerman and Ross[96] of lower plasma concentrations and increased rate of methaemoglobin production following intravenous administration of the R-enantiomer compared to either (S)- or racemic prilocaine to cats, it was suggested that the therapeutic use of the S-enantiomer would result in a safer product. However, the original report indicates that the rate, but not the extent of methaemoglobinaemia differs following administration of the three forms of the drug.[96] An examination of the plasma concentrations of the individual enantiomers following brachial plexus injection of the racemate to man indicated similar plasma profiles and areas under the plasma-concentration-time curves, with an enantiomeric ratio S/R of 1.06.[122] In contrast following oral drug administration the enantiomeric ratio (S/R) was at least eight with the concentrations of the R-enantiomer being close to the analytical limit of detection.[122]

## Inhalational Anaesthetics: Volatile Liquids

The pharmacological effects of the volatile liquid anaesthetics have been extensively examined but their mechanism of action has remained a matter of controversy as a result of the traditional view that they act by some non-specific perturbation of lipid membranes. That they ultimately act on neuronal ion channels is generally accepted[123] but whether this results via drug–protein interactions rather than as a secondary effect arising from drug–lipid interactions has been a matter of debate.[124]

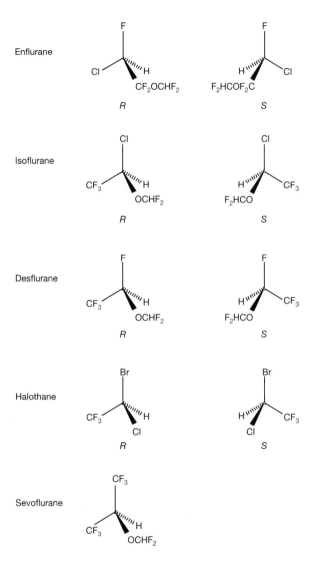

**Figure 6** Structures of the chiral volatile liquid anaesthetic agents and the achiral sevoflurane.

Five volatile liquid anaesthetic agents are listed in the current BNF (No. 43) of which four are chiral compounds and the fifth, sevoflurane, is achiral (fig. 6). Initial investigations concerned with the possible stereoselectivity of action of these agents were carried out in the early 1970s using enantiomerically enriched samples of halothane.[125,126] However, no selectivity in action was detected with what were relatively stereochemically impure compounds, the enantiomeric compositions being approximately 1:3 in each case.[125,126] However, in the early 1990s the enantiomers of halothane, enflurane and isoflurane were resolved by enantioselective gas chromatography using a chiral stationary phase[127] and Franks and Lieb[124] were able to demonstrate the stereoselectivity of action of the enantiomers of isoflurane on potassium channels in neurones of the molluscan CNS. The (+)-enantiomer was found to be ca. 2 fold more potent than (−)-isoflurane in activation of the anaesthetic-activated potassium current $I_K(A_n)$, and inhibition of the inward current mediated by neuronal nicotinic acetylcholine receptors. However, the (−)-enantiomer was slightly more potent than (+)-isoflurane in the inhibition of the less sensitive transient potassium current $I_A$.[124]

Although in the context of the molecular mechanism of general anaesthesia stereoselective interactions with the chiral components of lipid bilayers cannot be ruled out, previous investigations have demonstrated little chiral discrimination by phospholipids[128] and both isoflurane enantiomers are equally soluble in lipid bilayers.[129] In addition, both enantiomers have identical effects on the shift of the chain-melting phase transition temperature of dipalmitoyl lecithin (dipalmitoyl-L-α-phosphatidyl choline) a test of bilayer disruption.[124]

Initial *in vivo* studies with isoflurane were carried out following intraperitoneal administration of the individual enantiomers to mice and determination of sleeping time. Both enantiomers produced a dose-dependent increase in sleeping time with (+)-isoflurane being significantly more potent than the (−)-enantiomer.[130] Subsequent reports on the stereoselectivity of action of isoflurane have provided contradictory data. Lysko *et al.*[131] showed the (+)-S-enantiomer to be ca. 50% more potent than (−)-(R)-isoflurane with respect to minimum alveolar concentration (MAC) in rats, but others have found no significant differences between the enantiomers.[132] Whereas examination of loss in righting reflex and sleeping time in rats indicated the (+)-S-enantiomer to be 40–50% more potent than (−)-(R)-isoflurane.[133] Interestingly the racemic drug showed a potency similar to that of the (−)-enantiomer for loss of righting reflex.[133]

The stereoselectivity of isoflurane on the preservation of ATP concentrations in anoxic rat hepatocytes has also been examined.[134] The (−)-R-enantiomer was found to be approximately 2.5 fold greater in potency compared to (+)-(S)-isoflurane, thus the anaesthetic and biochemical effects of the two enantiomers are opposite which imply that the effects are independent of one another.[134]

As indicated above the majority of the available data on the stereoselectivity of action of these agents is derived from studies on isoflurane. However, some investigations have been carried out with the enantiomers of halothane.[135]

Using the immobilization of the nematode *Caenorhabditis elegans* as a model of anaesthetic action Sedensky *et al.*[135] have shown genetic differences with respect to the stereoselectivity of the action of halothane, the (+)-*R*-enantiomer being ca. 3 fold more potent than (−)-(*S*)-halothane in some genetic mutants, whereas in others the differences between the enantiomers were minimal.[135]

The stereoselectivity of disposition of some of these agents has been investigated following their administration to either animals or man. Following exposure of rats to racemic halothane in a constant volume chamber the drug concentration, and enantiomeric composition, were determined in the chamber atmosphere with time, providing an indirect estimation of the whole body pharmacokinetics of the drug.[136] The chamber drug concentrations decreased in a biphasic manner with an essentially constant enantiomeric ratio of one, indicative of minimal stereoselectivity in drug disposition. Similarly, the enantiomeric composition of isoflurane in rat brain, following intravenous administration of the racemate, was essentially unity.[133] The enantiomeric disposition of isoflurane has also been examined following administration to patients.[137,138] The enantiomeric composition *S*:*R* of the drug in blood varied between 51:49 to 54:46 in samples collected up to 8 days following administration,[137,138] indicating a lack of stereoselective distribution.

The oxidative metabolism of these agents, mediated by cytochrome P450 (CYP), involves formation of reactive acylhalide intermediates which bind covalently to liver protein and are associated with hepatotoxicity. In the case of halothane approximately 20% of patients experience mild liver dysfunction. In order to examine a possible association between halothane stereochemistry and hepatotoxicity the individual enantiomers and racemic drug were administered intraperitoneally to mice. Using immunoblotting techniques (*R*)-halothane was found to yield two to three times more covalently bound adducts than either the *S*-enantiomer or the racemate.[139] Similarly the metabolism of enflurane to difluoromethoxydifluoroacetic acid, the end product of the oxidative transformation, has been examined *in vitro* using both human liver microsomal preparations and microsomes containing cDNA-expressed human CYP2E1. The rate of formation of the acid from the *R*-enantiomer was approximately 2 fold that from (*S*)-enflurane, with the racemate yielding an intermediate value.[140] While these are obviously preliminary observations if the stereoselectivity of metabolism of these agents is associated with hepatotoxicity and there are relatively minor differences in anaesthetic potency then an argument could be made for the use of the single *S*-enantiomers of these drugs.[139]

While from the available literature there appears to be little argument for the use of single enantiomers of the volatile liquid anaesthetics from a pharmacodynamic viewpoint examination of their selectivity of action does contribute to our understanding of their mechanism of action. Such stereoselectivity in action should be viewed in the context of Lehman's statement that "the stereoselectivity displayed by pharmacological systems constitutes the best evidence that receptors exist and that they incorporate concrete molecular entities as integral components of their active sites."[21]

## Chiral Drugs and Regulation

The increased appreciation of the potential significance of the pharmacological differences between enantiomers, together with associated safety issues,[34] resulted in drug chirality and particularly the use of racemic mixtures vs single enantiomers, becoming an area of concern for the pharmaceutical industry and leading regulatory authorities.[141-144] Those advocating the use of single enantiomers stating that the use of racemates is essentially polypharmacy with the dosage being determined by chemical rather than therapeutic or pharmacological criteria and regarding racemates as drugs containing 50% impurity. In the lay press the issue was frequently addressed in emotive terms citing, unjustifiably,[32,141] the hypnotic–sedative–teratogenic agent thalidomide as an example where the use of a single enantiomer would have prevented the tragedy of the early 1960s.

There are a number of potential advantages associated with the use of single enantiomers including: a less complex more selective pharmacological profile; potential for an improved therapeutic index; a less complex pharmacokinetic profile; reduced potential for complex drug interactions, and a less complex relationship between plasma concentrations and effect.

The major regulatory authorities have addressed the issues associated with drug chirality and published guidelines or policy statements.[145-147] At present there is no absolute requirement from the regulatory authorities for the development of single enantiomer drugs, the choice of stereoisomeric form, i.e. single enantiomer or racemic mixture, residing with the compound sponsor, but the decision requires scientific justification based on quality, safety and efficacy criteria together with the risk-benefit ratio.[147]

As a result of regulatory attitudes the number of new chemical entities submitted for approval as single stereoisomers rather than racemates to various regulatory bodies over the last 10 years appears to have increased.[147-149] The most recent data, for the period 1996–1999, from the Medicines Control Agency, indicates that 24 of a total of 37 synthetic chiral new chemical entities submitted for evaluation were single stereoisomers.[147]

# Chiral Switch

In addition to new chemical entities a number of agents initially, or currently, marketed as racemates have been re-introduced as single enantiomer products undergoing the so-called Chiral Switch process.[9] The idea of evaluating single enantiomers following either developments in synthetic technology or the observation of unacceptable adverse effects with the racemate is not new and the examples of D-penicillamine,[150,151] L-dopa[152,153] and levonorgestrel may be cited. The Chiral Switch has resulted in a number of agents being re-marketed as single enantiomers including levobupivacaine, (S)-ketamine, cisatracurium, dexibuprofen and dexketoprofen, in a number of countries (table 4). These re-introductions have resulted in products containing both single enantiomer and racemic mixtures being available at the same time, hence the requirement for physicians to have an appreciation of stereochemical nomenclature to ensure that they know what they have in fact prescribed.

However, as noted in table 4, such re-evaluations/re-introductions are not without problems and in the case of dilevalol, the β-blocking stereoisomer of the combined α, β-blocking drug labetalol, the development of the drug was stopped as a result of hepatotoxicity;[34] the development of (R)-fluoxetine was terminated due to a small but significant increase in QTc prolongation at the highest dose examined;[154] both dex- and racemic fenfluramine were withdrawn following an association with valvular heart disease;[155] and the SWORD trial (Survival With Oral d-Sotalol) was terminated early due to increased mortality in the treatment compared to the placebo control group.[156] The above examples illustrate that removal

---

**Table 4** Single enantiomers from marketed racemates: the Chiral Switch

| Drug | Action/indication | Availability/comment |
|---|---|---|
| Dexfenfluramine | Anoretic | Withdrawn |
| Dilevalol | β-antagonist | Development stopped |
| Levofloxacin | Antimicrobial | Japan, UK, USA |
| Dexibuprofen | NSAID | Austria, Switzerland |
| Dexketoprofen | NSAID | Spain, UK |
| Levobupivacaine | Regional anaesthetic | UK |
| (S)-Ketamine | Anaesthetic | Germany |
| Esomeprazole | Proton-pump inhibitor | UK, USA |
| (R)-Salbutamol | β$_2$-agonist | USA |
| (R)-Fluoxetine | Selective serotonin re-uptake inhibitor | Development stopped |
| Cisatracurium | Neuromuscular blocker | UK, USA |
| Levocetirizine | Antihistamine | UK |
| (R,R)-Methylphenidate | Attention-deficit hyperactivity disorder | USA |
| Escitalopram | Selective serotonin re-uptake inhibitor | USA, UK |

of the 50% 'isomeric impurity' present in a racemate is by no means a trivial matter.

In addition to the agents cited in table 4 a number of other compounds are undergoing evaluation as potential single enantiomer products including (R,R)-formoterol for the treatment of asthma; (S)-fluoxetine for migraine prophylaxis; (S)-oxybutinin, for urinary incontinence; (S)-doxazosin for treatment of benign prostatic hyperplasia; the proton pump inhibitors (S)-lansoprazole and (−)-pantoprazole and (+)-norcisapride for the treatment of nocturnal heartburn.[9]

## Conclusions

This chapter has attempted to explain the terminology and pharmacological significance of stereochemistry, together with the current regulatory position regarding chiral pharmaceuticals. There can be no doubt that stereochemical considerations in pharmacology will continue and provide additional insights into the mechanisms of drug action and disposition. From a clinical perspective such investigations should contribute to improved drug use and the re-evaluation of 'old' racemates will in some instances result in single enantiomer products with an increase in both drug safety and efficacy.

### Note added in proof

The attention of interested readers is drawn to two recently published articles relevant to the topics addressed in this chapter.[157,158]

### References

1. Tucker G. The clinical relevance of chirality. Prescribers J 1991; 31: 189–197.
2. Shah RR. The influence of chirality on drug development. Future Prescriber 2000; 1: 14–17.
3. Mason S. The left hand of nature. New Scientist 1984; 101: 10–14.
4. Matteson D. Through the chemical looking glass. New Scientist 1991; 132: 35–39.
5. Amato I. Looking glass chemistry. Science, 1992; 256: 964–966.
6. Hawkes N. Lateral thinking. The Times Magazine, London, UK. June 5th, 1993.
7. Moran N. Drug firms sort their lefts from their rights. Independent on Sunday, London, UK. November 7th, 1993.
8. Ariëns EJ, Wuis EW, Veringa EJ. Stereoselectivity of bioactive xenobiotics. A pre-Pasteur attitude in medicinal chemistry, pharmacokinetics and clinical pharmacology. Biochem Pharmacol 1988; 37: 9–18.
9. Tucker GT. Chiral switches. Lancet 2000; 355: 1085–1087.
10. Controulis J, Rebstock MC, Crooks HM. Chloramphenicol (chloromycetin) V. Synthesis. J Am Chem Soc 1949; 71: 2463–2468.
11. Rebstock MC, Crooks HM, Controulis J, Bartz QR. Chloramphenicol (chloromycetin) IV. Chemical studies. J Am Chem Soc 1949; 71: 2458–2462.

12. Ceccarini G, Maione AM. Variations of optical rotation of naproxen: polarimetric determination in the presence of non-chiral basic compounds. J Pharm Sci 1989; 78: 1053–1054.

13. Stoschitzky K, Klein W, Stark G, Stark U, Zernig G, Graziadei I, Lindner W. Different stereoselective effects of (R)- and (S)- propafenone: clinical pharmacologic, electrophysiologic and radioligand binding studies. Clin Pharmacol Ther 1990; 47: 40–46.

14. Cahn RS, Ingold CK, Prelog V. The specification of asymmetric configuration in organic chemistry. Experientia 1956; 12: 81–94.

15. May P. The Chemistry of Synthetic Drugs. London, UK: Longmans, Green and Co; 1918: 34.

16. Cushny AR. Biological Relations of Optically Isomeric Substances. London: Bailliere, Tindall and Cox; 1926.

17. Easson LH, Stedman E. Studies on the relationship between chemical constitution and physiological action V. Molecular dissymmetry and physiological activity. Biochem J 1933; 27: 1257–1266.

18. Booth TD, Wahnon D, Wainer IW. Is chiral recognition a three-point process? Chirality 1997; 9: 96–98.

19. Mesecar AD, Koshland DE. A new model for protein stereospecificity. Nature 2000; 403: 614–615.

20. Lehman PAF, De Miranda JFR, Ariëns EJ. Stereoselectivity and affinity in molecular pharmacology. In: Jucker E, ed. Progress in drug research, Basel, Switzerland: Birkhauser Verlag. 1976; 20: 101–142.

21. Lehman PAF. Quantifying stereoselectivity or how to choose a pair of shoes when you have two left feet. Trend Pharmacol Sci 1982; 3: 103–106.

22. White PF, Ham J, Way WL, Trevor AJ. Pharmacology of ketamine isomers in surgical patients. Anesthesiology 1980; 52: 231–239.

23. Sasaki T, Andoh T, Watanabe I, Kamiya Y, Itoh H, Higashi T, Matsuura T. Nonstereoselective inhibition of neuronal nicotinic acetylcholine receptors by ketamine isomers. Anesth Analg 2000; 91: 741–748.

24. Caldwell J, Winter SM, Hutt AJ. The pharmacological and toxicological significance of the stereochemistry of drug disposition. Xenobiotica 1988; 18 (Suppl 1): 59–70.

25. Mason JP, Hutt AJ. Stereochemical aspects of drug metabolism. In: Aboul-Enein HY, Wainer IW, eds. The Impact of Stereochemistry on Drug Development and Use. New York: John Wiley 1997: 45–105.

26. Tucker GT, Lennard MS. Enantiomer specific pharmacokinetics. Pharmacol Ther 1990; 45: 309–329.

27. Levy RH, Boddy AV. Stereoselectivity in pharmacokinetics: a general theory. Pharm Res 1991; 8: 551–556.

28. Ariëns EJ. Stereochemistry, a basis for sophisticated nonsense in pharmacokinetics and clinical pharmacology. Eur J Clin Pharmacol 1984; 26: 663–668.

29. Evans AM, Nation RL, Sansom LN, Bochner F, Somogyi AA. Stereoselective drug disposition: potential for misinterpretation of drug disposition data. Br J Clin Pharmacol 1988; 26: 771–780.

30. Crossley R. Chirality and the Biological Activity of Drugs. Boca Raton: CRC Press. 1995.

31. Hutt AJ. Drug chirality and its pharmacological consequences. In: Smith HJ, ed. Introduction to the Principles of Drug Design and Action, 3rd edition: Reading: Harwood Academic; 1998: 97–166.

32. Hutt AJ, Tan SC. Drug chirality and its clinical significance. Drugs 1996; 52 (Suppl 5): 1–12.
33. Powell JR, Ambre JJ, Ruo TJ. The efficacy and toxicity of drug stereoisomers. In: Wainer IW, Drayer DE, eds, Drug Stereochemistry. Analytical Methods and Pharmacology. New York: Marcel Dekker; 1988: 245–270.
34. Shah RR, Midgley JM, Branch SK. Stereochemical origin of some clinically significant drug safety concerns: lessons for future drug development. Adverse Drug React Toxicol Rev 1998; 17: 145–190.
35. Eichelbaum M, Gross AS. Stereochemical aspects of drug action and disposition. In: Testa B, Meyer UA, eds. Advances in Drug Research, London: Academic 1996; 28: 1–64.
36. Portoghese PS. Stereoisomeric ligands as opioid receptor probes. Acc Chem Res 1978; 11: 21–29.
37. Hutt AJ, Caldwell J. The metabolic chiral inversion of 2-arylpropionic acids – a novel route with pharmacological consequences. J Pharm Pharmacol 1983; 35: 693–704.
38. Hutt AJ, Caldwell J. The importance of stereochemistry in the clinical pharmacokinetics of the 2-arylpropionic acid non-steroidal anti-inflammatory drugs. Clin Pharmacokin 1984; 9: 371–373.
39. Caldwell J, Hutt AJ, Fournel-Gigleux S. The metabolic chiral inversion and dispositional enantioselectivity of the 2-arylpropionic acids and their biological consequences. Biochem Pharmacol 1988; 37: 105–114.
40. Evans AM. Enantioselective pharmacodynamics and pharmacokinetics of chiral non-steroidal anti-inflammatory drugs. Eur J Clin Pharmacol 1992; 42: 237–256.
41. Brune K, Beck WS, Geisslinger G, Menzel-Soglowek S, Peskar BM, Peskar BA. Aspirin-like drugs may block pain independently of prostaglandin synthesis inhibition. Experientia 1991; 47: 257–261.
42. Malmberg AB, Yaksch TL. Antinociception produced by spinal delivery of the S and R enantiomer of flurbiprofen in the formalin test. Eur J Pharmacol 1994; 256: 205–209.
43. Brune K, Geisslinger G, Menzel-Soglowek S. Pure enantiomers of 2-arylpropionic acids: tools in pain research and improved drugs in rheumatology. J Clin Pharmacol 1992; 32: 944–952.
44. Buritova J, Besson J-M. Peripheral and/or central effects of racemic, S(+)- and R(−)-flurbiprofen on inflammatory nociceptive processes: a c-Fos protein study in the rat spinal cord. Br J Pharmacol 1998; 125: 87–101.
45. Lötsch J, Geisslinger G, Mohammadian P, Brune K, Kobal G. Effects of flurbiprofen enantiomers on pain-related chemosomatosensory evoked potentials in human subjects. Br J Clin Pharmacol 1995; 40: 339–346.
46. Wechter WJ, Bigornia AE, Murrey ED, Levine BH, Young IW. *Rac* – flurbiprofen is more ulcerogenic than its (S)-enantiomer. Chirality 1993; 5: 492–494.
47. Mahmud T, Somasundaram S, Sigthorsson G *et al.* Enantiomers of flurbiprofen can distinguish key pathophysiological steps of NSAID enteropathy in the rat. Gut 1998; 43: 775–782.
48. Heykants JPP, Meuldermans WEG, Michiels LJM, Lewi PJ, Janssen PAJ. Distribution, metabolism and excretion of etomidate, a short-acting hypnotic drug in the rat. Comparative study of (R)-(+) and (S)-(−) etomidate. Arch Int Pharmacodyn Ther 1975; 216: 113–129.
49. Ashton D, Wauquier A. Modulation of a GABA-ergic inhibitory circuit in the in vitro hippocampus by etomidate isomers. Anesth Analg 1985; 64: 975–980.
50. Tomlin SL, Jenkins A, Lieb WR, Franks NP. Stereoselective effects of etomidate optical isomers on gamma-aminobutyric acid type A receptors and animals. Anesthesiology 1998; 88: 708–717.

51. Oye I, Paulsen O, Maurset A. Effects of ketamine on sensory perception: evidence for a role of N-methyl-D-aspartate receptors. J Pharmacol Exp Ther 1992; 260: 1209–1213.

52. White PF, Way WL, Trevor AJ. Ketamine – its pharmacology and therapeutic uses. Anesthesiology 1982; 56: 119–136.

53. Kohrs R, Durieux ME. Ketamine: teaching an old drug new tricks. Anesth Analg 1998; 87: 1186–1193.

54. Marietta MP, Way WL, Castagnoli N, Trevor AJ. On the pharmacology of the ketamine enantiomorphs in the rat. J Pharmacol Exp Ther 1977; 202: 157–165.

55. Ryder S, Way WL, Trevor AJ. Comparative pharmacology of the optical isomers of ketamine in mice. Eur J Pharmacol 1978; 49: 15–23.

56. Meliska CJ, Greenberg AJ, Trevor AJ. The effects of ketamine enantiomers on schedule-controlled behaviour in the rat. J Pharmacol Exp Ther 1980; 212: 198–202.

57. Muir WW, Hubbell JA. Cardiopulmonary and anesthetic effects of ketamine and its enantiomers in dogs. Am J Vet Res 1988; 49: 530–534.

58. Deleforge J, Davot JL, Boisrame B, Delatour P. Enantioselectivity in the anaesthetic effect of ketamine in dogs. J Vet Pharmacol Ther 1991; 14: 418–420.

59. Zeilhofer HU, Swandulla D, Geisslinger G, Brune K. Differential effects of ketamine enantiomers on NMDA receptor currents in cultured neurons. Eur J Pharmacol 1992; 213: 155–158.

60. Hustveit O, Maurset A, Oye I. Interactions of the chiral forms of ketamine with opioid, phencyclidine, sigma and muscarinic receptors. Pharmacol Toxicol 1995; 77: 355–359.

61. Sekino N, Endou M, Hajiri E, Okumura F. Nonstereospecific actions of ketamine isomers on the force of contraction, spontaneous beating rate and $Ca^{2+}$ current in the guinea pig heart. Anesth Analg 1996; 83: 75–80.

62. Durieux ME. Inhibition by ketamine of muscarinic acetylcholine receptor function. Anesth Analg 1995; 81: 57–62.

63. Durieux ME, Nietgen GW. Synergistic inhibition of muscarinic signaling by ketamine stereoisomers and the preservative benzethonium chloride. Anesthesiology 1997; 86: 1326–1333.

64. Schüttler J, Stanski DR, White PF, Trevor AJ, Horai Y, Verotta D, Sheiner LB. Pharmacodynamic modeling of the EEG effects of ketamine and its enantiomers in man. J Pharmacokin Biopharm 1987; 15: 241–253.

65. Hong SC, Davidson JN. Stereochemical studies of demethylated ketamine enantiomers. J Pharm Sci 1982; 71: 912–914.

66. Edwards SR, Mather LE. Tissue uptake of ketamine and norketamine enantiomers in the rat. Indirect evidence for extrahepatic metabolic inversion. Life Sci 2001; 69: 2051–2066.

67. Ebert B, Mikkelsen S, Thorkildsen C, Borgbjerg FM. Norketamine, the main metabolite of ketamine, is a non-competitive NMDA receptor antagonist in the rat cortex and spinal cord. Eur J Pharmacol 1997; 156: 177–180.

68. Christensen HD, Lee IS. Anesthetic potency and acute toxicity of optically active disubstituted barbituric acids. Toxicol Appl Pharmacol 1973; 26: 495–503.

69. Ho IK, Harris RA. Mechanism of action of barbiturates. Ann Rev Pharmacol Toxicol 1981; 21: 83–111.

70. Schombert VI, Scheider-Affeld F, Büch HP. Zur gewebsverteilung von racemischer S-(+)- und R-(−)- MPPB (1-methyl-5-phenyl-5-propylbarbitursäure) bei der ratte. Arzneim Forsch 1979; 29: 38–44.

71. Downes H, Perry RS, Ostlund RE, Karler R. A study of the excitatory effects of barbiturates. J Pharmacol Exp Ther 1970; 175: 692–699.

72. Chandler MMH, Scott SR, Blouin RA. Age associated stereoselective alterations in hexobarbital metabolism. Clin Pharmacol Ther 1988; 43: 436–441.

73. Hooper WD, Qing MS. The influence of age and gender on the stereoselective metabolism and pharmacokinetics of mephobarbital in humans. Clin Pharmacol Ther 1990; 48: 633–640.

74. Smith DA, Chandler MHH, Shedlofsky SI, Wedlund PJ, Blouin RA. Age-dependent stereoselective increase in the oral clearance of hexobarbitone isomers caused by rifampicin. Br J Clin Pharmacol 1991; 32: 735–739.

75. Ebling WF, Danhof M, Stanski DR. Pharmacodynamic characterization of the electroencephalographic effects of thiopental in rats. J Pharmacokin Biopharm 1991; 19: 123–143.

76. Gustafsson LL, Ebling WF, Osaki E, Stanski DR. Quantitation of depth of thiopental anesthesia in the rat. Anesthesiology 1996; 84: 415–427.

77. Bührer M, Maitre PO, Hung OR, Ebling WF, Shafer SL, Stanski DR. Thiopental pharmacodynamics: defining the pseudo steady state serum concentration-EEG relationship. Anesthesiology 1992; 77: 23–44.

78. Hung OR, Varvel JR, Shafer SL, Stanski DR. Thiopental pharmacodynamics II. Quantitation of clinical and electroencephalographic depth of anesthesia. Anesthesiology 1992; 77: 237–244.

79. Mather LE, Edwards SR, Duke CC. Electroencephalographic effects of thiopentone and its enantiomers in the rat. Life Sci 2000; 66: 105–114.

80. Cordato DJ, Chebib M, Mather LE, Herkes GK, Johnston GAR. Stereoselective interaction of thiopentone enantiomers with the GABA$_A$ receptor. Br J Pharmacol 1999; 128: 77–82.

81. Mather LE, Edwards SR, Duke CC. Electroencephalographic effects of thiopentone and its enantiomers in the rat: correlation with drug tissue distribution. Br J Pharmacol 1999; 128: 83–91.

82. Mather LE, Edwards SR, Duke CC, Cousins MJ. Enantioselectivity of thiopental distribution into the central neural tissue of rats: an interaction with halothane. Anesth Analg 1999; 89: 230–235.

83. Mather LE, Upton RN, Huang JL, Ludbrook GL, Gray E, Grant C. The systemic and cerebral kinetics of thiopental in sheep: enantiomeric analysis. J Pharmacol Exp Ther 1996; 279: 291–297.

84. Mark LC, Brand L, Perel JM, Carroll FI. Barbiturate stereoisomers: direction for the future? Excepta Medica Int. Congress Series 1976; No 399: 143–146.

85. Cook CE, Seltzman TB, Tallant CR, Lorenzo B, Drayer DE. Pharmacokinetics of pentobarbital enantiomers as determined by enantiospecific radioimmunoassay after administration of racemate to humans and rabbits. J Pharmacol Exp Ther 1987; 241: 779–785.

86. Nguyen KT, Stephens DP, McLeish MJ, Crankshaw DP, Morgan DJ. Pharmacokinetics of thiopental and pentobarbital enantiomers after intravenous administration of racemic thiopental. Anesth Analg 1996; 83: 552–558.

87. Cordato DJ, Gross AS, Herkes GK, Mather LE. Pharmacokinetics of thiopentone enantiomers following intravenous injection or prolonged infusion of *rac*-thiopentone. Br J Clin Pharmacol 1997; 43: 355–362.

88. Cordato DJ, Mather LE, Gross AS, Herkes GK. Pharmacokinetics of thiopental enantiomers during and following prolonged high-dose therapy. Anesthesiology 1999; 91: 1693–1702.

89. Ruetsch YA, Böni T, Borgeat A. From cocaine to ropivacaine: the history of local anesthetic drugs. Curr Top Med Chem 2001; 1: 175–182.

90. Burke D, Bannister J. Left-handed local anaesthetics. Curr Anaesth Crit Care 1999; 10: 262–269.

91. McClellan KJ, Faulds D. Ropivacaine. An update of its use in regional anaesthesia. Drugs 2000; 60: 1065–1093.

92. Foster RH, Markham A. Levobupivacaine. A review of its pharmacology and use as a local anaesthetic. Drugs 2000; 59: 551–579.

93. Ekatodramis G, Borgeat A. The enantiomers: revolution or evolution. Curr Top Med Chem 2001; 1: 205–206.

94. Åkerman B, Persson H, Tegnéer C. Local anaesthetic properties of the optically active isomers of prilocaine (Citanest). Acta Pharmacol Toxicol 1967; 25: 233–241.

95. Luduena FP. Duration of local anesthesia. Ann Rev Pharmacol 1969; 9: 503–520.

96. Åkerman B, Ross S. Stereospecificity of the enzymatic biotransformation of the enantiomers of prilocaine (Citanest). Acta Pharmacol Toxicol 1970; 28: 445–453.

97. Åberg G. Toxicological and local anaesthetic effects of optically active isomers of two local anaesthetic compounds. Acta Pharmacol Toxicol 1972; 31: 273–286.

98. Aps C, Reynolds E. An intradermal study of the local anaesthetic and vascular effects of the isomers of bupivacaine. Br J Clin Pharmacol 1978; 6: 63–68.

99. Khodorova AB, Strichartz GR. The addition of dilute epinephrine produces equieffectiveness of bupivacaine enantiomers for cutaneous analgesia in the rat. Anesth Analg 2000; 91: 410–416.

100. Bernard CM, Ulma GA, Kopacz DJ. The meningeal permeability of *R*- and *S*-bupivacaine are not different. Evidence that pharmacodynamic differences between the enantiomers are not the result of differences in bioavailability. Anesthesiology 2000; 93: 896–897.

101. Nau C, Vogel W, Hempelmann G, Bräu ME. Stereoselectivity of bupivacaine in local anesthetic-sensitive ion channels of peripheral nerve. Anesthesiology 1999; 91: 786–795.

102. Valenzuela C, Synders DJ, Bennett PB, Tamargo J, Hondeghem LM. Stereoselective block of cardiac sodium channels by bupivacaine in guinea pig ventricular myocytes. Circulation 1995; 92: 3014–3024.

103. Valenzuela C, Delpón E, Tamkun MM, Tamargo J, Snyders DJ. Stereoselective block of a human cardiac potassium channel (Kv 1.5) by bupivacaine enantiomers. Biophys J 1995; 69: 418–427.

104. Franqueza L, Longobardo M, Vicente J, Delpón E, Tamkun MM, Tamargo J, Synders DJ, Valenzuela C. Molecular determinants of stereoselective bupivacaine block hKv 1.5 channels. Circ Res 1997; 81: 1053–1064.

105. Franqueza L, Valenzuela C, Eck J, Tamkun MM, Tamargo J, Synders DJ. Functional expression of an inactivating potassium channel (Kv 4.3) in a mammalian cell line. Cardiovasc Res 1999; 41: 212–219.

106. Zapata-Sudo G, Trachez MM, Sudo RT, Nelson TE. Is comparative cardiotoxicity of $S(-)$ and $R(+)$ bupivacaine related to enantiomer-selective inhibition of L-type $Ca^{2+}$ channels? Anesth Analg 2001; 92: 496–501.

107. Cox CR, Faccenda KA, Gilhooly C, Bannister J, Scott NB, Morrison LMM. Extradural $S(-)$-bupivacaine: comparison with racemic *RS*-bupivacaine. Br J Anaesth 1998; 80: 289–293.

108. Cox CR, Checketts MR, MacKenzie N, Scott NB, Bannister J. Comparison of $S(-)$ bupivacaine with racemic $(RS)$-bupivacaine in supraclavicular brachial plexus block. Br J Anaesth 1998; 80: 594–598.

109. Burke D, Henderson DJ, Simpson AM, Faccenda KA, Morrison LMM, McGrady EM, McLeod GA, Bannister J. Comparison of 0.25% S(−)-bupivacaine with 0.25% RS-bupivacaine for epidural analgesia in labour. Br J Anaesth 1999; 83: 750–755.

110. Lyons G, Colomb MO, Wilson RC, Johnson RV. Epidural pain relief in labour: relative potencies of bupivacaine and levobupivacaine. Br J Anaesth 1998; 81: 989–991.

111. Albright GA. Cardiac arrest following regional anesthesia with etidocaine or bupivacaine. Anesthesiology 1979; 51: 285–286.

112. Heath ML. Deaths after intravenous regional anaesthesia. Br Med J 1982; 285: 913–914.

113. Crandell JT, Kotelco DM. Cardiotoxicity of local anaesthetics during late pregnancy. Anesth Analg 1985; 64: 204.

114. Bardsley H, Gristwood R, Baker H, Watson N, Nimmo W. A comparison of the cardiovascular effects of levobupivacaine and rac-bupivacaine following intravenous administration to healthy volunteers. Br J Clin Pharmacol 1998; 46: 245–249.

115. Vanhoulte F, Vereeke J, Verbeke N, Carmeliet E. Stereoselective effects of the enantiomers of bupivacaine on the electrophysiological properties of the guinea-pig papillary muscle. Br J Pharmacol 1991; 103: 1275–1291.

116. Denson DD, Behbehani MM, Gregg RV. Enantiomer-specific effects of an intravenously administered arrhythmogenic dose of bupivacaine on neurons of the nucleus tractus solitarius and the cardiovascular system in the anesthetized rat. Reg Anesth 1992; 17: 311–316.

117. Graf BM, Martin E, Bosnjak ZJ, Stowe DF. Stereospecific effect of bupivacaine isomers on atrioventricular conduction in the isolated perfused guinea pig heart. Anesthesiology 1997; 86: 410–419.

118. Huang YF, Pryor ME, Mather LE, Veering BT. Cardiovascular and central nervous system effects of intravenous levobupivacaine and bupivacaine in sheep. Anesth Analg 1998; 86: 797–804.

119. Burm AGL, Van der Meer AD, Van Kleef JW, Zeijlmans PWM, Groen K. Pharmacokinetics of the enantiomers of bupivacaine following intravenous administration of the racemate. Br J Clin Pharmacol 1994; 38: 125–129.

120. Fawcett JP, Kennedy J, Kumar A, Ledger R, Zacharias M. Stereoselective urinary excretion of bupivacaine and its metabolites during epidural infusion. Chirality 1999; 11: 50–55.

121. Rosenberg PH, Heavner JE. Acute cardiovascular and central system toxicity of bupivacaine and desbutylbupivacaine in the rat. Acta Anaesthesiol Scand 1992; 36: 138–141.

122. Tucker GT, Mather LE, Lennard MS, Gregory A. Stereoisomers of prilocaine after administration of the racemate: implications for toxicity. Br J Anaesth 1990; 65: 333–336.

123. Franks NP, Lieb WR. Molecular and cellular mechanisms of general anaesthesia. Nature 1994; 367: 607–614.

124. Franks NP, Lieb WR. Stereospecific effects of inhalational general anesthetic optical isomers on nerve ion channels. Science 1991; 254: 427–430.

125. Kendig JJ, Trudell JR, Cohen EN. Halothane stereoisomers: lack of stereospecificity in two model systems. Anesthesiology 1973; 39: 518–524.

126. Laasberg LH, Hedley-Whyte J. Optical rotatory dispersion of hemoglobin and polypeptides. Effect of halothane. J Biol Chem 1971; 246: 4886–4893.

127. Meinwald J, Thompson WR, Pearson DL, König WR, Runge T, Francke W. Inhalational anesthetics stereochemistry: optical resolution of halothane, enflurane and isoflurane. Science 1991; 251: 560–561.

128. Arnett EM, Gold GM, Harvey N, Johnson EA, Whitesell LG. Stereoselective recognition in phospholipid monolayers. Adv Biol Med 1988; 238: 21–36.

129. Dickinson R, Franks NP, Lieb WR. Can the stereoselective effects of the anesthetic isoflurane be accounted for by lipid solubility. Biophys J 1994; 66: 2019–2023.

130. Harris B, Moody E, Skolnick P. Isoflurane anesthesia is stereoselective. Eur J Pharmacol 1992; 217: 215–216.

131. Lysko GS, Robinson JL, Casto R, Ferrone RA. The stereospecific effects of isoflurane isomers in vivo. Eur J Pharmacol 1994; 263: 25–29.

132. Eger E, Koblin DD, Laster MJ, Schurig V, Juza M, Ionescu P, Gong D. Minimum alveolar anesthetic concentration values for the enantiomers of isoflurane differ minimally. Anesth Analg 1997; 85: 188–192.

133. Dickinson R, White I, Lieb WR, Franks NP. Stereoselective loss of righting reflex in rats by isoflurane. Anesthesiology 2000; 93: 837–843.

134. Pohorecki R, Howard BJ, Matsushita M, Stemmer PM, Becker GL, Landers DF. Isoflurane isomers differ in preservation of ATP in anoxic rat hepatocytes. J Pharmacol Exp Ther 1994; 268: 625–628.

135. Sedensky MM, Cascorbi HF, Meinwald J, Radford P, Morgan PG. Genetic differences affecting the potency of stereoisomers of halothane. Proc Natl Acad Sci USA 1994; 91: 10054–10058.

136. Mather LE, Fryirs BL, Duke C, Cousins MJ. Lack of whole-body pharmacokinetic differences of halothane enantiomers in the rat. Anesthesiology 2000; 92: 190–195.

137. Juza M, Jakubetz H, Hettesheimer H, Schurig V. Quantitative determination of isoflurane enantiomers in blood samples during and after surgery via headspace gas chromatography–mass spectrometry. J Chromatogr B 1999; 735: 93–102.

138. Schmidt R, Wahl HG, Häberle H, Dieterich H-J, Schurig V. Headspace gas chromatography–mass spectrometry analysis of isoflurane enantiomers in blood samples after anesthesia with the racemic mixture. Chirality 1999; 11: 206–211.

139. Martin JL, Meinwald J, Radford P, Liu Z, Graf MLM, Pohl LR. Stereoselective metabolism of halothane enantiomers to trifluoroacetylated liver proteins. Drug Metab Rev 1995; 27: 179–189.

140. Garton KJ, Yuen P, Meinwald J, Thummel KE, Kharasch ED. Stereoselective metabolism of enflurane by human liver cytochrome P4502E1. Drug Metab Dispos 1995; 23: 1426–1430.

141. De Camp WH. The FDA perspective on the development of stereoisomers. Chirality 1989; 1: 2–6.

142. Cayen MN. Racemic mixtures and single stereoisomers: industrial concerns and issues in drug development. Chirality 1991; 3: 94–98.

143. Nation RL. Chirality in new drug development. Clinical pharmacokinetic considerations. Clin Pharmacokin 1994; 27: 249–255.

144. Rauws AG, Groen K. Current regulatory (draft) guidance on chiral medicinal products: Canada, EEC, Japan, United States. Chirality 1994; 6: 72–75.

145. FDAs Policy statement for the development of new stereoisomeric drugs. Chirality 1992; 4: 338–340.

146. Daniels JM, Nestmann ER, Kerr A. Development of stereoisomeric (chiral) drugs: a brief review of scientific and regulatory considerations. Drug Info J 1997; 31: 639–646.

147. Branch S. International regulation of chiral drugs. In: Subramanian G, ed. Chiral Separation Techniques: A Practical Approach, 2nd edition. Weinheim: Wiley-VCH. 2001: 319–342.

148. Shindo H, Caldwell J. Development of chiral drugs in Japan: an update on regulatory and industrial opinion. Chirality 1995; 7: 349–352.

149. Caldwell J. Through the looking glass in chiral drug development. Modern Drug Discovery 1999 July/August; 51–60.

150. Walshe JM. Penicillamine, a new oral therapy for Wilson's disease. Am J Med 1956; 21: 487–254.

151. Walshe JM. Chirality of penicillamine. Lancet 1992; 339: 254.

152. Cotzias GC, Papavasiliou PS, Gellene R. Modification of Parkinsonism – chronic treatment with L-dopa. New Engl J Med 1969; 280: 337–345.

153. Cotzias GC, Van Woert MH, Schiffer LM. Aromatic amino acids and modification of Parkinsonism. New Engl J Med 1967; 276: 374–379.

154. Thayer A. Eli Lilly pulls the plug on prozac isomer drug. Chem Eng News 2000 October 30; 8.

155. Connolly MH, Cary CL, McGoon MD. Valvular heart disease associated with fenfluramine-phentamine. New Engl J Med 1997; 337: 581–558.

156. Waldo AL, Camm AJ, de Ruyter H, Friedman PL, MacNeil DJ, Pauls JF, Pitt B, Pratt CM, Schwartz PJ, Veltri EP. Effect of d-sotalol on mortality in patients with left ventricular dysfunction after recent and remote myocardial infarction. Lancet 1996; 348: 7–12.

157. Nau C, Strichartz GR. Drug chirality in anesthesia. Anesthesiology 2002; 97: 497–502.

158. Agranat I, Caner H, Caldwell J. Putting chirality to work: The strategy of chiral switches. Nature Reviews Drug Discovery 2002; 1: 753–768.

G.A. McLeod

CHAPTER

# 3

# New local anaesthetics

The impetus to develop new local anaesthetic agents followed reports of sudden cardiac arrest, prolonged resuscitation and a disproportionately high number of deaths in pregnant women receiving epidural bupivacaine and etidocaine for caesarean section.[1] The subsequent, prompt changes in anaesthetic practice such as slow incremental dosing and the use of test doses undoubtedly reduced mortality but, nevertheless, failed to eliminate the cause of toxicity – accidental intravascular injection.

Recent reports suggest that local anaesthetic toxicity still remains a problem. A recent survey[2] reported 16 seizures in over 21,000 patients undergoing limb blocks. The regulatory studies for the two new safer local anaesthetics, ropivacaine and laevobupivacaine corroborate this evidence. Of the 4,500 patients recruited world-wide in clinical studies comparing the new drugs to bupivacaine, nine showed symptoms of toxicity due to inadvertent intravascular injection, two of whom progressed to convulsions.[3]

Increased awareness of the benefits of high quality prolonged post-surgical pain relief has spurred the search for ultra long acting local anaesthetics. Long duration pain relief is already obtainable with insertion of epidural or nerve sheath catheters. Unfortunately, even with high technical success rates of catheter insertion, patients do not often receive optimal pain relief because service provision falls down and catheters have a tendency to fall out, leak, break and migrate.[4]

Recent evidence has highlighted the many diverse actions of local anaesthetics. Not only do they block sodium and potassium ion channels, but interact with

G-coupled receptor proteins,[5] muscarinic receptors[6] and endothelial nitric oxide (NO).[7]

This review will present the evidence for the improved safety profile and potency of the enantiomers, ropivacaine and laevobupivacaine and will introduce the reader to some novel ultra long acting local anaesthetics as well as an insight into the possible future applications of local anaesthetics on the endothelium, coagulation system and the inflammatory response via inter-actions with G-coupled receptor proteins.

## Voltage-Gated Ion Channels

Before discussing new local anaesthetic agents, it is useful to be aware of some new advances in molecular biology. Visualisation of the sodium receptor and understanding of the molecular mechanisms of sodium channel binding and gating has the potential to not only advance local anaesthesia and pain relief but also the treatment of epilepsy and cardiac dysrhythmias.[8]

The unique anatomical features of nervous tissue provide long distance conduction of electrical signals without loss of information. Clustered within the Nodes of Ranvier are voltage-gated sodium and potassium channels where electrical impulses are regenerated for propagation down the nerve. These channels are embedded in the lipid bilayer cell membrane that surrounds the axoplasm and cover the entire width of the nerve cell membrane.

### Sodium channel

Cryo-electron microscopy and image reconstruction has recently revealed the three-dimensional structure of the sodium channel.[9,10] As viewed parallel to the membrane surface, the sodium-channel protein is bell-shaped with four transmembrane domains arrayed symmetrically around a central pore that splits into four passages that communicate between the intra and extracel-lular spaces (fig. 1).

The four homologous domains (I–IV) contain six transmembrane alpha helices (S1–S6) and an inactivating particle connecting domains III and IV. The S5 and S6 segments and the short loops between them form the pore (fig. 2). The fourth helix (S4) has positively charged arginine or lysine residues at every third position and is regarded as the 'voltage-sensitive' region of the sodium channel. The cationic sites on S4 are postulated to be paired with anionic sites that may reside on nearby transmembrane helices (S1–S3 or S5–S6).

Three major conformational states of the sodium channel exist, i.e. resting, open, and inactivated. In the resting state, the membrane potential is negative

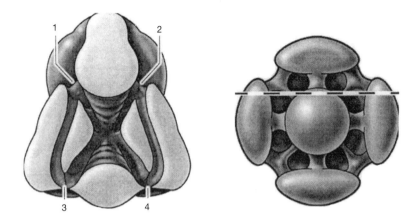

**Figure 1** A three-dimensional representation of the voltage-gated sodium channel. The first image shows the central ion-conducting pore and its intracellular and extracellular connections. The peripheral areas 1–4 indicate 'gating' pores, containing the S4 segments, and their connections to the central pore. The dashed lines show the position at which the cross-section was take.

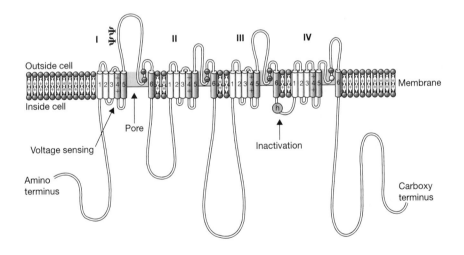

**Figure 2** Map of the voltage-gated sodium channel, showing how it folds over and crosses the plasma membrane. It is composed of four homologous domains (I–IV) each of which contains six transmembrane segments (cylinders 1–6).

inside because of the presence of large concentrations of sodium ions outside the cell and relatively large concentration of potassium ions inside the cell. The S4 segments are in the 'down' position, making the channel non-conductive.

Outward movement and spiral rotation of the S4 segments through special, narrow-waisted pores in each domain, moves positive gating charges across the membrane's electric field and opens the ion channel. Subsequent channel inactivation involves the closure of a hydrophobic inactivation gate or motif called IFMT (isoleucine, phenylalanine, methionine, threonine), between domains III and IV.[11] The gate has little affinity for the mouth of the channel when all S4 segments are down. When they are in the up position, the affinity of the inactivating particle for the mouth increases and it docks in, inducing inactivation.

## Potassium channels

In contrast to voltage-gated sodium channels, potassium channels are a very diverse family of membrane proteins with many subtypes although their distribution in nerve cells is still not clear. They fulfil a number of roles in peripheral nerves such as establishing the resting membrane potential and accomplishing repolarisation.

The hallmark of potassium channels is their ability to allow potassium ions to pass uninterrupted while presenting a formidable barrier to sodium ions. Unlike sodium channels, the potassium channel only contains the equivalent of one domain that folds over. The pore presents a wide, non-polar intracellular opening, and narrows on the extracellular side.[12] This region of the pore acts as a 'selectivity filter' by allowing only the passage of potassium ions in single file across the cell membrane. As with sodium channels, the S4 transmembrane segment, is the voltage sensor and the inactivation gate 'swings in', binds to the S4–S5 loop and blocks the channel.

## Local anaesthetic blockade of ion channels

Local anaesthetic binding to the sodium receptor is achieved by the ionised moiety of the anaesthetic molecule in a reversible and concentration-dependent manner. Recent molecular cloning studies give an insight into the affinity of recombinant sodium-channel isoforms for local anaesthetics. Parts of the local anaesthetic binding sites have been identified in IV-S6 as phenylalanine (F1764) and tyrosine (Y1771) of rat brain IIA sodium channels (rIIA), residues that correspond to F1760 and Y1767 in human heart (hH1).[13] It is phenylalanine (F) in position F1760 in hH1 sodium channels that binds with the positively charged moiety of bupivacaine but the whereabouts of a proposed hydrophobic binding site for local anaesthetics remains elusive.

The affinity of the sodium receptor for local anaesthetics is higher in the open or inactivated states compared to the resting state. Binding of anaesthetics to open sodium channels increases with the frequency of nerve depolarisation and is described as use-dependant or phasic block. Local anaesthetics that bind with more affinity to open or inactivated channels or that dissociate more slowly (such as bupivacaine) will generate a more potent block than local anaesthetics such as lidocaine, which dissociates four times faster. Consequently, bupivacaine accumulation during diastole is likely to delay recovery of cardiac sodium channels, prolong conduction and induce re-entry-induced dysrhythmias.

Potassium channel blockade further enhances local anaesthetic blockade. Potassium block broadens the action potential and encourages the open and inactivated sodium channel states thereby enhanced the binding of local anaesthetic.[14]

Local anaesthetics show a slightly higher potency to block cardiac than nerve sodium channels. Investigators have attributed this to a greater affinity of cardiac sodium channel for local anaesthetics[15] or a larger proportion of heart (hH1) channels in the inactivated (i.e. high-affinity) state at physiological resting potentials ($-100$ to $-90\,mV$).[16]

The most likely answer lies within the electrophysiological differences between nerve and heart. Nerves undergo a very brief depolarisation due to rapid flux of sodium ions and neural blockade, probably of resting state sodium channels at a potential of $-70$ to $-80\,mV$, and need relatively high concentrations of bupivacaine for blockade.

In contrast, cardiac depolarisation lasts 200–400 ms due to an initial sodium flux followed by a longer lasting influx of calcium that prolongs the duration of the action potential and produces a characteristic long plateau phase. As a result, blockade is produced by much lower drug concentrations binding frequently to more available and higher affinity inactivated sodium channels.[17]

## New Safer Local Anaesthetics

### Stereoselective blockade of ion channels

Bupivacaine exists in two forms called enantiomers, which are mirror images of each other. Although structurally identical, stereoisomers can exhibit pharmacodynamic and pharmacokinetic differences which manifest clinically as differences in potency or in side effects. The discovery, 30 years ago, of a stereoselective blockade of cardiac sodium channels by the enantiomers of bupivacaine[18] and advances in chiral chemistry have spurned the development of two new local anaesthetics ropivacaine and S-bupivacaine. The underlying principle of development was that if a significant difference in cardiotoxicity between the enantiomers of ropivacaine and between the enantiomers of bupivacaine was coupled with equivalent potency for nerve block, the added gain in therapeutic index warranted their clinical use.

Before discussing the evidence of stereoselective myocardial toxicity it is necessary to explain the confusing nomenclature surrounding chiral compounds (table 1). A chiral molecule has no internal plane of symmetry and is non-superimposable on its mirror image (fig. 3). Even after rotating one of the molecules it remains different from its partner in the same way a right hand will not fit properly into a left handed glove. Enantiomers can be classified according to their ability to rotate the plane of polarised light through a polarimeter. This is described as optical activity. Right handed or clockwise rotation is called dextrorotatory, 'd' or '+' and left handed or counterclockwise rotation is called laevorotatory, 'l', or '−'. A solution that contains a mixture of the two optical isomers will not change the plane of plane polarised light, because the effects of the two isomers cancel each other out.

The S and R descriptors are based on the configuration of the four asymmetrical groups around the central carbon atom (fig. 4).[19] An accurate description is determined by the following sequence rules (a) put the lowest priority towards the back by rotating the molecule (b) look at the direction of highest to lowest: if clockwise, then R (rectus), otherwise it is S (sinister). For the purposes of this review S-, l, (+) and laevo (bupivacaine) and R-, d, (−) and dextro (bupivacaine) are considered the same and are interchangeable.

**Table 1** Chiral terminology[19]

| | |
|---|---|
| Chirality | Spatial arrangement of atoms, non-superimposable on its mirror image |
| Isomer | A molecular entity with the same atomic composition but different stereochemical formulae and hence different physical or chemical properties |
| Stereoisomers | Isomers that possess identical constitution but which differ in the arrangement of their atoms in space |
| Enantiomers | One of a pair of molecular entities which are mirror images of each other and non-superimposable |
| Racemate | An equimolar mixture of a pair of enantiomers |

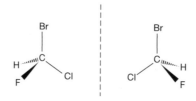

**Figure 3** Schematic representation of a chiral compound. Both enantiomers are non-superimposable.

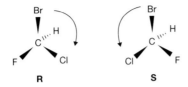

**Figure 4** Sequence notation of chiral compound. First put the lowest priority towards the back by rotating the molecule then look at the direction of highest to lowest: if clockwise, then **R** (rectus), otherwise it is **S** (sinister).

**Table 2** Physicochemical characteristics of local anaesthetics

|  | pKa | Protein binding | $Vd_{ss}$ (L) | $t_{1/2}$ (min) | Clearance (l min$^{-1}$) |
|---|---|---|---|---|---|
| Lidocaine[84] | 7.9 | 75 | 91 | 96 | 0.88 |
| Bupivacaine | 8.1 | 95 | 73 | 210 | 0.58 |
| Ropivacaine[85] | 8.1 | 94 | 59 | 111 | 0.72 |
| Laevobupivacaine[86] | 8.1 | 95.5 | 54 | 157 | 0.32 |
| Dextrobupivacaine[86] | 8.1 | 93.4 | 84 | 210 | 0.40 |

pKa – constant.
$Vd_{ss}$ – Volume of distribution at steady state.

Bupivacaine is an amino-amide local anaesthetic and is a member of the homologous series of *n*-alkyl substituted pipecholyl xylidines first synthesised by Ekenstam in 1957. Ropivacaine is a single enantiomer, structurally similar to bupivacaine but with a propyl side chain replacing the butyl group. The smaller side chain contributes less lipid solubility, less toxicity and an increased separation of sensory and motor blockade compared to bupivacaine. Laevobupivacaine, an enantiomer of bupivacaine, shares the same molecular structure as bupivacaine but due to its different spatial configuration has a different pharmacokinetic and pharmacodynamic profile. The physicochemical properties of laevobupivacaine and ropivacaine are compared in table 2 to bupivacaine and other commonly used local anaesthetics.

## Reduced Toxicity

In order to demonstrate any reduced cardiotoxicity of the new stereoisomers compared to bupivacaine, many *in vitro* and *in vivo* animal toxicity, human volunteer and clinical studies have been conducted on ropivacaine and laevobupivacaine. The following text describes the impact of these new drugs on ion channel blockade, myocardial electrophysiological and contractility changes, convulsive and dysrhythmogenic thresholds, resuscitation from cardiac arrest, vasoactivity and clinical potency.

## Ion channel blockade

Stereoselectivity of the inactivated state of the sodium channel has been demonstrated by use of the whole-cell voltage clamp technique in isolated guinea-pig ventricular myocytes[20] and recently in human cardiac sodium channels.[13] In both, dextrobupivacaine was more potent than laevobupivacaine. Potency is attributable to a more stable and longer interaction (dwell time) with the binding site and is expressed as the dissociation constant ($K_D$). No stereoselectivity was exhibited with the activated or open state of the channel.

Potassium channel blockade enhances block of the inactivated state of the sodium channel. Stereoselective inhibition of cloned human ventricle delayed rectifier potassium channels (hKv1.5) has been demonstrated for both the enantiomers of both bupivacaine and ropivacaine. $K_D$ of 27.3 µM and 4.1 µM were calculated for dextrobupivacaine and laevobupivacaine, indicating dextrobupivacaine to be sevenfold more potent in blocking the potassium channel than laevobupivacaine.[21] The corresponding concentration-dependant block induced by R-ropivacaine yielded a $K_D$ value of 32 µM, two and a half times more potent than S-ropivacaine.[22] Unlike sodium and potassium channels, no stereoselectivity has been observed for calcium channels.

## Electrophysiology and contractility

The maximum upstroke velocity ($V_{max}$) of the action potential using a standard microelectrode technique in isolated guinea-pig papillary muscle also depicts the inhibitory effect of local anaesthetics on the sodium channel current. Using this methodology, Moller et al., showed that $V_{max}$ and duration of block were significantly decreased in the presence of bupivacaine compared to ropivacaine and lidocaine.[23] Similarly, $V_{max}$ was reduced to a greater extent in the presence of dextrobupivacaine than laevobupivacaine over a range of stimulation frequencies, indicating a more profound blockade of sodium channels and slowing of cardiac conduction with dextrobupivacaine.[24]

Excessive shortening of action potential duration (APD) can precipitate re-entrant dysrhythmias and lengthening of action potential duration may prolong the QT interval in the clinical ECG. Harding et al., compared the effects on $V_{max}$ and action potential duration of laevobupivacaine, racemic bupivacaine and ropivacaine.[25] At 30 µM bupivacaine reduced $V_{max}$ 50% more than laevobupivacaine and ropivacaine and a significant increase in action potential duration was seen with ropivacaine that was not apparent with laevobupivacaine. After a 40 min-washout period, $V_{max}$ recovered fully with laevobupivacaine and ropivacaine but not for bupivacaine suggesting that any toxicity induced by these new enantiomers may be easier to reverse.

The *in vitro* studies have shown that both ropivacaine and laevobupivacaine are less likely to dwell on myocardial sodium channels, have much less potency at potassium channels and are less likely to impair myocardial electrical conduction and contractility compared to bupivacaine.

## Interaction of central nervous system (CNS) and cardiovascular system (CVS)

Observation of the CNS and CVS side effects of ropivacaine and laevobupivacaine has been possible in large animal models by injection into the systemic and coronary circulation. Chronically instrumented sheep were injected intravenous boluses of lidocaine bupivacaine and ropivacaine.[26] The mean convulsive doses were 110 mg, 60 mg and 45 mg for lidocaine, ropivacaine and bupivacaine. Ventricular fibrillation caused death in two sheep after bupivacaine (80 mg) and in two sheep after ropivacaine (90 and 120 mg) administration.

A similar investigation was undertaken by the same group in order to examine the cardiac effects of sub-convulsive and convulsive intravenous doses of laevobupivacaine and bupivacaine.[27] At subconvulsive doses, bupivacaine and laevobupivacaine produced depression of left ventricular systolic contractility ($dP/dt_{max}$) which was reversed following the onset of convulsions. The mean (SD) dose at which convulsions occurred was significantly higher with laevobupivacaine 103 (18) mg than with bupivacaine 85 (11) mg. Significantly fewer and less deleterious dysrrhythmias were induced by laevobupivacaine. Three animals died after 150, 150, and 200 mg respectively of bupivacaine from the sudden onset of ventricular fibrillation. These doses of laevobupivacaine produced non-fatal dysrrhythmias that automatically returned to sinus rhythm.

A further study was conducted to explore the effects of higher doses.[28] Eight chronically-instrumented conscious female sheep were intravenously infused with laevobupivacaine and bupivacaine. Doses were given over 3 min, with 50 mg increments, starting at 200 mg. The mean fatal dose of laevobupivacaine (277 mg) was almost twice that of bupivacaine (156 mg). This compares to a mean dose of 263 mg with ropivacaine found in a previous study.[26]

Unfortunately, onset of convulsions and their haemodynamic sequelae masks the direct CVS effects of local anaesthetic drugs. A means of obviating this is by direct administration of study drug into coronary arteries. Two studies by Reiz *et al.*, regarded prolongation of the QRS-interval of pigs as a measure of electrophysiological toxicity. In the first, the electrophysiological toxicity ratio for bupivacaine, ropivacaine and lidocaine was 15, 6.7, 1.0.[29] The respective toxicity ratios for bupivacaine, laevobupivacaine and ropivacaine in the second study were 2.1, 1.4, 1.0.[30]

A further study[31] injected bupivacaine, laevobupivacaine or ropivacaine over a three minute period into the left main coronary arteries of conscious ewes. This investigation used equimolar doses in order to negate differences in molecular weight or presentation as base or hydrochloric acid. Interestingly, there were no differences between all three drugs. Cardiovascular changes, QRS widening, fatal doses and survival rates were similar suggesting that all three drugs possess comparable capacity for cardiac toxicity when given into the left intracoronary artery.

What, therefore accounts for differences in cardiac toxicity between bupivacaine and the new chiral compounds? Perhaps the answer lies within the CNS. Dextrobupivacaine and laevobupivacaine given intravenously in a rat model at an dysrrhythmogenic dose[32] reduced the cell firing rate of the nucleus tractus solitarus. Dextrobupivacaine produced severe bradycardia, progressive hypotension, apnoea and death in all animals, whereas laevobupivacaine produced a mild bradycardia in only one third of the animals. Further investigation is needed regarding the interaction of the CNS and CVS in local anaesthetic toxicity.

## Human volunteer toxicity

Although the animal studies have assiduously demonstrated reduced cardiac toxicity for both ropivacaine and laevobupivacaine, the circumstance of accidental intravenous injection needs to be replicated in human beings as much as possible. Fortunately, a means of exhibiting local anaesthetic toxicity exists in human volunteers. Acute tolerance of intravenous infusion of $10 \, mg \, min^{-1}$ of bupivacaine, ropivacaine and laevobupivacaine has been studied in four crossover, randomised, double-blind studies in volunteers previously acquainted with the CNS effects of lidocaine. Changes in conductivity and myocardial contractility were monitored using the ECG (PR interval, QRS duration, QTc, QTd), echocardiography or thoracic bioimpedance. QTc dispersion is a marker of dysrhythmogenesis and is calculated, on a 12 lead ECG, from the difference between smallest and largest QT interval, and is corrected for time.

Bupivacaine impaired myocardial contractility, extended QRS duration and was less likely to be tolerated than ropivacaine.[33,34] The threshold for CNS toxicity was apparent at a mean free plasma concentration of $0.6 \, mg^{-1}$ for ropivacaine and $0.3 \, mg^{-1}$ for bupivacaine. Using thoracic bioimpedance, laevobupivacaine had significantly less effect on stroke index, acceleration index and ejection fraction.[35] In a further study of 22 volunteers, those who received over 75 mg of drug had significantly less QTc dispersion with laevobupivacaine.[36] The mean (SD) increase in QTc dispersion for bupivacaine was 24 ms (17 ms) compared to mean (SD) increase of 3 ms (11 ms) for laevobupivacaine.

## Reversibility and resuscitation

There is no information comparing the ability to reverse the cardiotoxic effects associated with incremental overdosage of bupivacaine, laevobupivacaine or ropivacaine, nor indeed, any evidence regarding best drugs to use. Anaesthetised rats[37] and dogs[38] were given local anaesthetic until the point of cardiovascular collapse at which point epinephrine and open-chest massage was started. In rats, the doses of laevobupivacaine and ropivacaine that produced seizures were similar and were greater than bupivacaine but the number of successful resuscitations did not differ among groups. In dogs, mortality from bupivacaine, laevobupivacaine, ropivacaine and lidocaine was 50%, 30%, 10% and 0%, respectively. Epinephrine-induced ventricular fibrillation occurred more frequently in bupivacaine-intoxicated dogs. The unbound plasma concentrations at collapse were larger for ropivacaine compared with bupivacaine after resuscitation.

## Sensory motor split and potency

An early *in vitro* study was the first indication that ropivacaine's intermediate lipid solubility between that of lidocaine and bupivacaine could translate into a preferential blockade of sensory to motor fibres. The response of compound action potentials in A and C nerve fibers to different concentrations of ropivacaine and bupivacaine was measured in isolated rabbit vagus nerves.[39] The results showed that the depressant effect of bupivacaine was 16% greater than that of ropivacaine on motor fibres, but only 3% greater on sensory fibres. The enhanced differential between sensory and motor blockade was given further standing from an epidural infusion study on volunteers using 0.1%, 0.2%, 0.3% ropivacaine, 0.25% bupivacaine or saline.[40] Over the 21-hour study period, sensory block and isometric quadriceps function were measured. The results showed that ropivacaine 0.2% and 0.3% were associated with less motor block than 0.25% bupivacaine. However, the extent of sensory spread was concentration-dependent for ropivacaine and receded much more quickly than bupivacaine.

The results of this study triggered a key question in regional anaesthesia. Are patients given ropivacaine less likely to suffer motor blockade and lower limb weakness compared to patients given the same dose of bupivacaine or does the limited sensory *and* motor spread of ropivacaine indicate less potency? The question is crucial because any reduction in potency narrows the therapeutic window between clinical efficacy and adverse side effects because more drug is required.

A comparison of the potency of ropivacaine and laevobupivacaine from standard regulatory studies is impossible because many are statistically powered to show equivalence of effect rather than differences between drugs and, as such, the vast majority of patients lie at the flat top of the dose response curve for analgesia and any difference between drugs manifests as side effects. Many of these studies have been highlighted in table 3.

In order to compare the analgesic potency of two drugs, one must come down the analgesic dose response curve to the point at which half the patient population responds, the EC50. The minimum effective local analgesic concentration (MLAC) for epidural analgesia in the first stage of labour remains the only valid means of measuring clinical potency. Patients are administered a standard 20 ml volume local anaesthetic and the pain of contractions measured using a 100 mm visual analogue pain ruler. A score of ≤10 mm within 30 min is defined as effective. The concentration of local anaesthetic given to each patient is increased or decreased according to the response of the previous patient (up-down sequential allocation). Using this methodology, the EC50 of ropivacaine has been calculated in two studies to be 0.111(95% CI: 0.100–0.122)%[41] and 0.156(95% CI: 0.136–0.176)%[42] compared to 0.067(95% CI: 0.052–0.082)%[41] and 0.093 (95% CI: 0.076–0.110)%[42] for bupivacaine. The corresponding EC50 for laevobupivacaine is 0.083(95% CI: 0.065–0.101)% compared to 0.081(95% CI: 0.055–0.108)% for bupivacaine.[43]

Thus, the potency of ropivacaine is six tenths that of bupivacaine 0.60 (95% CI: 0.47–0.75) and the potency of laevobupivacaine no different to that of bupivacaine 0.98 (95% CI: 0.67–1.41). European regulations insist on presentation of new drugs as base rather than the hydrochloride. The result, in the case of laevobupivacaine, is that 13% more active drug has been given in most clinical studies. Despite this, and taking the extra drug into account, 'the molar ratio of laevobupivacaine is 0.87 (95% CI: 0.60–1.25) compared to a molar ratio of 0.57 (95% CI: 0.45–0.72) for ropivacaine.[42] As the decrement in potency is still less than the overall 25–30% reduction in cardiac toxicity determined by preclinical studies, laevobupivacaine remains a safer drug than bupivacaine.

The MLAC methodology has been criticised because the ED5 and ED95 points each represent a single patient. Nevertheless, a study[44] in volunteers receiving epidural boluses of ropivacaine or bupivacaine in increments of 0.02% then measuring, at the L2 dermatome, sensory thresholds by $CO_2$ laser and isometric quadriceps function has confirmed the findings from EMLAC. A 50% higher concentration of ropivacaine than bupivacaine was required to produce onset of both superficial and deep analgesia giving a potency ratio of 0.67. The motor blocking ratio was also 0.67 indicating that both drugs have identical motor-sensory separation. Interestingly, the authors concluded that deep analgesia could not be obtained without motor blockade.

**Table 3** Examples of clinical studies assessing efficacy and safety of laevobupivacaine (L) and ropivacaine (R)

| | Laevobupivacaine (n) | Results | Ropivacaine (n) | Results |
|---|---|---|---|---|
| Infiltration anaesthesia for inguinal hernia | 0.25% L (33) 0.25% B (33) 50 ml | Similar postoperative pain scores over 48 h[87] | 0.125% R (26) 0.25% R (25) 0.5% R (27) Saline (24) 30 ml | 0.25% and 0.5% equally effective[88] |
| Opthalmic anaesthesia Peribulbar block | 0.75% L (25) 0.75% B (25) | No differences in volume (11 vs 10 ml), time to satisfactory block (13 vs 11 min) or perioperative pain scores[89] | 1% R (45) 0.75% B/2% L mixture (45) | Both provided similar anaesthesia at 8 min[90] |
| Upper limb block | 0.25% L (25) 0.5% L (26) 0.5% B (23) 0.4 ml kg⁻¹ Supraclavicular block | Sensory block duration (min) 0.25% L, 892 min, 0.5% L, 1039 min 0.5% B, 896 min Motor block duration (min) 0.25% L, 847 min, 0.5% L, 1050 min 0.5% B, 933 min[91] | 0.5% R (15) 0.75% R (15) 1% R (15) 2% M (15) Interscalene block | Readiness for surgery greater with 1% R Duration of analgesia >10 h with all concentrations of R[92] |
| Lower limb block | 0.5% L (15) 0.5% R (15) 0.5% B (15) Sciatic nerve block | Onset of block 0.5% L, 15 min, 0.5% R, 15 min 0.5% B, 30 min Duration of analgesia (h) 0.5% L, 16 h, 0.5% R, 17 h; 0.5% B, 14 h[93] | 0.75% R (12) 0.5% B (12) Sciatic nerve block | Onset of block 0.75% R, 27.5 min 0.5% B, 25 min Duration 0.75% R, 13.4 h; 0.5% B, 15.8 h[94] |
| Lumbar epidural block for surgery | 0.75% L (29) 0.5% L (30) 0.5% B (29) | Duration of sensory block 0.75% L, 460 min 0.5% L, 377 min, 0.5% B, 345 min[95] | 0.5% R (32) 0.5% B (35) | 0.5% R, 3.5 h 0.5% B, 3.4 h[96] |
| Postoperative analgesia | 0.125% L (21) 0.125% L and 4 µg/ml F (22) 4 µg/ml F (22) PCEA basal rate 4 ml h⁻¹, 2 ml bolus, 10 min lockout | Pain scores lower and longer time to first request in the combination group than in the plain fentanyl group at 6 h and 12 h[97] | 0.2% R (60) 0.2% R, 1 mg ml⁻¹ F(59) 0.2% R, 2 mg ml⁻¹ F(62) 0.2% R, 4 µg/ml F(63) Infusion up to 14 ml/h for 72 h | >90% no motor block after 24 h. Better analgesia with 4 µg/ml fentanyl[98] |
| Spinal anaesthesia | 0.5% L (40) 0.5% B (40) 3.5 ml Plain solutions | Duration of sensory blockade L, 228 min, B, 237 min Duration of motor blockade L, 280 min, B, 284 min[99] | 0.5% R with 1% dextrose (20) 0.5% R with 5% dextrose (20) | No difference in spread or sensory regression (150–330 min)[100] |

B = bupivacaine; F = fentanyl; M = mepivacaine.

## Vasoactivity

The vascular effects of local anaesthetics are important determinants of their therapeutic activity. Drugs that vasoconstrict have the potential clinical advantages of limited systemic uptake, increased neural uptake[45] and prolonged duration of effect. Skin blood flow after intradermal injection of bupivacaine, ropivacaine[46,47] and laevobupivacaine[7] in various anaesthetic and analgesic concentrations has been evaluated by laser Doppler flowmetry[46,47] and perfusion imaging[48] following injection in volunteers. All three drugs show a biphasic dose-response relationship with profound vasodilitation with anaesthetic dosages and relative vasoconstriction compared to saline control at analgesic concentrations over a 60 min study period. Laevobupivacaine is significantly less vasodilatory than bupivacaine at the 0.75% concentration and this inherent vasoactivity probably accounts for its increased duration of action.[49]

Vasoconstriction may increase the neuronal uptake of a local anaesthetic drug.[17] As ropivacaine and laevobupivacaine are both more vasoconstrictor than bupivacaine, it has been hypothesised that more local anaesthetic can enter the nerve and prolong the duration and quality of block thus cancelling out any intrinsic advantage in potency of the racemate or other enantiomer on nerve blockade.

# Long Acting Local Anaesthetics

## Slow release formulations of bupivacaine

Prolonged excellent postoperative analgesia can be achieved by continuous or repeated administration via indwelling catheters for regional, epidural, or spinal anaesthesia. However, complications associated with catheterisation are not uncommon and include leakage, intravascular injection, catheter migration and infection.

A long acting anaesthetic placed accurately has the potential to provide long-lasting pain relief and eliminate technical problems. Strategies in the search for prolonged postoperative analgesic have focused on drug delivery systems for slow release of local anaesthetics held in lipid emulsion, liposomes, microspheres or in suspension.

## Lipid emulsions

The rationale for development of lipid emulsions of local anaesthetics is based on the relative solubility of the ionised and free base forms of bupivacaine in aqueous and lipid solutions. Ionisation is limited to those molecules at the lipid/aqueous interface, thus slowly releasing active drug. A formulation of bupivacaine in an emulsion of soya bean oil, triglycerides of C8–C10 fatty acids and egg lecithin has been administered as a sciatic nerve block to Sprague Dawley rats and epidurally to dogs. The emulsion induced complete, reversible motor and sensory blockade, while increasing the duration of the anaesthetic effect by one third compared with the standard bupivacaine aqueous solution.[50,51]

## Liposomes

Liposomes are amphipathic lipid molecules with a polar head and two hydrophobic hydrocarbon tails which form lipid bilayers not unlike a cell membrane when suspended in an aqueous solution. Liposomal function is dictated by size[52] structure, and composition. The larger liposomes tend to remain at the site of action and multilamellar (multilayer) vesicles release drug more slowly. Permeability is determined by the incorporation of other components in the bilayer, such as cholesterol. Possession of both aqueous and lipid environments enables both water and lipid soluble drugs to be carried.

The likelihood of tissue toxicity being induced by liposome constituents is low[52,53] as they are biodegradable. However, much research requires to be done to ensure that the preparation stays at the site of action, deliver a predictable concentration of drug over a prolonged period of time and to produce adequate sensory block without motor block[54] or toxicity. Bupivacaine 0.25% encapsulated by multilamellar liposomes was administered epidurally to a patient suffering pain associated with lung cancer and the effect compared with a plain bupivacaine solution of the same concentration. Complete analgesia was produced for 4 h with the plain solution and 11 h with the liposomal formulation. No motor blockade or haemodynamic instability was observed with the liposome-associated bupivacaine.[55]

## Polymer microspheres

Biodegradable polylactic and lactic-glycolic acid polymers are widely used in drug delivery of implantable contraceptives and sutures. Polylactic-co-glycolic acid (PLGA) is a random co-polymer polymerised from lactic and glycolic acids. The ratios 75/25, 65/35, and 50/50 refer to the molar ratios of lactic to glycolic acid repeating units.

Previous clinical uses of microspheres has applied mainly to high potency drugs, which require release of µg per day, and therefore have drug/polymer weight ratios less than 10–12%. Local anaesthetics are comparatively low potency drugs, and require several mg/h$^{-1}$ to maintain blockade of nerves. Thus, to make clinically useful microspheres with local anaesthetics, it has become necessary to develop microsphere formulations with previously unattainably high drug loadings, that is, 50–75% drug to polymer weight to weight ratio.

In the most studied formulation, 65/35 polylactic-co-glycolic acid, roughly 20% of the bupivacaine was released in the first 24 h, and approximately 7% released daily thereafter up to approximately day 10. Even with doses of 600 mg/kg, more than 30–150 times the convulsant dose for aqueous bupivacaine hydrochloride, toxicity was not seen.

Incorporation of dexamethasone into bupivacaine microspheres has prolonged blockade by eight to 13 times compared with bupivacaine microspheres alone.[56,57] This would appear to be a local and not a systemic effect of dexamethasone as injections at other remote sites has no effect on duration of blockade.[58] Moreover, inhibition of the action of dexamethasone by the glucocorticoid antagonist cortexolone suggests blockade of glucocorticoid receptors.[58] Phase II, dose finding studies on ilio-inguinal and intercostal block are currently underway.

### Suspensions

Suspensions of local anaesthetics in polysorbate-80 offer the potential for long duration of action by slow, continuous dissolution of otherwise short-acting drugs. An example is 9.1% *n*-butyl-*p*-aminobenzoate (BAB, butamben) which is an amino ester derivative of benzene with atypical physicochemical characteristics: a very low pKa of 2.6, a very low partition coefficient and very low water solubility. Slow release from the particles of the suspension is controlled by the physicochemical properties of butamben and by the characteristics of the suspension (particle size and size-distribution, pH, additives). The epidural administration of the butamben suspension to rats,[59] dogs[60] and human beings with chronic pain resulted in ultralong-lasting pain relief up to six months, without motor block.

## New Long Acting Local Anaesthetics

### Structure activity relationships

When designing a new long-lasting local anaesthetic, what are the most important requirements? Knowledge of both receptor topology, the physicochemical properties of local anaesthetics and their diffusion into surrounding tissues are required to design drugs which can rapidly access ion channels and exert their effects reversibly and without local and systemic toxicity in a range of nerve fibres that differ in size and function.

The structure of local anaesthetics can be considered amphipathic, possessing an aromatic (hydrophobic) benzene ring connected to a tertiary amine (hydrophilic) group by a short alkyl chain and a hydrophilic bond (amide, ester). The lipophilic, aromatic ring aids the penetration of the molecule through the perineurium and nerve cell membrane where dissociation occurs into the ionic and the non-ionic form of the tertiary amine. The relative proportion of ionised and ionised forms is determined by the pH of solution and pKa of local anaesthetic. The benzene ring restricts the movement of the amide (hydrophilic) group to an axis perpendicular to the aromatic ring helping direct it towards the sodium receptor. Substitutions on the ring or tertiary amine portion of the local anaesthetic molecule alter its pKa, lipid solubility and protein binding, determining respectively the speed of onset, potency and duration of action.

Replacement of the tertiary amine by a piperidine ring increases lipid solubility and duration of action. The size of the nitrogen (N)-substituent on the piperidine ring is critical. Generally, the greater the number of carbon atoms and branching the greater the potency (and toxicity) up to 3–4 carbon atoms. After this, the activity drops off, since the analogues are too lipid soluble.

## IQB-9302

An example of small structural change sufficient to alter function is replacement of the N-substituent butyl chain of bupivacaine for a cyclopropylmethyl group while retaining the same number of carbon atoms. The effect of this structural change was investigated in human cardiac potassium channels.[61,62] Bupivacaine was 2.5 times more potent than IQB-9302 to block hKv1.5 channels EC50 8.9 (1.4) vs. 21.5 (4.7) µmol. Stereoselective block was also demonstrated with the dextro enantiomer being over three times more potent than the laevo enantiomer.

## Quaternary amines

Many other structural modifications of local anaesthetics have involved replacement of the tertiary amine with an ionised quaternary amine. Potent and long-lasting quaternary derivatives of cocaine, tetracaine, and cinchocaine, albeit with a protracted onset and offset of action, were described 30 years ago. Derivatives of tetraethylammonium ions (alkyl triethyl quaternary ammonium ions) have also been synthesised in which one ethyl group was replaced by a side chain of up to 16 carbon atoms. All produced sensory block of the rat infraorbital nerve lasted 17–20 days.[63] Later studies, however, revealed that this type of compound resulted in loss of myelinated axons, and axonal oedema within four weeks of treatment. It is important to

note that systemic toxicity with quaternary ammonium-type local anaesthetics may include, in addition to or instead of the typical patterns of
cardiac and CNS toxicity of tertiary amine type local anaesthetics, effects on
peripheral nicotinic acetylcholine receptors manifesting as ganglionic or
neuromuscular block.

### Tonicaine

New data suggesting that the local anaesthetic binding site has two large
hydrophobic domains that can accommodate up to a 12-hydrocarbon chain,
that the neutral tertiary amine is less potent and that permanently charged
amphipathic local anaesthetics can be easily trapped within the cell,
prompted investigators to add a hydrophobic phenyl ethyl moiety to the
tertiary amine of lignocaine creating a new ionised quaternary ammonium
compound called tonicaine. The advantage of this local anaesthetic is that
its amphipathic nature allows a much faster onset than traditional quaternary compounds, probably because the additional hydrophobic arm shields
the positive charge.

The permanently charged amphipathic molecule is a more potent sodium
channel blocker than its parent drug as it is trapped within the cytoplasm,
prolonging the duration of local anaesthetic blockade. For example, tonicaine produced sciatic nerve blockade as assessed by withdrawal response to
pinching that lasted over nine times longer than the blockade produced by
lidocaine. Intruigingly, sensory blockade was more three-fold longer than
proprioception or motor blockade.[64] This ratio is important for the management of postoperative and obstetric anaesthesia, because it confers sensory
blockade without the hindrance of motor blockade, thus allowing patient
mobility. In addition, a recent study using prolonged nerve block (12–16 h)
in a rat model with tonicaine prevented the development of long-lasting (3–5
days) inflammatory hyperalgesia not only with a prolonged pre-injury block
but also with a prolonged postinjury block when hyperalgesia was already
present.[65] Unfortunately, direct clinical application is unlikely as tonicaine
has a relatively small therapeutic range and new evidence has demonstrated
some neurotoxicity.[66] Nevertheless, an opportunity now exists using tonicaine to further investigate, in the laboratory, the molecular determinants of
sensory-motor split and mechanisms of hyperalgesia.

### Amitriptyline

The tricyclic antidepressant, amitriptyline, is prescribed as an analgesic in
patients with neuropathic pain. Recent evidence suggests that the pain relieving
properties of amitriptyline are due to antagonism of N-methyl-D-aspartate
(NMDA).[67] The structure of amitriptyline suggests it may be useful as a local
anaesthetic. A recent study using amitriptyline for peripheral nerve blockade

rats *in vivo* and *in vitro* has shown amitriptyline to be a more potent blocker of neuronal sodium channels than bupivacaine. Using whole-cell voltage clamping of cultured rat GH3 cells, amitriptyline was five times more potent than bupivacaine in binding to the resting channels (50% inhibitory concentration (IC50) of 39.8 (2.7) vs. 189.6 (22.3) μmol and 10 times more potent in binding to the inactivated sodium channels (IC50) of 0.9 (0.1) vs. 9.6 (0.9) μmol). Use-dependent blockade increased blockade by 14% for bupivacaine and by 50% for amitriptyline.[68] *In vivo*, complete sciatic nerve blockade for nociception was 454 (38) min amitriptyline vs. 90 (13) min bupivacaine. Time to full recovery of nociception for amitriptyline 656 (27) min (10 mmol) vs. 155 (9) min for bupivacaine.

### N-phenylethyl amitriptyline

The principles of local anaesthetic structural modification used with lignocaine have also been applied to amitriptyline in order to extend its duration of action. A quaternary ammonium derivative, N-phenylethyl amitriptyline was synthesised[69] and assessed using the same *in vitro* and *in vivo* techniques described above. N-phenylethyl amitriptyline was found to be a highly potent sodium channel blocker *in vitro* and its potency was estimated to be eight times higher than the parent drug. The duration of full recovery from sciatic nerve block using 2.5 mmol N-phenylethyl amitriptyline was 30.3 (2.1) h, seven times longer than that of the parent drug amitriptyline and 12 times longer than bupivacaine.

### Tetrodotoxin (TTX)

Voltage-gated sodium channels are the molecular targets for a broad range of neurotoxins that act at six or more receptor sites on the channel protein. These toxins fall into three groups according to their site of action – block the pore, alter voltage-dependent gating of sodium channels through binding to intramembranous or extracellular receptor sites.[70]

Tetrodotoxin is a poison found in puffer fish (fugu) and acts by selectively blocking sodium channels at a site and by an action that differs from that of lidocaine. Despite these desirable characteristics, tetrodotoxin has not achieved clinical use as a local anaesthetic because of its perceived systemic toxicity culminating in diaphragmatic paralysis leading to respiratory arrest and death. In light of the discovery that tetrodotoxin does not cause local neurotoxicity (sakura) and the lack of enduring central nervous or cardiac sequelae (unlike bupivacaine), tetrodotoxin has been investigated as a potential long-lasting local anaesthetic.

Tetrodotoxin, when given alone to rats, resulted in an increase in thermal nocifensive and withdrawal latency in the contralateral limb almost as large as the injected leg.[71] This is suggestive of systemic toxicity and is attributable to distribution of toxin to systemic nerves and muscles rather than an action on the CNS.

Addition of epinephrine reduced the EC50 and a five-fold increase in the duration of tetrodotoxin-induced nerve blockade (13.3 h for 50 mmol tetrodotoxin in 55 mM, 1 in 100,000 epinephrine) compared to 15.4 mmol (0.5%) bupivacaine alone. The addition of epinephrine increased the therapeutic index (the LD50:EC50 ratio) of tetrodotoxin four-fold.

Addition of bupivacaine to tetrodotoxin increased duration of block synergistically. Blocks lasting 11 (1.28) h were obtained with 50 mmol tetrodotoxin combined with 15.4 mmol bupivacaine. However, no additional benefit was obtained by all three drugs in combination, suggesting the benefits of bupivacaine and epinephrine act via the same mechanism. Bupivacaine possesses vasoconstrictive properties at concentrations of 0.25% and less[48] and, like epinephrine, slows the resorption of tetrodotoxin from the site of injection. All these blocks were achieved with no deaths or signs of respiratory distress or systemic toxicity as indicated by contralateral limb dysfunction. Rabbits receiving all three concentrations of tetrodotoxin did not demonstrate any ocular irritation, corneal thickening, or signs of systemic toxicity. At a dose of 10 mmol, tetrodotoxin produced an anaesthetic effect lasting up to 8 h.[72]

### Capsaicin

Evidence from animal models and studies of human sensory nerves demonstrate that tetrodotoxin-resistant sodium channels are found primarily in small-diameter nociceptor afferent neurons and play an important role in pain conduction and chronic pain. Capsaicin, the pungent ingredient in chilli peppers, is a vanilloid with noxious and analgesic effects that inhibits tetrodotoxin-resistant sodium currents. Sciatic nerve block with capsaicin in male Sprague-Dawley rats produced selective anaesthesia with an increase in thermal latency but no effect on motor strength.[73] The combination of capsaicin and 0–120 μmol tetrodotoxin was synergistic prolonging both nociceptive and motor block, with the effect of capsaicin reversed by the vanilloid antagonist capsazepine. Similar interactions were found between tetrodotoxin and resiniferatoxin (another vanilloid), but much less so between bupivacaine and capsaicin.

### Prenylamine

The investigations into long acting local anaesthetic compounds have identified the ideal compound as one possessing two large hydrophobic regions. Prenylamine, a known calcium channel blocker, fulfills these structural criteria but its clinical development has been hindered by reports of the torsade de pointes syndrome. In cultured rat neuronal GH3 cells during whole-cell voltage clamp conditions[74] prenylamine elicited both use-dependent and tonic block of both resting and inactivated sodium channels. In addition, *in vivo* data show that prenylamine produced a complete sciatic nerve block that lasted over 24 h. Although it is unlikely that prenylamine will be developed for clinical use, knowledge gained from laboratory experiments using these compounds such as this will bring us closer to developing a local anaesthetic which offers both safety and a prolonged duration of action.

## Local Anaesthetics and the Inflammatory Response

Although local anaesthetics are better known for their ability to block sodium and potassium ion channels, recent work has uncovered interactions with other cellular systems, particularly the G protein-coupled receptors mediating inflammatory responses (lysophosphatidic acid and thromboxane A2), m1 muscarinic acetylcholine receptors and endothelial NO synthase.

### G-coupled receptor proteins

Interaction of an agonist with its enzyme-activating receptor coupled to a guanosine triphosphate (GTP)-binding protein or G-protein initiates a cascade of events within the cell called the 'cellular conduction pathway' leading to a physiological response (fig. 5). The membrane receptors coupled to the GTP-binding proteins form a very large family of proteins estimated to contain as many as 1,000 proteins. Each of the three G-protein subunits $\alpha$, $\beta$ and $\gamma$ can occur in various isoforms ($20\alpha$, $6\beta$ and $12\gamma$). However, there are four main classes of G-proteins of known function. $G_s$ activates adenylyl cyclase, $G_i$ inhibits adenylyl cyclase, $G_t$ activates photoreceptor cyclic guanosine monophosphate (cGMP) phosphodiesterase and $G_q$ activates phospholipase C. It is the latter which hydrolyses the membrane phospholipid called phosphatidylinositol-4,5-bisphosphate ($PIP_2$) into inositol triphosphate ($IP_3$) and diacylglycerol (DAG). This is termed the inositol phospholipid signaling pathway. One of the products of this pathway, diacylglycerol activates protein kinase C which activates gene-specific transcription factor and $IP_3$ stimulates $Ca^{2+}$ release from the endoplasmic reticulum.

### The inflammatory response

The inflammatory response to surgical trauma induces polymorphonuclear granulocytes, macrophages and monocytes to migrate into the injured area where they engulf pathogens by phagocytosis. Due to their ability to phagocytose and kill bacteria, polymorphonuclear granulocytes represent a major

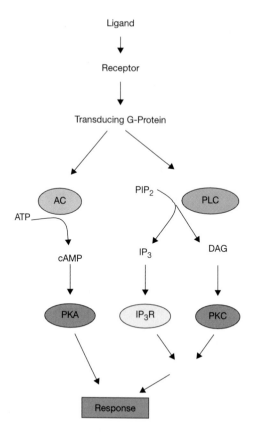

**Figure 5** Schematic diagram showing the roles of protein kinases A (PKA) and C (PKC) in signal transduction following the ligand (L) interaction with the receptor (R). AC is adenylyl cyclase; PLC is phospholipase C; cAMP is cyclic 3',5'-adenosine monophosphate; The membrane phospholipid phosphatidylinositol-4,5-bisophosphate ($PIP_2$) is hydrolysed into inositol triphosphate ($IP_3$) and diacylglycerol (DAG). This is termed the inositol phospholipid signaling pathway. One of the products of this pathway, DAG, activates PC which activates gene-specific transcription factor and $IP_3$ attaches to its receptor ($IP_3R$) and stimulates calcium ($Ca^{2+}$) release from the edoplasmic reticulum.

defense mechanism in the circulating blood. Polymorphonuclear granulocytes attach to endothelial cells (margination and adhesion), squeeze between endothelial cells (diapedesis), migrate to the pathogen (chemotaxis), are primed (switched to an activated state with increased surface expression of plasma membrane receptors) enabling production of oxygen free radicals.

Attachment of local anaesthetics to G-coupled receptor proteins linked to lysophosphatilic acid[75] attenuates neutrophil, macrophage and monocyte function.[76,77] More specifically, local anaesthetics have been shown *in vitro* to inhibit adhesion to endothelium by reducing surface expression on polymorphonuclear granulocytes of the adhesion molecule CD11b-CD18,[78] reduce priming of polymorphonuclear granulocytes[76] by tumour necrosis factor (TNF)-α, platelet-activating factor or IL-8, inhibit chemotaxis[5] by leukotriene B4 and IL-1, reduce lysozyme release and decrease free radical[76] production. These pathways are protein lipase C and protein kinase C-dependent and $G_q$-mediated.

Does the encouraging effect of local anaesthetics on cellular mechanisms in the laboratory translate into humans. Two studies suggest it may do. The first study investigated the reasons why regional anaesthesia is associated with reductions in thromboembolic complications by assessing the impact of epidural anaesthesia on platelet-mediated hemostasis time, clotting time and collagen-induced thrombus formation in 41 patients after hip surgery.[79] The results in the general anaesthesia group showed a significant decrease in all parameters by up to one third compared to preoperative values whereas epidural anaesthesia had no significant impact. This study has demonstrated that general anaesthesia induces a hypercoagulable state without affecting physiologic aggregation and coagulation processes.

The second study investigated the specific cellular pathways of vascular regulation in 10 young, healthy, male volunteers.[7] Three solutions, prilocaine 1%, prilocaine 1% with L-NAME (Nω-nitro-L-arginine methyl ester), and saline alone were injected intradermally and the resulting change in skin blood flow at each injection site was measured by laser Doppler imaging. L-NAME is an NO-synthase inhibitor. Injection of prilocaine increased skin blood flow significantly greater than that caused by saline alone. Addition of L-NAME, however, significantly reduced the prilocaine response by 25% and suggests that NO is involved in the vasodilitation of local anaesthetics.

## Conclusion

Two new safer local anaesthetics are now in clinical use after providing evidence in pre-clinical studies that they exhibit less cardiovascular and CNS toxicity than bupivacaine. The use of regional anaesthesia will continue to expand in clinical practice over the next decade; limb plexus blockade for limb surgery and thoracic epidural anaesthesia for gastrointestinal, thoracic and cardiac surgery. Clinical demand already exists for a 0.75% obstetric preparation of laevobupivacaine for emergency caesarian section and studies are ongoing. One must be aware, however, that the mode of action of local anaesthetics is also the mode of toxicity – blockade of sodium and potassium ion channels – and that inadvertent intravascular injection can and will occur. If given intravenously, in high enough doses,[80] all local anaesthetics can have perilous consequences.[81–83] Clinical vigilance will always be necessary when using these drugs.

The longer acting compounds remain at the experimental stage but two different approaches offer a solution. Slow release preparations of bupivacaine have the potential of providing extended pain relief, particularly for infiltration local anaesthesia after day case surgery and intercostal block after thoracic surgery. Of course, their slow onset of action will necessitate the concomitant use of laevobupivacaine or ropivacaine. New local anaesthetics, devised from analysis of structure and function relationships at ion channels, have shown promise of long acting pain relief but invariably many have fallen by the wayside as a result of their neural toxicity. However, for every study more knowledge is gained. Eventually one compound with the ability to reversibly and safely block nerves, with even perhaps an impact on spinal cord hyperalgesia, will emerge.

The mechanisms of action of local anaesthetics on the triad of endothelium function, coagulation system and the inflammatory response is only now emerging. From this, structure – function studies will shape the development of novel compounds to be used in clinical studies and open the possibility of using local anaesthetics in the future not simply for pain relief or selective sympathetic blockade but perhaps as therapeutic agents with an influence on the perioperative inflammatory response.

## References

1. Albright GA. Cardiac arrest following regional anesthesia with etidocaine or bupivacaine. Anesthesiol 1979; 51: 285–287.
2. Auroy Y, Narchi P, Messiah A, Litt L, Rouvier B, Samii K. Serious complications related to regional anesthesia: Results of a prospective survey in France. Anesthesiol 1997; 87: 479–486.
3. McLeod GA, Burke D. Laevobupivacaine. Anaesthesia 2001; 56: 331–341.
4. McLeod G, Davies H, Munnoch N, Bannister J, MacRae W. Postoperative pain relief using thoracic epidural analgesia: outstanding success and disappointing failures. Anaesthesia 2001; 56: 75–81.
5. Hollmann MW, Difazio CA, Durieux ME. Ca-signaling G-protein-coupled receptors: a new site of local anesthetic action? Reg Anesth Pain Med 2001; 26: 565–571.
6. Hollmann MW, Fischer LG, Byford AM, Durieux ME. Local anesthetic inhibition of m1 muscarinic acetylcholine signaling. Anesthesiol 2000; 93: 497–509.
7. Sur E, Newton DJ, Khan F, McLeod GA, Belch JJF. Nitric oxide release contributes to the vasoactive properties of prilocaine. Scottish Medical Journal 2002; 47: 17–18.
8. Catterall WA. Molecular mechanisms of gating and drug block of sodium channels. Novartis Found Symp 2002; 241: 206–218.
9. Sato C, Ueno Y, Asai K, Takahashi K, Sato M et al. The voltage-sensitive sodium channel is a bell-shaped molecule with several cavities. Nature 2001; 409: 1047–1051.
10. Catterall WA. A 3D view of sodium channels. Nature 2001; 409: 988–989, 991.
11. McPhee JC, Ragsdale DS, Scheuer T, Catterall WA. A critical role for the S4-S5 intracellular loop in domain IV of the sodium channel alpha-subunit in fast inactivation. J Biol Chem 1998; 273: 1121–1129.

12. Doyle DA, Morais Cabral J, Pfuetzner RA, Kuo A, Gulbis JM, Cohen SL *et al.* The structure of the potassium channel: molecular basis of $K^+$ conduction and selectivity. Science 1998; 280: 69–77.

13. Nau C, Wang SY, Strichartz GR, Wang GK. Block of human heart hH1 sodium channels by the enantiomers of bupivacaine. Anesthesiol 2000; 93: 1022–1033.

14. Drachman D, Strichartz G. Potassium channel blockers potentiate impulse inhibition by local anesthetics. Anesthesiol 1991; 75: 1051–1061.

15. Wang DW, Nie L, George Jr AL, Bennett PB. Distinct local anesthetic affinities in $Na^+$ channel subtypes. Biophys J 1996; 70: 1700–1708.

16. Wright SN, Wang SY, Kallen RG, Wang GK. Differences in steady-state inactivation between Na channel isoforms affect local anesthetic binding affinity. Biophys J 1997; 73: 779–788.

17. Vladimirov M, Nau C, Mok WM, Strichartz G. Potency of bupivacaine stereoisomers tested in vitro and in vivo: biochemical, electrophysiological, and neurobehavioral studies. Anesthesiol 2000; 93: 744–755.

18. Aberg G. Toxicological and local anesthetic effects of optically active isomers of two local anesthetic compounds. Acta Pharmacol Toxicol 1972; 31: 273–286.

19. McNaught AD, Wilkinson A. IUPAC Compendium of Chemical Terminology 2nd edn. 1997.

20. Valenzuela C, Snyders DJ, Bennett PB, Tamargo J, Hondeghem LM. Stereoselective block of cardiac sodium channels by bupivacaine in guinea pig ventricular myocytes. Circulation 1995; 92: 3014–3024.

21. Valenzuela C, Delpon E, Tamkun MM, Tamargo J, Snyders DJ. Stereoselective block of a human cardiac potassium channel (Kv1.5) by bupivacaine enantiomers. Biophys J 1995; 69: 418–427.

22. Longobardo M, Delpon E, Caballero R, Tamargo J, Valenzuela C. Structural determinants of potency and stereoselective block of hKv1.5 channels induced by local anesthetics. Mol Pharmacol 1998; 54: 162–169.

23. Moller R, Covino BG. Cardiac electrophysiologic properties of bupivacaine and lidocaine compared with those of ropivacaine, a new amide local anesthetic. Anesthesiol 1990; 72: 322–329.

24. Vanhoutte F, Vereecke J, Verbeke N, Carmeliet E. Stereoselective effects of the enantiomers of bupivacaine on the electrophysiological properties of the guinea-pig papillary muscle. Br J Pharmacol 1991; 103: 1275–1281.

25. Harding DP, Collier PA, Huckle RM, Gristwood R, Spridgen E. Comparison of the cardiotoxic effects of bupivacaine, laevobupivacaine and ropivacaine: An in vitro study in guinea-pig and human cardiac muscle. Br J Pharmacol 1998: 125: 127P.

26. Rutten AJ, Nancarrow C, Mather LE, Ilsley AH, Runciman WB, Upton RN. Hemodynamic and central nervous system effects of intravenous bolus doses of lidocaine, bupivacaine, and ropivacaine in sheep. Anesth Analg 1989; 69: 291–299.

27. Huang YF, Pryor ME, Mather LE, Veering BT. Cardiovascular and central nervous system effects of intravenous laevobupivacaine and bupivacaine in sheep. Anesth Analg 1998; 86: 797–804.

28. Chang DH, Ladd LA, Wilson KA, Gelgor L, Mather LE. Tolerability of large-dose intravenous laevobupivacaine in sheep. Anesth Analg 2000; 91: 671–679.

29. Reiz S, Haggmark S, Johansson G, Nath S. Cardiotoxicity of ropivacaine – a new amide local anaesthetic agent. Acta Anaesthesiol Scand 1989; 33: 93–98.

30. Morrison SG, Dominguez JJ, Frascarolo P, Reiz S. A comparison of the electrocardiographic cardiotoxic effects of racemic bupivacaine, laevobupivacaine, and ropivacaine in anesthetized swine. Anesth Analg 2000; 90: 1308–1314.

31. Chang DH, Ladd LA, Copeland S, Iglesias MA, Plummer JL, Mather LE. Direct cardiac effects of intracoronary bupivacaine, laevobupivacaine and ropivacaine in the sheep. Br J Pharmacol 2001; 132: 649–658.

32. Denson DD, Behbehani MM, Gregg RV. Enantiomer-specific effects of an intravenously administered arrhythmogenic dose of bupivacaine on neurons of the nucleus tractus solitarius and the cardiovascular system in the anesthetized rat. Reg Anesth 1992; 17: 311–316.

33. Scott DB, Lee A, Fagan D, Bowler GM, Bloomfield P, Lundh R. Acute toxicity of ropivacaine compared with that of bupivacaine. Anesth Analg 1989; 69: 563–569.

34. Knudsen K, Beckman Suurkula M, Blomberg S, Sjovall J, Edvardsson N. Central nervous and cardiovascular effects of i.v. infusions of ropivacaine, bupivacaine and placebo in volunteers. Br J Anaesth 1997; 78: 507–514.

35. Bardsley H, Gristwood R, Baker H, Watson N, Nimmo W. A comparison of the cardiovascular effects of laevobupivacaine and rac-bupivacaine following intravenous administration to healthy volunteers. Br J Clin Pharmacol 1998; 46: 245–249.

36. Wyld PJA. Comparison of the effects of laevobupivacaine and racemic bupivacaine on QT dispersion and signal averaged ECG in healthy male volunteers. Chiroscience study 012105.

37. Ohmura S, Kawada M, Ohta T, Yamamoto K, Kobayashi T. Systemic toxicity and resuscitation in bupivacaine-, laevobupivacaine-, or ropivacaine-infused rats. Anesth Analg 2001; 93: 743–748.

38. Groban L, Deal DD, Vernon JC, James RL, Butterworth J. Cardiac resuscitation after incremental overdosage with lidocaine, bupivacaine, laevobupivacaine, and ropivacaine in anesthetized dogs. Anesth Analg 2001; 92: 37–43.

39. Bader AM, Datta S, Flanagan H, Covino BG. Comparison of bupivacaine- and ropivacaine-induced conduction blockade in the isolated rabbit vagus nerve. Anesth Analg 1989; 68: 724–727.

40. Zaric D, Nydahl PA, Philipson L, Samuelsson L, Heierson A, Axelsson K. The effect of continuous lumbar epidural infusion of ropivacaine (0.1%, 0.2%, and 0.3%) and 0.25% bupivacaine on sensory and motor block in volunteers: a double-blind study. Reg Anesth 1996; 21: 14–25.

41. Polley LS, Columb MO, Naughton NN, Wagner DS, van de Ven CJ. Relative analgesic potencies of ropivacaine and bupivacaine for epidural analgesia in labor: implications for therapeutic indexes. Anesthesiol 1999; 90: 944–950.

42. Capogna G, Celleno D, Fusco P, Lyons G, Columb M. Relative potencies of bupivacaine and ropivacaine for analgesia in labour. Br J Anaesth 1999; 82: 371–373.

43. Lyons G, Columb M, Wilson RC, Johnson RV. Epidural pain relief in labour: potencies of laevobupivacaine and racemic bupivacaine. Br J Anaesth 1998; 81: 899–901.

44. Egli G, Morrison S, Vial A, Trojan D, Reiz S. Analgesic potency and motor-sensory separation of lumbar epidural bupivacaine (B) and ropivacaine (R). Br J Anaesth 1999; 82: 105.

45. Strichartz G. Pathways and obstacles to local anesthesia, a personal account: the 2000 Gaston Labat lecture. Reg Anesth Pain Med 2000; 25: 447–451.

46. Cederholm I, Evers H, Lofstrom JB. Skin blood flow after intradermal injection of ropivacaine in various concentrations with and without epinephrine evaluated by laser Doppler flowmetry. Reg Anesth 1992; 17: 322–328.

47. Cederholm I, Akerman B, Evers H. Local analgesic and vascular effects of intradermal ropivacaine and bupivacaine in various concentrations with and

without addition of adrenaline in man. Acta Anaesthesiol Scand 1994; 38: 322–327.

48. Newton DJ, Burke D, Khan F, McLeod GA, Belch JJ, McKenzie M et al. Skin blood flow changes in response to intradermal injection of bupivacaine and laevobupivacaine, assessed by laser Doppler imaging. Reg Anesth Pain Med 2000; 25: 626–631.

49. Kopacz DJ, Allen HW, Thompson GE. A comparison of epidural laevobupivacaine 0.75% with racemic bupivacaine for lower abdominal surgery. Anesth Analg 2000; 90: 642–648.

50. Lazaro JJ, Franquelo C, Navarro X, Castellano B, Verdu E, Cristofol C et al. Prolongation of nerve and epidural anesthetic blockade by bupivacaine in a lipid emulsion. Anesth Analg 1999; 89: 121–127.

51. Franquelo C, Toledo A, Manubens J, Cristofol C, Valladares JE, Arboix M. Prolongation of epidural anaesthesia in dogs with bupivacaine in a lipid emulsion. Vet Rec 2000; 147: 477–480.

52. Umbrain V, Alafandy M, Bourgeois P, D'Haese J, Boogaerts JG, Goffinet G et al. Biodistribution of liposomes after extradural administration in rodents. Br J Anaesth 1995; 75: 311–318.

53. Boogaerts JG, Declercq AG, Lafont ND, Benameur H, Akodad EM, Dupont JC et al. Toxicity of bupivacaine encapsulated into liposomes and injected intravenously: comparison with plain solutions. Anesth Analg 1993; 76: 553–555.

54. Boogaerts JG, Lafont ND, Declercq AG, Luo HC, Gravet ET, Bianchi JA et al. Epidural administration of liposome-associated bupivacaine for the management of postsurgical pain: a first study. J Clin Anesth 1994; 6: 315–320.

55. Lafont ND, Legros FJ, Boogaerts JG. Use of liposome-associated bupivacaine in a cancer pain syndrome. Anaesthesia 1996; 51: 578–579.

56. Curley J, Castillo J, Hotz J, Uezono M, Hernandez S, Lim JO et al. Prolonged regional nerve blockade. Injectable biodegradable bupivacaine/polyester microspheres. Anesthesiol 1996; 84: 1401–1410.

57. Drager C, Benziger D, Gao F, Berde CB. Prolonged intercostal nerve blockade in sheep using controlled-release of bupivacaine and dexamethasone from polymer microspheres. Anesthesiol 1998; 89: 969–979.

58. Castillo J, Curley J, Hotz J, Uezono M, Tigner J, Chasin M et al. Glucocorticoids prolong rat sciatic nerve blockade in vivo from bupivacaine microspheres. Anesthesiol 1996; 85: 1157–1166.

59. Grouls RJ, Meert TF, Korsten HH, Hellebrekers LJ, Breimer DD. Epidural and intrathecal n-butyl-p-aminobenzoate solution in the rat. Comparison with bupivacaine. Anesthesiol 1997; 86: 181–187.

60. Korsten HH, Hellebrekers LJ, Grouls RJ, Ackerman EW, van Zundert AA, van Herpen H et al. Long-lasting epidural sensory blockade by n-butyl p-aminobenzoate in the dog: neurotoxic or local anesthetic effect? Anesthesiol 1990; 73: 491–498.

61. Gonzalez T, Longobardo M, Caballero R, Delpon E, Tamargo J, Valenzuela C. Effects of bupivacaine and a novel local anesthetic, IQB-9302, on human cardiac $K^+$ channels. J Pharmacol Exp Ther 2001; 296: 573–583.

62. Gonzalez T, Longobardo M, Caballero R, Delpon E, Sinisterra JV, Tamargo J et al. Stereoselective effects of the enantiomers of a new local anaesthetic, IQB-9302, on a human cardiac potassium channel (Kv1.5). Br J Pharmacol 2001; 132: 385–392.

63. Scurlock JE, Curtis BM. Tetraethylammonium derivatives: ultralong-acting local anesthetics? Anesthesiol 1981; 54: 265–269.

64. Wang GK, Quan C, Vladimirov M, Mok WM, Thalhammer JG. Quaternary ammonium derivative of lidocaine as a long-acting local anesthetic. Anesthesiol 1995; 83: 1293–1301.

65. Kissin I, Lee SS, Bradley Jr EL. Effect of prolonged nerve block on inflammatory hyperalgesia in rats: prevention of late hyperalgesia. Anesthesiol 1998; 88: 224–232.

66. Gerner P, Nakamura T, Quan CF, Anthony DC, Wang GK. Spinal tonicaine: potency and differential blockade of sensory and motor functions. Anesthesiol 2000; 92: 1350–1360.

67. Watanbe Y, Saito H, Abe, K. Tricyclic antidepressants block NMDA receptor-mediated synaptic responses and induction of long-term potentiation in rat hippocampal slices. Neuropharmacology 1993; 32: 479–486.

68. Gerner P, Mujtaba M, Sinnott CJ, Wang GK. Amitriptyline versus bupivacaine in rat sciatic nerve blockade. Anesthesiol 2001; 94: 661–667.

69. Sudoh Y, Gerner P, Mustafa M, Khan M, Wang GK. N-Phenylethyl amitripyline acts as a long acting local anesthetic in rat. Anesthesiol 2001: A-988.

70. Cestele S, Catterall WA. Molecular mechanisms of neurotoxin action on voltage-gated sodium channels. Biochimie 2000; 82: 883–892.

71. Kohane DS, Yieh J, Lu NT, Langer R, Strichartz GR, Berde CB. A re-examination of tetrodotoxin for prolonged duration local anesthesia. Anesthesiol 1998; 89: 119–131.

72. Schwartz DM, Fields HL, Duncan KG, Duncan JL, Jones MR. Experimental study of tetrodotoxin, a long-acting topical anesthetic. Am J Ophthalmol 1998; 125: 481–487.

73. Kohane DS, Kuang Y, Lu NT, Langer R, Strichartz GR, Berde CB. Vanilloid receptor agonists potentiate the in vivo local anesthetic activity of percutaneously injected site 1 sodium channel blockers. Anesthesiol 1999; 90: 524–534.

74. Mujtaba MG, Gerner P, Kuo Wang G. Local anesthetic properties of prenylamine. Anesthesiol 2001; 95: 1198–1204.

75. Nietgen GW, Chan CK, Durieux ME. Inhibition of lysophosphatidate signaling by lidocaine and bupivacaine. Anesthesiol 1997; 86: 1112–1119.

76. Hollmann MW, Gross A, Jelacin N, Durieux ME. Local anesthetic effects on priming and activation of human neutrophils. Anesthesiol 2001; 95: 113–122.

77. Welters ID, Menzebach A, Langefeld TW, Menzebach M, Hempelmann G. Inhibitory effects of S(−)- and R(+)- bupivacaine on neutrophil function. Acta Anaesthesiol Scand 2001; 45: 570–575.

78. Hollmann MW, Durieux ME. Local anesthetics and the inflammatory response: a new therapeutic indication? Anesthesiol 2000; 93: 858–875.

79. Hollmann MW, Wieczorek KS, Smart M, Durieux ME. Epidural anesthesia prevents hypercoagulation in patients undergoing major orthopedic surgery. Reg Anesth Pain Med 2001; 26: 215–222.

80. Ala-Kokko TI, Lopponen A, Alahuhta S. Two instances of central nervous system toxicity in the same patient following repeated ropivacaine-induced brachial plexus block. Acta Anaesthesiol Scand 2000; 44: 623–626.

81. Abouleish EI, Elias M, Nelson C. Ropivacaine-induced seizure after extradural anaesthesia. Br J Anaesth 1998; 80: 843–844.

82. Mardirosoff C, Dumont L. Convulsions after the administration of high dose ropivacaine following an interscalenic block. Can J Anaesth 2000; 47: 1263.

83. Kopacz DJ, Allen HW. Accidental intravenous laevobupivacaine. Anesth Analg 1999; 89: 1027–1029.

84. Burm AG, de Boer AG, van Kleef JW, Vermeulen NP, de Leede LG, Spierdijk J et al. Pharmacokinetics of lidocaine and bupivacaine and stable isotope labelled analogues: a study in healthy volunteers. Biopharm Drug Dispos 1988; 9: 85–95.

85. Lee A, Fagan D, Lamont M, Tucker GT, Halldin M, Scott DB. Disposition kinetics of ropivacaine in humans. Anesth Analg 1989; 69: 736–738.

86. Burm AG, van der Meer AD, van Kleef JW, Zeijlmans PW, Groen K. Pharmacokinetics of the enantiomers of bupivacaine following intravenous administration of the racemate. Br J Clin Pharmacol 1994; 38: 125–129.

87. Bay-Nielsen M, Klarskov B, Bech K, Andersen J, Kehlet H. Laevobupivacaine vs bupivacaine as infiltration anaesthesia in inguinal herniorrhaphy. Br J Anaesth 1999; 82: 280–282.

88. Mulroy MF, Burgess FW, Emanuelsson BM. Ropivacaine 0.25% and 0.5%, but not 0.125%, provide effective wound infiltration analgesia after outpatient hernia repair, but with sustained plasma drug levels. Reg Anesth Pain Med 1999; 24: 136–141.

89. McLure HA, Rubin AP. Comparison of 0.75% laevobupivacaine with 0.75% racemic bupivacaine for peribulbar anaesthesia. Anaesthesia 1998; 53: 1160–1164.

90. Nicholson G, Sutton B, Hall GM. Ropivacaine for peribulbar anesthesia. Reg Anesth Pain Med 1999; 24: 337–340.

91. Cox CR, Checketts MR, Mackenzie N, Scott NB, Bannister J. Comparison of S(−)-bupivacaine with racemic (RS)-bupivacaine in supraclavicular brachial plexus block. Br J Anaesth 1998; 80: 594–598.

92. Casati A, Fanelli G, Aldegheri G, Berti M, Colnaghi E, Cedrati V et al. Interscalene brachial plexus anaesthesia with 0.5%, 0.75% or 1% ropivacaine: a double-blind comparison with 2% mepivacaine. Br J Anaesth 1999; 83: 872–875.

93. Santorsola R, Casati A, Cerchierini E, Moizo E, Fanelli G. Laevobupivacaine for peripheral blocks of the lower limb: a clinical comparison with bupivacaine and ropivacaine. Minerva Anestesiol 2001; 67(9 Suppl 1): 33–36.

94. Connolly C, Coventry DM, Wildsmith JA. Double-blind comparison of ropivacaine 7.5 mg ml⁻¹ with bupivacaine 5 mg ml⁻¹ for sciatic nerve block. Br J Anaesth 2001; 86: 674–677.

95. Cox CR, Faccenda KA, Gilhooly C, Bannister J, Scott NB, Morrison LM. Extradural S(−)-bupivacaine: comparison with racemic RS-bupivacaine. Br J Anaesth 1998; 80: 289–293.

96. McGlade DP, Kalpokas MV, Mooney PH, Buckland MR, Vallipuram SK, Hendrata MV et al. Comparison of 0.5% ropivacaine and 0.5% bupivacaine in lumbar epidural anaesthesia for lower limb orthopaedic surgery. Anaesth Intensive Care 1997; 25: 262–266.

97. Kopacz DJ, Sharrock NE, Allen HW. A comparison of laevobupivacaine 0.125%, fentanyl 4 μg/mL, or their combination for patient-controlled epidural analgesia after major orthopedic surgery. Anesth Analg 1999; 89: 1497–1503.

98. Scott DA, Blake D, Buckland M, Etches R, Halliwell R, Marsland C et al. A comparison of epidural ropivacaine infusion alone and in combination with 1, 2, and 4 μg/mL fentanyl for seventy-two hours of postoperative analgesia after major abdominal surgery. Anesth Analg 1999; 88: 857–864.

99. Glaser C, Marhofer P, Zimpfer G, Heinz MT, Sitzwohl C, Kapral S et al. Laevobupivacaine versus racemic bupivacaine for spinal anesthesia. Anesth Analg 2002; 94(1): 194–198.

100. Whiteside JB, Burke D, Wildsmith JA. Spinal anaesthesia with ropivacaine 5 mg ml in glucose 10 mg ml or 50 mg ml. Br J Anaesth 2001; 86: 241–244.

*L. Cormican   J. Rees*

# Asthma

The definition of asthma has changed significantly over the last 50 years. In the 1950s it was defined as a disease of airway smooth muscle such that it contracted excessively on minimal stimulation.[1] With a greater understanding of the pathogenesis of the disease the definition has now extended to encompass the contribution of bronchial wall inflammation, bronchial hyper-reactivity and airflow obstruction. A current definition is of a 'chronic inflammatory disorder of the airways in which many cells play a role, in particular mast cells, eosinophils, T-lymphocytes, neutrophils, macrophages and epithelial cells'. In susceptible individuals, the inflammation causes recurrent episodes of wheezing, breathlessness, chest tightness and coughing, particularly at night or the early morning. These episodes are usually associated with widespread but variable airflow obstruction, that is often reversible either spontaneously or with treatment. The inflammation also causes an associated increase in the existing bronchial hyper-responsiveness to a variety of stimuli.[2]

## Epidemiology

The prevalence of asthma has substantially increased in western countries over the past 30 years in both adult and paediatric populations. In the USA the prevalence of asthma among 6–11 year olds was 4.8% between the years 1971–1974, and had increased to 7.6% between 1976 and 1980 in the same population.[3] Similarly in Australia and New Zealand, the prevalence of asthma among 8–11 year olds in 1982 was 12.9%, but by 1992 had soared to a staggering 29.4%.[4] The International Study of Asthma and Allergies in

Childhood (ISAAC) Steering Committee study[5] in 1998, found that the prevalence of asthma in the 13–14 year old population of the UK was among the highest in the world.

In association with an increase in the international prevalence of the disease there is evidence of an increase in mortality from asthma throughout the world. An increase in asthma death rate from 5.3 to 10.5 per million in the 5–34 year age group during the period 1974–1984 in England and Wales has been reported.[6,7] In the United States the asthma death rate increased from 8 to 20 per million in the period 1977–1997.[8] Similar findings have also been noted by So *et al.*, in Hong Kong,[9] and more recently by Pritchard *et al.*, in Ireland.[10]

### Increased prevalence and the hygiene hypothesis

Epidemiological studies have given some insight into potential causes for the increase in the prevalence. An atopic predisposition is the biggest risk factor for the development of asthma[11] and data has shown that the prevalence of atopy in the population is proportional to the prevalence of asthma. However the reason for the increase in the prevalence[5] of atopy is also still poorly understood. A number of possible explanations have been proposed.

Asthma and atopy are regarded as diseases of civilisation.[12] Evidence is at hand which supports the hypothesis that development of these two conditions may be due to a lack of sufficient antigenic stimulation in early childhood. The frequency of serious infections in childhood is reduced in the western world because of vaccination programmes, increased use of antibiotics, fewer parasitic infestations, fewer children per household and fewer shared bedrooms.

In an interesting study comparing two sex- and age-matched paediatric cohorts from Munich and Leipzig, Von Mutius[13] has demonstrated a much higher prevalence of asthma and atopic disease among children from Munich. Both populations were ethnically, geographically and climatically similar but in the course of history between 1945 and 1989, they had differed vastly in terms of affluence and their surrounding environment. The children from the former East German industrial town of Leipzig were less likely to develop asthma and atopy and the authors postulated that this was because of the degree of protection afforded by immune stimulation in childhood. This is the 'hygiene hypothesis', and is supported by additional reports in the literature. Children from itinerant families in Ireland are noted to have a much lower prevalence of atopy and asthma than their counterparts from the settled communities.[14] Children from farming communities are less likely to develop asthma and atopy than their counterparts from non-farming communities.[15]

Another factor, which supports the rise of atopy and asthma in westernised societies, is the increased number of nuclear families.[16] Children from larger families are less likely to develop upper respiratory symptoms due to atopy.[17] It is postulated that repeated exposure to viral and bacterial infection in larger families skews the cytokine repertoire of the T-lymphocyte population and prevents the development of asthma. There is some evidence that previously common childhood infections such as Toxoplasma gondi and hepatitis A have a protective role against the development of atopy and asthma.[18] The basis of this phenomenon involves the T-helper type 1/T-helper type 2 (Th-1/Th-2) paradigm: antigenic stimulation resulting in a Th-1 mediated CD4+ T-lymphocyte response results in a humoral reaction with the production of IgM and IgG1, macrophage activation, cellular immunity and eventually tolerance of the antigen. However antigenic stimulation resulting in a Th-2 mediated CD4+ T-lymphocyte response produces an immediate type 1 hypersensitivity reaction as occurs in allergic disease.[19,20,21]

Furthermore, children growing up in western societies are also more likely to be exposed to large quantities of allergens such as house dust mites. Modern homes with central heating, poor ventilation and an abundance of soft furnishings, carpets and curtains provide the optimal conditions for the proliferation of dust mite populations.[22]

The immune system of the pregnant mother, the embryo and the neonate is programmed to respond in a Th-2 like manner to antigenic stimulation producing immediate hypersensitivity-like reactions. At some point, the neonatal immune system changes its pattern of T-lymphocyte reactivity from Th-2 to Th-1 with the production of interleukin-2 (IL-2), interferon-gamma (IFN-$\gamma$), and the development of immunological 'tolerance'.[23,24] This change is believed to be mediated by the antigenic stimulation of the neonatal immune system by repeated exposure to viral and bacterial antigens. Failure to do so could result in a persistently Th-2 polarised T-lymphocyte population, and repeated immediate type hypersensitivity reactions facilitated by an environment rich in allergens.

## Genetics of Asthma

The genetics of asthma are complex. Asthma is not inherited in the standard Mendelian pattern but demonstrates a pattern of polygenic inheritance in common with other diseases such as hypertension and atherosclerosis.

Specific areas of the genome harbour genes that contribute to asthma and atopy. Independent investigators have implicated five different loci, C5q, C6p21, C11q13, C12q and C13q.

The β-adrenergic receptor gene (BADR) has been located in the C5q region. A number of haplotypes have been identified which alter receptor function. The most important are Arg-16 → Gly and Gln-27 → Glu polymorphisms, which influence the downregulation of the receptor in response to agonist. These polymorphisms have been associated with several characteristics of asthma including bronchial hyper-responsiveness,[25] bronchial reversibility[26] and some measures of asthma severity.[27]

The IL-4 gene is also located in the C5q region and IL-4 production/level is closely related to serum IgE concentrations. A polymorphism has been iden-tified (IL-4 C-589T) in a region of the gene that binds transcription factors and may increase gene expression.[28] A number of association studies have demonstrated an increased prevalence of this polymorphism in individuals who have asthma or atopy.[28,29] The gene for the CD14 receptor is also located within the C5q region. The CD14 receptor mediates the cellular response to endotoxin. A polymorphism of the CD14 gene has been identi-fied and associated with increased concentrations of IgE.[30] It is believed that the link between IgE and CD14 is governed by the Th-1/Th-2 balance. Binding of endotoxin to the CD14 receptor during infection may stimulate the expression of the Th-1 cytokines, steering the immune system away from the Th-2 predominance that exists *in utero*. If the CD14 polymorphism attenu-ates the strength of this immune modulation, it could encourage the persist-ence of a Th-2 phenotype.

Mutations of the FcεRIβ (High affinity IgE receptor) gene (leu 81) on the C11q13 region have also been found in association with atopy[31] and asthma.[32] Mutations of this gene may function by increasing the secretion of IL-4 due to increased signal transduction after allergen binds to IgE.

The IL-4 receptor α gene (IL4Rα) has been located in a linked region of C16q. One variant of the IL-4 gene (Gln576-Arg) has been associated with increased signal transduction and elevated serum IgE including the Hyper IgE Syndrome.[33] These examples show the complexity of the genetics of asthma.

The aspiration of such research is to identify specific genotypic variants of the disease and ultimately to develop therapies targeted against 'rogue genes' and hence manipulate the pathogenesis or the pharmacological responses of the disease.

# Pathophysiology of Asthma

## Chronic inflammation in asthma

While the eosinophils of the asthmatic bronchial wall are believed to be responsible for the production of asthmatic symptoms, the T-cell population regulates control over the eosinophil population.[34–39] Strong support for this hypothesis came from the observation that, compared to controls, the numbers of activated T (CD4+, CD25+) cells in peripheral blood were markedly elevated in patients admitted to hospital with acute severe asthma[34] and the finding of a correlation between numbers of activated peripheral blood T-cells and airway narrowing as measured by peak expiratory flow rate.[35] Further support comes from the demonstration by immunohisto-chemistry of increased numbers of activated T-cells (CD25+ cells),[36] associated with an increase in the numbers of eosinophils in the asthmatic bronchial wall.

Subsequently increased concentrations of the cytokines IL-4 and IL-5 (by immunohistochemistry), and mRNA for IL-4 and IL-5 (by reverse transcriptase-polymerase chain reaction – RT-PCR) have been demonstrated in asthmatic bronchial wall biopsy[39,40] and bronchoalveolar lavage[41] respectively.

The CD4+ T-lymphocytes produce a large number of cytokines. The most important in the immunopathogenesis of asthma are IL-4, IL-5, IL-2 and IFN-γ. Murine and human studies have enabled the differentiation of the CD4+ cell population into two general phenotypes based on the profile of cytokines they elaborate. The Th-1 CD4+ subset produces IL-2 and IFN-γ upon antigenic stimulation. The Th-2 CD4 subset produces IL-4 and IL-5 upon antigenic stimulation.[42,43]

The CD4+ T-lymphocyte can be regarded as the essential orchestrator of both the humeral and cellular events of the asthmatic bronchial wall immune response. Reciprocal regulatory roles of IFN-γ and IL-4 on the development of the Th-1 and Th-2 clones have been demonstrated in animals and human beings. Maggi et al.,[44] have demonstrated the capacity of IFN-γ to inhibit the development of Der P specific T-cell clones into a functional Th-2 phenotype in an atopic subject. The addition of IL-4 to the IFN-γ and IL-2 producing, human T-cell Th-1 clones increased the production of IL-4 and IL-5 by these cells.

Therefore the balance of T-cell sub-populations is under the control of the cytokines present in the surrounding microenvironment. The findings have been extended to the inflammatory processes involving the asthmatic bronchial wall, where alterations in the Th-1/Th-2 balance appear to be central to the development of the clinical syndrome of asthma.

## Airway Remodelling

This term refers to some of the structural changes associated with asthma in the bronchial wall. Airway walls thicken from increases in the quantity of submucosal tissue, basement membrane and smooth muscle by hyperplasia and hypertrophy. Enhanced subepithelial fibrosis by collagen deposition is postulated to be due to increased myofibroblast activity. The precise mechanisms underlying these changes are unclear but are believed to be related to persistent airway inflammation. This phenomenon also occurs in the bronchial wall in some patients suffering from chronic obstructive pulmonary disease (COPD), allergic rhinitis and eosinophilic bronchitis. In the asthmatic population, this process contributes to a greater rate of decline of the predicted $FEV_1$ per year in comparison to the non-asthmatic population and hence irreversible loss of airway function. There is some evidence that adequate treatment to reduce inflammation will limit airway remodelling and prevent the development of irreversible damage.

## Treatment of Chronic Asthma and the Goals of Therapy

International guidelines favour a stepwise approach to the treatment of chronic asthma. Therapy is started at an appropriate level and stepped up or down according to an algorithm with the intention of achieving disease control and minimising side effects. A modified algorithm based on that recommended by the British Thoracic Society,[45] which incorporates the availability and efficacy of leukotriene receptor antagonists is outlined as follows. Newer guidelines are currently in preparation (British Thoracic Society Website: www.brit-thoracic.org.uk)

| | |
|---|---|
| Step 1 | Short acting β-agonist as required |
| Step 2 | Above + inhaled corticosteroid 200–800 μg/day |
| Step 3 | Above + long acting β-agonist or if not tolerated, another *add-on* drug; such as leukotriene receptor antagonist or theophylline |
| Step 4 | Above + add any or all of the following as determined by empirical trial<br>Increase inhaled steroid to 2000 μg/day<br>Long acting β-agonist<br>Theophylline<br>Leukotriene receptor antagonist |
| Step 5 | Above + daily oral steroid or regular booster courses of oral steroid |

The aims of treatment are:

- to minimise/have no chronic symptoms
- to minimise exacerbations
- to have no emergency visits
- to have no/less than once daily PRN short term β-agonist use

Once control is achieved, a step down approach can be considered. There is controversy over the optimal period of disease control which should be achieved prior to stepping down treatment. A period of 3–6 months is considered sensible. However, airway hyper-reactivity can continue to improve for up to 2 years of treatment and it is important not to step down prematurely.


## Anaesthesia and Asthma

Asthma contributes to morbidity and mortality in the practice of anaesthesia. Bronchospasm accounts for up to 2% of all malpractice claims according to the closed claims project of the American Society of Anesthesiologists. Eighty percent of cases occurred during general anaesthesia and the remainder during regional anaesthesia. Bronchospasm related to anaesthesia occurred during induction and intubation in 69% of cases and in 25% of cases during actual anaesthesia.[46]


## Preoperative Considerations

The factors which need to be considered in an asthmatic patient undergoing anaesthesia are disease severity, adequacy of disease control as indicated by the frequency of exacerbations and degree of reversibility to bronchodilators and occurrence of recent upper respiratory tract disease.

A detailed history is of central importance to document the frequency, severity of exacerbations, precipitating factors, treatment and actual response to treatment. Some experts divide the asthmatic population undergoing anaesthesia into three groups. Asymptomatic and inactive asthmatics are those who are asymptomatic at the time of presentation and without any episodes of bronchospasm for the previous 2 years. No further investigations are required in this group but the anaesthetic technique and drugs least likely to precipitate bronchospasm should be selected as the majority of these patients will still have evidence of inflammation in the airway wall and of bronchial hyper-reactivity.[47]

Those who are asymptomatic at the time of presentation but with a history of active disease as indicated by persistent symptoms or an episode of bronchospasm in the last 2 years should have a preoperative evaluation where possible to include lung function tests with documentation of reversibility to $\beta_2$-agonists. Elective surgery should be scheduled for a time when disease is well controlled, and not within 6 weeks of an upper respiratory infection, as this may precipitate an exacerbation[48]. Reversibility of greater than 30% of $FEV_1$ following bronchodilator inhalation indicates that disease is not optimally controlled.[49]

In those with active disease who are symptomatic, surgery should be rescheduled when possible until disease is properly controlled with inhaled corticosteroids and or the use of add-on drugs such as long acting $\beta_2$- agonists, leukotriene receptor antagonists or theophyllines.[45,49] Preoperative systemic glucocorticoids may have some role in such patients in addition to standard efforts at disease control with inhaled corticosteroids. The potential benefits of corticosteroids are the upregulation of $\beta_2$-adrenergic receptor number and function, a reduction in bronchial hyper-reactivity, reduction in bronchial wall inflammation, frequency and severity of disease exacerbation.[50,51,52]

One study demonstrated that systemic steroid therapy for 1 week prior to general anaesthesia and surgery did not increase the risk of impaired wound healing, postoperative infection or the incidence of hypoadrenalism.[53] The perioperative pulmonary complication rate was 5.4%[53] while another study reported a perioperative pulmonary complication rate of 24% in a similar population who received no systemic corticosteroids preoperatively.[54]

Short courses of systemic corticosteroids can be immediately discontinued postoperatively without tapering and without any adverse effects. Assessment should take into account individual patient characteristics of the adequacy of control, history of exacerbations, usual treatment and intended surgery.

## Intraoperative Considerations

### Effect of anaesthetic drugs on airway tone

*Induction agents*

Thiobarbiturates (e.g. thiopentol) are known to trigger mast cell histamine release at clinical concentrations and may present as airway obstruction and hypotension.[55] There is conflicting evidence as to whether thiobarbiturates are associated with an increased risk of bronchospasm in comparison to other induction agents. However one study has demonstrated higher incidence of wheezing among patients treated with thiopentol in comparison to the non-barbiturate propofol.[56]

Propofol is associated with a lower incidence of wheezing[56] as an induction agent and also reduces airway resistance when given as a continuous infusion.[57]

Ketamine is occasionally used as an induction agent and has well-known bronchodilator effects. Inhibition of the re-uptake of noradrenaline at sympathetic nerve endings is the most likely mode of its bronchodilatory action as the effect can be prevented by a β-adrenoceptor blocker such as propranolol.[58] At higher than normal clinical concentrations, ketamine may contribute to the reduction in airway tone and reactivity by direct smooth muscle relaxation and inhibition of the vagal reflex pathway.[59]

Etomidate, does not have a significant effect on mast cell histamine release and there are no reports of adverse effects when used in asthma.[60] Like ketamine it produces less respiratory depression than other induction agents.

### Non-depolarising neuromuscular blocking agents

Agents such as gallamine and pancuronium can potentiate bronchospasm. Both drugs bind to M2 and or M3 muscarinic receptors on airway smooth muscle cells and nerves. Blockade of M2 receptors can potentiate vagally mediated bronchospasm while M3 receptor blockade inhibits it, thus the net effect of each of these drugs depends on their relative potency at each site. Gallamine is now infrequently used as it can precipitate bronchospasm and tachycardia. Pancuronium has less potential to do so.[61,62]

Other non-depolarising neuromuscular blockers such as mivacurium[63] and atracurium[64] can result in the release of histamine from mast cells.

### Opioids

Opioids carry the risk of respiratory depression. Codeine and morphine in high doses can precipitate histamine release from mast cells and can precipitate bronchospasm in asthmatic patients. However fentanyl lacks this property.[65]

## Developments in the Pharmacological Management of Acute Asthma

### Theophyllines

Aminophylline has a controversial role in the treatment of asthma. It is less effective than β2-agonists as a single agent in the treatment of acute asthma.[66] There is debate as to whether it has a clinically synergistic effect with β2-agonists.[67] Theophyllines also have the potential benefit of increasing the cardiac output, increasing diaphragmatic contraction and possible anti-inflammatory effects.[68,69] The toxic effects include nausea, vomiting, headaches, restlessness, life threatening dysrhythmias and convulsions. Even though not generally recommended for the treatment of acute asthma, it may confer benefit in patients failing to respond to conventional treatment with $\beta_2$-agonists and corticosteroids. A loading dose of 3 mg/kg is recommended in patients not receiving maintenance theophyllines as outpatients, and it is followed by an infusion of 0.5 mg/kg/h.[69,70] Serum concentrations need to be checked within 1–2 and then 12 h after initiation of the maintenance infusion and then daily thereafter. The dose needs to be reduced in patients suffering from congestive cardiac failure and there is an interaction with a number of drugs including cimetidine, erythromycin and ciprofloxacin.

## Magnesium

Magnesium is postulated to be of benefit in the treatment of acute asthma. This was initially based on anecdotal evidence without objective spirometric demonstration of a benefit. Magnesium sulphate in addition to adrenaline was an accepted part of the armamentarium for the treatment of acute asthma prior to the advent of selective $\beta_2$-agonist use. In the 1980s and 1990s there was increased interest in the use of magnesium sulphate ($MgSO_4$) as an adjunct to the standard treatment of acute asthma. Its mechanism of action is poorly understood. Magnesium sulphate is believed to act as an antagonist of voltage gated calcium channels. In airway smooth muscle, increased cytosolic calcium leads to the activation of the contractile system. Increases in cytosolic calcium are believed to be dependent on release from intracellular compartments and on calcium influx through voltage dependent channels.[71]

A recent systematic review of the use of magnesium in acute asthma, has analysed five adult and three paediatric randomised controlled clinical trials (RCCTs) involving a total of 665 patients.[72] Addition of magnesium sulphate to the standard treatment of acute asthma overall was not associated with a reduction in the hospital admission rate. However subgroup analysis demonstrated that patients with an $FEV_1$ <30% predicted, failure of $FEV_1$ to improve to >60% predicted within the first 1 h in the emergency department or failure to respond to initial standard treatment had a better improvement in peak expiratory flow rate and a reduced hospital admission rate following treatment with magnesium sulphate.[72]

Magnesium sulphate has also been compared with normal saline as an addition to salbutamol delivered by nebuliser in acute asthma in one RCCT.[73] In this study the magnesium sulphate limb was associated with a significantly better PEFR after 10 min. No adverse effects were noted with its use by nebuliser.

Currently magnesium sulphate appears to be safe and beneficial in the treatment of acute asthma, but it is not needed in most patients who respond to conventional therapy.

## Helium

Helium in the form of a helium/oxygen mixture (Heliox) reduces inspired gas density, turbulence and airway resistance, hence decreasing the work of breathing and potentially increasing the distribution of nebulised bronchodilators within the lung.[74] Its role in acute asthma is not well established at the moment, but it may serve as an adjunct to treatment in a deteriorating patient in an effort to avert the need for invasive ventilation or to aid the invasive ventilation of a persistently difficult patient.

## Ketamine

Ketamine, as noted above can be used as a bronchodilator.[58,75] The use of ketamine is of benefit in the maintenance of general anaesthesia in the mechanical ventilation of the lungs of a severe asthmatic. Ketamine is used in conjunction with additional sedatives such as benzodiazipines because of the high incidence of visual and auditory hallucinations and out of body experiences. Ketamine must be used with caution in those with pre-existing hypertension and ischaemic heart disease.

**Other drugs.** These include calcium antagonists, nitrates, clonidine and IV glucagon have been shown to ameliorate bronchospasm to some degree but are not recommended for the treatment of acute severe asthma.

# Developments in the Pharmacological Management of Chronic Asthma

## Long acting $\beta_2$-agonists

The introduction of long acting $\beta_2$-agonists has been a major therapeutic development and has led to a fundamental reappraisal of $\beta_2$-agonist use in asthma management. Their use is recommended in patients suffering from persistently symptomatic asthma despite being established on low dose inhaled corticosteroids according to internationally accepted guidelines.[45] Salmeterol and formoterol are the two long acting $\beta_2$-agonists available for prescription in the UK and are highly selective with bronchodilatory effects lasting for 12 h after a single inhalation.[76,77]

Several studies have demonstrated that in a combination with inhaled short acting $\beta_2$-agonists, long acting $\beta_2$-agonists are clinically inferior to inhaled corticosteroids as a maintenance treatment for persistent asthma.[78,79,80] This is in keeping with the current understanding of asthma as an inflammatory disorder. However many patients will be insufficiently controlled on a low to moderate dose of inhaled corticosteroid. For this group an alternative is to increase the dose of inhaled corticosteroids, but it is recognised that inhaled corticosteroids display a flat dose response curve when disease control is measured using measures of disease severity such as symptom score, peak flow rate and $FEV_1$. In a population of moderately severe asthmatics, Greening has shown that the addition of salmeterol to low dose beclomethasone produced significantly better disease control in terms of improvement in symptoms and peak flow.[81] Woolcock[82] has shown that the addition of long acting $\beta_2$-agonists to inhaled corticosteroids produced significantly better disease control in persistently symptomatic asthma than doubling the dose of inhaled corticosteroids as measured by symptoms, peak flow and lung function changes. Current evidence also demonstrates that long acting $\beta_2$-agonists produce better disease control when added onto inhaled corticosteroids in persistently symptomatic patients than the addition of a theophylline or leukotriene receptor antagonist.[83,84]

An area of concern was that long acting $\beta_2$-agonists as an add-on treatment might mask underlying inflammation. However markers of inflammation such as induced sputum eosinophil counts and disease exacerbation rates are similar in patients treated with low dose inhaled corticosteroids plus long acting $\beta_2$-agonists or high dose inhaled corticosteroids alone.

The addition of long acting $\beta_2$-agonists also allows the dose of inhaled corticosteroids to be reduced without losing disease control in mild to moderate asthma. The implementation of and compliance with treatment with long acting $\beta_2$-agonists and inhaled corticosteroids is postulated to be further improved by combinations of the two drugs in the same inhaler device.[85] Despite the theoretical advantages over separate inhaler therapy, conclusive evidence of superiority in compliance or effect does not yet exist.

The currently available combinations are Seretide® which contains salmeterol 50 µg and fluticasone propionate 125, 250 or 500 µg per inhalation, and Symbicort® which contains formoterol 4.5 µg and budesonide 80 or 160 µg per inhalation.

## Arachidonic acid metabolism and leukotriene receptor antagonists

The cysteinyl leukotrienes (LT) CD and E4 are the products of the metabolism of arachidonic acid by the 5-lipoxygenase (5-LO) pathway.[86]

They elicit bronchoconstriction in human beings at concentrations of 1:10,000 that required of histamine or methacholine.[87] Additionally, leukotrienes and other products of the 5-Lipoxygenase pathway induce pathophysiological changes similar to those associated with asthma. Specifically they can produce tissue oedema, eosinophil migration and can stimulate the increased production of airway secretions. The cysteinyl leukotrienes also stimulate smooth muscle proliferation and cell cycling.[88] Two types of cysteinyl leukotriene receptors have been identified, Cys LT1 and Cys LT2. Most of the actions of cysteinyl leukotrienes are mediated through Cys LT1, these actions include human airway smooth muscle contraction, chemotaxis and increased vascular permeability.[88]

Leukotriene receptor antagonists have been developed which antagonise the Cys LT1 receptor. This class of drug has been given the generic suffix -lukast, and three of them have proven to be effective treatments for asthma. Two of these three, zafirlukast and montelukast sodium, are available for prescription in the United Kingdom. They are given orally. Cysteinyl leukotrienes are implicated in the early and late phase asthmatic responses post allergen inhalation.[89] They also have been recovered from the urine of patients with exercise induced asthma in some studies.[90] Cysteinyl leukotriene receptor antagonists have a role in exercise induced asthma, but the benefits vary between patients.[91]

Leukotriene receptor antagonists have an important role in the treatment of aspirin and non-steroidal anti-inflammatory sensitive asthma. In 3–8% of asthmatic patients, the initiation of these drugs can sometimes cause severe and life threatening bronchoconstriction.[92] Pre-treatment with leukotriene receptor antagonists has been shown to ameliorate aspirin induced bronchospasm and longer term treatment has been shown to improve lung function in patients with aspirin sensitive asthma even in the absence of an aspirin challenge.[88]

In chronic persistent/symptomatic asthma the addition of leukotriene receptor antagonists orally may improve lung function, decrease the need for rescue treatment with short acting $\beta_2$-agonists, relieve the symptoms of asthma and reduce the frequency of disease exacerbations.[93] Oral leukotriene receptor antagonists also have an acute bronchodilatory onset in 1–3 h of the order of 8–20% in some studies. The bronchodilator effects are maximal in those with the greatest degree of airways obstruction but are about half the response obtained from $\beta_2$-agonists.[93,94]

The benefits of leukotriene receptor antagonists in the treatment of chronic asthma vary considerably, and it has not been possible to identify specific subgroups most likely to benefit from this treatment. Overall they provide an alternative to increasing the dose of ICS but have less effect and less evidence behind them at present.

### Inhaled corticosteroids

Corticosteroids are the most potent anti-inflammatory drugs used in the treatment of asthma.[80,95] Since the early 1990's inhaled corticosteroids are recommended as first line therapy for patients with persistent asthma. This is supported by clinical studies of inhaled corticosteroids in patients with asthma of disease severity from mild to severe. In concert with improvements in lung function[96,97] and symptom scores,[50] attenuation of bronchial reactivity[98] and inflammatory cell recruitment[50,96,97,99] are all hallmarks of inhaled corticosteroid usage.

Corticosteroids have effects on airway inflammation through the increase and decrease in transcription of many anti- and pro-inflammatory genes, respectively. Corticosteroids increase the synthesis of lipocortin-1, a protein that has an inhibitory effect on the production of lipid mediators, and recombinant lipocortin-1 has acute anti-inflammatory properties.[100] Corticosteroids can inhibit the activity of NF-κB, which plays a pivotal role in inflammation. This effect is mediated through the increased transcription of inhibitory protein IκB which binds NF-κB in the cytoplasm.[101]

Corticosteroids are very effective in downregulating airway wall inflammation in asthma. They reduce the number and activation status of inflammatory cells in the airway wall.[50,96,97,99,102–104] Reductions are seen in eosinophil numbers and eosinophil cationic protein concentration[105,106] and in the numbers of activated CD4+ cells (CD4+, CD25+) in BALF.[107] The effect of inhaled corticosteroid therapy is also evident in studies of induced sputum where eosinophil numbers and eosinophilic cationic protein (ECP) concentration are reduced following treatment with inhaled corticosteroids,[108,109] while the apoptosis of eosinophils is increased.[110] Conversely, reducing the dosage of steroid results in an increase in sputum eosinophils and a worsening of asthmatic symptoms.[111]

Corticosteroids have been shown to reduce bronchial hyper-reactivity, improve clinical parameters and reduce disease severity.[50,51] These factors have been shown to be time dependent[96,98,112] but controversy exists as to whether they are particularly dose dependent.[113] Bronchial hyper-reactivity has been shown to return to normal levels after a year of treatment in some patients.[114,115] However, cessation of corticosteroid therapy results in a return of airway hyper-responsiveness to pre-treatment levels within a few weeks.[51,98,116]

The mechanism underlying the efficacy of corticosteroids in ameliorating bronchial hyper-reactivity presumably relates to their ability to control or alter the different aspects of bronchial wall inflammation.

### Anti-IgE therapy

Recombinant humanised monoclonal antibody against IgE (rhuMAb-E25) has been tested in moderate to severe asthma and atopic rhinitis. This medication is still experimental and is not available for prescription. The monoclonal antibody is designed so that it interacts with the Fc portion of the IgE antibody preventing binding with the IgE receptor (FcεRI) on mast cells, basophils, thus preventing the activation of these cells by cross-linking of bound IgE.[117] A randomised double blind placebo control trial over a period of 21 weeks examined the benefits of intravenous rhuMAb-E25 given once every 2 weeks in addition to standard therapy in a population with atopic asthma of moderate to severe disease severity.[118] Anti-IgE therapy improved symptom scores, decreased serum IgE concentrations and permitted more subjects to safely reduce their oral and ICS intake than placebo. The treatment was also well tolerated. Anti-IgE therapy may have an important role to play as a steroid sparing agent in steroid dependent asthma, but further studies are required in larger numbers of patients to validate this new and exciting therapy.

## Alteration of the Th-1/Th-2 Balance

'Vaccination' against asthma is the aspiration of many scientists and clinicians throughout the world. Potential mechanisms would involve the manipulation of the Th-1/Th-2 balance of the CD4+ lymphocyte population in early childhood. Potential methods of doing so could involve DNA-like proteins.[119] However such an attempt would have to be cautiously approached as a skewing of the immune system from Th-2 reactivity could facilitate the development of Th-1 mediated diseases such as diabetes mellitus or Crohn's disease. Other approaches could involve drugs that alter the Th-1/Th-2 balance or manipulation through their cytokine products. Attempts have been made to alter the synthesis, release or effect of beneficial cytokines such as IL-10 or IL-12, or potentially harmful ones such as IL-4, IL-5 or IL-13.

## Conclusion

Coupled with a better understanding of the epidemiology, genetics and immunopathology of asthma should be the ability to develop novel and targeted methods to manipulate the factors which predispose the population to develop this disease. Furthermore improved understanding of these aspects of asthma will allow the development of new and effective treatments for the disease. The basic information from the last decade is beginning to produce exciting therapeutic possibilities that may change our treatment over the next few years. However the majority of patients with asthma can have their disease controlled with the appropriate use of current therapy.

## References

1. Ciba Foundation guest symposium. Terminology, definitions and classification of chronic pulmonary emphysema and related conditions. Thorax 1959; 14: 286–299.
2. NHBLI. Guidelines for the diagnosis and management of asthma. NIH Publication No. 97-4051A 1997: 17–47.
3. Gergen P, Mullally D, Evans I. National survey of asthma among children in the United States. Pediatrics 1988; 81: 1–7.
4. Peat J, Haby M, Spikjer J, Berry G, Woolcock A. Has the prevalence of adult asthma increased? Results of two population studies conducted at nine year intervals in Busselton, Western Australia. Br Med J 1992; 305: 1326–1329.
5. The International Study of Asthma and Allergies in Childhood (ISAAC) Steering Committee. Worldwide variation in prevalence of symptoms of asthma, allergic rhinoconjunctivitis, and atopic eczema: ISAAC. Lancet 1998; 351: 1225–1232.
6. Burney P. Asthma mortality: England and Wales. J Allergy Clin Immunol 1987; 80(3): 379–382.
7. Burney P. Asthma mortality in England and Wales: evidence for a further increase, 1974–84. Lancet 1986(August 9): 323–326.
8. Sly R. Decreases in asthma mortality in the United States. Ann Allergy Asthma Immunol. 2000; 85: 121–127.
9. So S, Ng N, Ip M, Lam W. Rising asthma mortality in young males in Hong Kong, 1976–1985. Respiratory Medicine 1990; 84: 457–461.
10. Sinclair H, Allwright S, Pritchard J. Secular trends in mortality from asthma in children and young adults: Republic of Ireland, 1970–91. Irish Journal of Medical Science 1995: 45–47.
11. Holt P. Key factors in the development of asthma: Atopy. Am J Respir Crit Care Med 2000; 161: S172–S175.
12. Holgate S, Finnerty J. Recent advances in understanding the pathogenesis of asthma and its clinical implications. Q J Med 1998; 249: 5–19.
13. von Mutius E, Martinez F, Fritzsch C, Nicolai T, Roell G, Thiemann H. Prevalence of asthma and atopy in two areas of West Germany and East Germany. Am J Respir Crit Care Med 1994; 149: 358–364.
14. Kearney PM, Kearney PJ. The prevalence of asthma in schoolboys of travellers' families. Ir Med J 1998; 91: 203–206.
15. Braun-Fahrlander C, Gassner M, Grize L. Prevalence of hay fever and allergic sensitisation in farmers children and their peers living in the same rural community. Clin Exp Allergy 1999; 29: 28–34.
16. Strachan D. Hay fever, hygiene and household size. BMJ 1989; 353: 450–454.
17. Strachan D. Allergy and family size, a riddle worth solving. Clin Exp Allergy 1997; 27: 235–236.
18. Matricardi P, Roamini F, Riondino S, Fortini M, Ferrigno L, Rapicetta M et al. Exposure to foodborne and orofecal microbes versus airborne viruses in relation to atopy and allergic asthma: epidemiological study. BMJ 2000; 320: 412–417.

19. Mosmann T, Cherwinski H, Bond M, Giedlin M, Coffmann R. Two types of murine helper T cell clone. Definition according to profiles of lymphokine activities and secreted proteins. J Immunol 1986; 136(7): 2348–2357.

20. Mosmann T, Coffman R. Heterogeneity of cytokine secretion patterns and functions of helper T cells. Adv Immunol 1989; 46: 111–147.

21. Mosmann T, Coffman R. Different patterns of lymphokine secretion lead to different functional properties. Annu Rev Immunol 1989; 7: 145–173.

22. Lordan J, Holgate S. Recent developments in the pathogenesis and epidemiological trends of asthma. J R Coll Physicians Lond 1999; 33: 418–425.

23. Holt P. Immunoregulation of the allergic reaction in the respiratory tract. Eur Respir J 1996; 9 (Suppl. 22): 85s–89s.

24. Holt P. Current concepts in pulmonary immunology: regulation of primary and secondary T-cell responses to inhaled antigens. Eur Resp J 1996; 6(36): 128–135.

25. D'Amato M, Vitiani L, Petrelli G, Ferrigno L, di Pietro A, Trezza R et al. Association of persistent bronchial hyperresponsiveness with 2-adrenoceptor (ADRB2) haplotypes a population study. Am J Respir Crit Care Med 1998; 158: 1968–1973.

26. Aziz I, Hall I, McFarlane L, Lipworth BJ. Beta 2-Adrenoceptor regulation and bronchodilator sensitivity after regular treatment with formoterol in subjects with stable asthma. J Allergy Clin Immunol 1998; 101: 337–341.

27. Weir T, Mallek N, Sandford T, Bai T, Awadh N, FitzGerald JM et al. Beta 2-Adrenergic receptor haplotypes in mild, moderate and fatal/near fatal asthma. Am J Respir Crit Care Med 1998; 158: 787–791.

28. Rosenwasser L, Klemm D, Dresback J, Inamura H, Mascali J, Klinnert M et al. Promoter polymorphisms in the chromosome 5 gene cluster in asthma and atopy. Clin Exp Allergy 1995; 25: 74–78.

29. Dizier M, Sandford A, Walley A, Philippi A, Cookson W, Demenais F. Indication of linkage of serum IgE levels to the interleukin-4 gene exclusion of the contribution of the (590 C to T) interleukin-4 promoter polymorphism to IgE variation. Genet Epidemiol 1999; 16: 84–94.

30. Baldini M, Lohman C, Halonen M, Erickson R, Holt P, Martinez F. A polymorphism in the 5′ flanking region of the CD 14 gene is associated with circulating soluble CD 14 levels and with total serum immunoglobulin E. Am J Respir Cell Mol Biol 1999; 20: 976–983.

31. Shirakawa T, Dubowitz W, Dekker J, Shaw A, Faux J, Ra C et al. Association between atopy and variants of the subunit of the high-affinity immunoglobulin E receptor. Nature Genet 1994; 7: 125–129.

32. Hijazi Z, Haider M, Khan M, Al-Dowaisan A. High frequency of IgE receptor FcRI variant (Leu 181/Leu 183) in Kuwaiti Arabs and its association with asthma. Clin Genet 1998; 53: 149–152.

33. Hershey G, Friedrich M, Esswein L, Thomas M, Chatila T. The association of atopy with a gain-of-function mutation in the subunit of the interleukin-4 receptor. N Engl J Med 1997; 337: 1720–1725.

34. Corrigan C, Hartnell A, Kay A. T lymphocyte activation in acute severe asthma. Lancet 1988; 1: 1129–1132.

35. Jeffrey P, Wardlaw A, Nelson F, Collins J, Kay A. Bronchial biopsies in asthma: an ultrastructural, quantitative study and correlation with bronchial hyperreactivity. Am Rev Respir Dis 1989; 140: 1745–1753.

36. Azzawi M, Bradley B, Jeffrey P, Frew A, Wardlaw A, Knowles G et al. Identification of activated T lymphocytes and eosinophils in bronchial biopsies in stable atopic asthma. Am Rev Respir Dis 1990; 142: 1407–1413.

37. Hamid Q, Barkans J, Robinson D, Durham S, Kay A. Co-expression of CD25 and CD3 in atopic asthma and allergy. Immunology 1992; 75: 659–663.

38. Robinson D, Bentley A, Hartnell A, Kay A, Durham S. Activated memory T helper cells in bronchoalveolar lavage from patients with atopic asthma: relationship to asthma symptoms, lung function and bronchial responsiveness. Thorax 1993; 48: 26–32.

39. Cormican L, O'Sullivan S, Gunaratnam C, Burke C, Poulter L. Selective increase in the apoptosis of IFN-g+ as opposed to IL-4+ cells in the asthmatic bronchial wall. Clinical and Experimental Allergy 2001; 31: 731–739.

40. Ying S, Durham S, Corrigan C, Hamid Q, Kay A. Phenotype of cells expressing mRNA for Th2-type (interleukin 4 and interleukin 5) and TH1-type (interleukin-2 and interferon-gamma) cytokines in bronchoalveolar lavage and bronchial biopsies from atopic asthmatic and normal control subjects. Am J Respir Cell Mol Biol 1995; 12(5): 477–487.

41. Robinson D, Hamid Q, Ying S, Tsicopoulos A, Barkans J, Bentley A et al. Predominant Th2-like bronchoalveolar T-lymphocyte population in atopic asthma. N Engl J Med 1992; 326: 298–304.

42. Powrie F, Coffman R. Cytokine regulation of T cell function: potential for therapeutic intervention. Immunol Today 1993; 14: 270.

43. Corry D, Kheradmand F. Induction and regulation of the IgE response. Nature 1999; 402 (Suppl. 6760): B18–B23.

44. Maggi E, Parronchi P, Manetti R, Simonelli C, Piccinni M, Rugiu F et al. Reciprocal regulatory effects of IFN gamma and IL4 on the in-vitro development of human Th1 and Th2 clones. J Immunol 1992; 148: 2142–2147.

45. British Thoracic Society. The British guidelines on asthma management. Thorax 1997; 52 (Suppl 1): S1–S21.

46. Cheney F, Posner K, Caplan K. Adverse respiratory events frequently leading to malpractice suits. Anaesthesiology 1991; 75: 932–939.

47. Martin A, Landau L, Phelan P. Lung function in young adults who had asthma in childhood. Am Rev Respir Dis 1980; 122: 609–616.

48. Nicholson K, Kent J, Ireland D. Respiratory viruses and exacerbations of asthma in adults. B Med J 1993; 307: 982–986.

49. National Asthma Education Program. Guidelines for the diagnosis and management of asthma. Bethesda, Md. National Heart, Lung and Blood Institute, National Institutes of Health, 1991.

50. Djucanovic R, Wilson J, Britten K, Wilson S, Falls A, Roche W et al. Effect of an inhaled corticosteroid on airway inflammation and symptoms in asthma. Am Rev Respir Dis 1992; 145: 669–674.

51. Vathenen A, Knox A, Wisniewski A, Tattersfield A. Time course of change in bronchial hyperreactivity with an inhaled corticosteroid in asthma. J Immunol 1991; 143: 1317–1321.

52. Barnes PJ. Mechanism of action of glucocorticoids in asthma. Am J Respir Crit Care Med 1996; 154: S21–S27.

53. Pien L, Grammer L, Patterson R. Minimal complications in a surgical population with severe asthma receiving propholactic corticosteroids. J Allergy Clin Immunol 1988; 82: 696–700.

54. Gold M, Helrich M. A study of complications related to anaesthesia in asthmatic patients. Anestg Analg 1963; 42: 283–293.

55. Hirshman C, Edelstein R, Ebertz J, Hanifin J. Thiobarbiturate induced histamine release in human skin mast cells. Anaesthesiology 1985; 63: 353–356.

56. Pizov R, Brown R, Weiss Y. Wheezing during induction of general anaesthesia with and without asthma: a randomised blinded trial. Anaesthesiology 1995; 82: 1111–1116.

57. Conti G, De'utri D, Vilardi V, De Blasi RA, Pelaia P, Antonelli M *et al.* Propofol induces bronchodilation in mechanically ventilated chronic obstructive pulmonary disease patients. Acta Anaesthesiol Scand 1993; 37: 105–109.

58. Hirshman C, Downes H, Farbood A, Bergman N. Ketamine block of bronchospasm in experimental canine asthma. Br J Anaesth 1979; 51: 713–718.

59. Nedergaard O. Cocaine like effect of ketamine on vascular adrenergic neurons. Eur J Pharmacol 1973; 23: 153–161.

60. Urdinovic S, Karoussos K. Experience with etomidate: a hypnotic for induction of anaesthesia. J Int Med Res 1978; 6: 452–454.

61. Fryer A, Maclagan J. Pancuronium and gallamine are antagonists for pre and post junctional muscarinic receptors in the guinea pig lung. Naunyn Schmiedebergs Arch Pharmacol 1987; 335: 367–371.

62. Oklanami O, Fryer A, Hirshman C. Pancuronium and pipecuronium are antagonists for M2 and M3 muscarinic receptors in guinea pig heart and lung. Crit Care Med 1993; 21: S221.

63. Lloyd T. Reflex effects of lung inflation and inhalation of halothane, ether and ammonia. J Appl Physiol 1978; 45: 212–218.

64. Mehr E, Hirshman C, Lindeman K. Mechanism of action of atracurium on airways. Anaesthesiology 192; 76: 448–454.

65. Roscow C, Moss J, Philbin D. Histamine release during morphine and fentanyl anaesthesia. Anaesthesiology 1982; 56: 93–96.

66. Rossing T, Fanta C, Goldstein D, Snapper J, Mc Fadden Jr E. Emergency therapy of asthma: comparison of the acute effects of parenteral and inhaled sympathomimetics and infused aminophylline. Am Rev Respir Dis 1980; 122: 365–371.

67. Ward M, MacFarlane J, Davies D. Treatment of acute asthma with intravenous aminophulline and nebulised ipratropium after salbutamol. Thorax 1982; 37: 785.

68. Aubier M, DeTroyer A, Sampson M, Macklem P, Roussos C. Aminophylline improves diaphragmatic contractility. N Engl J Med 1981; 305: 249–252.

69. Pauwells R. New aspects of the therapeutic potential of theophylline in asthma. J Allergy Clin Immunol 1989; 83: 548–553.

70. Mitenko P, Ogilvie R. Rational intravenous doses of theophylline. N Engl J Med 1973; 289: 600.

71. Putney J, Bird G. The signal for capacitative calcium entry. Cell 1993; 75: 199–201.

72. Rowe B, Bretzlaff J, Bourdon C, Bota G, Camargo CJ. Magnesium sulphate for treating exacerbations of acute asthma in the emergency department. Cochrane Database Syst Rev 2000; 2: CD001490.

73. Nannini LJ, Pendino J, Corna R, Mannarino S, Quispe R. Magnesium sulphate as a vehicle for nebulised salbutamol in acute asthma. Am J Med 2000; 108: 193–197.

74. Manthous C, Hall J, Caputo M, Walter J, Klocksieben J, Schmidt G *et al.* Heliox improves pulsus paradoxus and peak expiratory flow in nonintubated patients with severe asthma. Am J Resp Crit Care Med 1995; 151: 310–314.

75. Fisher M. Ketamine hydrochloride in severe bronchospasm. Anaesthesia 1977; 32: 771–772.

76. Ullman A, Svedmyr N. Salmeterol, a new long acting inhaled beta 2 adrenoceptor agonist: comparison with salbutamol in adult asthmatic patients. Thorax 1988; 43: 674–678.

77. Lofdahl CG, Svedmyr N. Formoterol fumarate, a new beta 2-adrenoceptor agonist: acute studies of selectivity and duration of effect after inhaled and oral administration. Allergy 1989; 44: 264–271.

78. Haahtela T, Jarvinen M, Kava T, Kiviranta K, Koskinen S, Lehtonen K. Comparison of a beta 2-agonist, terbutaline, with an inhaled corticosteroid, budesonide, in newly detected asthma. N Engl J Med 1991; 325: 388–392.

79. van-Essen-Zandvliet E, Hughes M, Waalkens H, Duiverman E, Pocock S, Kerrebijn K. Effects of 22 months of treatment with inhaled corticosteroids and/or beta-2-agonists on lung function, airway responsiveness, and symptoms in children with asthma. The Dutch Chronic Non-specific Lung Disease Study Group. Am Rev Respir Dis 1992; 146: 547–554.

80. Project IAM. International Consensus Report on Diagnosis and Management of Asthma. Allergy 1992; 47: 1–61.

81. Greening A, Ind P, Northfield M, Shaw G. Added salmeterol versus higher-dose corticosteroid in asthma patients with symptoms on existing inhaled corticosteroid. Lancet 1994; 344: 219–224.

82. Woolcock A, Lundback B, Ringdal N, Jacques L. Comparison of addition of salmeterol to inhaled steroids with doubling of the dose of inhaled steroids. Am J Respir Crit Care Med 1996; 153: 1481–1488.

83. Busse W, Nelson H, Wolfe J, Kalberg C, Yancey S, Rickard K. Comparison of inhaled salmeterol and oral zafirlukast in patients with asthma. J Allergy Clin Immunol 1999; 103: 1075–1080.

84. Davies B, Brooks G, Devoy M. The efficacy and safety of salmeterol compared to theophylline: meta-analysis of nine controlled studies. Respir Med 1998; 92: 256–263.

85. Zetterstrom O, Buhl R, Mellem H, Perpina M, Hedman J, O'Neill S. Improved asthma control with budesonide/formoterol in a single inhaler, compared with budesonide alone. Eur Respir J 2001; 18: 262–268.

86. Radmark O. The molecular biology and regulation of 5-lipoxygenase. Am J Respir Crit Care Med 2000; 161: S11–S15.

87. Adelroth E, Morris M, Hargreave F, O'Byrne P. Airway responsiveness to leukotrienes C4 and D4 and to methacholine in patients with asthma and normal controls. N Eng J Med 1986; 315: 480–484.

88. Drazen J, Israel E, O'Byrne P. Treatment of asthma with drugs modifying the leukotriene pathway. N Engl J Med 1999; 240: 197–206.

89. Manning P, Rokach J, Malo J, Ethier D, Cartier A, Girard Y et al. Urinary leukotriene E4 levels during early and late asthmatic responses. J Allergy Clin Immunol 1990; 86: 211–220.

90. Kikawa Y, Miyanomae T, Inoue Y, Saito M, Nakai A, Shigematsu Y et al. Urinary leukotriene E4 after exercise challenge in children with asthma. J Allergy Clin Immunol 1992; 89: 1111–1119.

91. Leff JA, Busse W, Pearlman D, Bronsky E, Kemp J, Hendeles L et al. Montelukast, a leukotriene-receptor antagonist, for the treatment of mild asthma and exercise-induced bronchoconstriction. N Engl J Med 1998; 339: 147–152.

92. Murray J, Nadel J. Respiratory Medicine, 2nd ed. Philadelphia: W.B. Saunders Company, 1994.

93. Liu M, Dube L, Lancaster J. Acute and chronic effects of a 5-lipoxygenase inhibitor in asthma: a six month randomised multicentre trial. J Allergy Clin Immunol 1996; 98: 859–871.

94. Hui K, Barnes N. Lung function improvement in asthma with a cysteinyl leukotriene receptor antagonist. Lancet 1991; 337: 1062–1063.

95. Barnes PJ. Inhaled glucocorticoids for asthma. N Engl J Med 1995; 332: 868–875.

96. Faul J, Leonard C, Burke C, Tormey V, Poulter L. Fluticasone propionate induced alterations to lung function and immunopathology of asthma over time. Thorax 1998; 53: 753–761.

97. Burke C, Power C, Norris A, Poulter L. Lung function and immunopathological changes after inhaled corticosteroid therapy in asthma. Eur Respir J 1992; 5: 73–79.

98. Bel E, Timmers M, Hermans J, Dijkman J, Sterk P. The long term effects of nedocromil sodium and beclomethasone dipropionate on bronchial responsiveness to methacholine in non-asthmatic subjects. Am Rev Respir Dis 1990; 141: 21–28.

99. Wilson JW, Djukanovic R, Howarth PH, Holgate ST. Inhaled beclomethasone dipropionate downregulates airway lymphocyte activation in atopic asthma. Am J Respir Crit Care Med 1994; 149: 86–90.

100. Flower R, Rothwell N. Lipocortin-1: cellular mechanisms and clinical relevance. Trends Pharmacol Sci 1994; 15: 71–76.

101. Auphan N, DiDonato J, Rosette C, Helmberg A, Karin M. Immunosuppression by glucocorticoids: inhibition of NF-κβ activity through induction of IκB synthesis. Science 1995; 270: 283–286.

102. Sont J, van Krieken J, Evertse C, Hooijer R, Willems L, Sterk P. Relationship between the inflammatory infiltrate in bronchial biopsy specimens and clinical severity of asthma in patients treated with inhaled steroids. Thorax 1996; 51: 496–502.

103. Trigg C, Monolitsas N, Wang J, Calderon M, McAuley A, Jordan S et al. Placebo controlled immunopathologic study of four months of inhaled corticosteroids in asthma. Am J Respir Crit Care Med 1994; 150: 17–22.

104. Corrigan C, Haczku A, Gemou-Engesaeth V, Doi S, Kikuchi Y, Takatsu K et al. CD4 T-lymphocyte activation in asthma is accompanied by increased serum concentrations of Interleukin-5. Effect of glucocorticoid therapy. Am Rev Respir Dis 1993; 147(3): 540–547.

105. Adelroth E, Rosenhall L, Johansson S, Linden M, Venge P. Inflammatory cells and eosinophilic activity in asthmatics investigated by bronchoalveolar lavage. Am Rev Respir Dis 1990; 142: 91–99.

106. Duddridge M, Ward C, Hendrick DJ, Walters EH. Changes in bronchoalveolar lavage inflammatory cells in asthmatic patients treated with high dose inhaled beclomethasone dipropionate. Eur Respir J 1993; 6: 489–497.

107. Laitinen LA, Laitinen A, Haahtela T. A comparative study of the effects of an inhaled corticosteroid, budesonide, and a 2-agonist, terbutaline, on airway inflammation in newly diagnosed asthma: a randomized, double-blind, parallel-group controlled trial. J Allergy Clin Immunol 1992; 90: 32–42.

108. Claman DM, Boushey HA, Liu J, Wong H, Fahy JV. Analysis of induced sputum to examine the effects of prednisone on airway inflammation in asthmatic subjects. J Allergy Clin Immunol 1994; 94: 861–869.

109. Keatings VM, Jatakanon A, Worsdell YM, Barnes PJ. Effects of inhaled and oral glucocorticoids on inflammatory indices in asthma and COPD. Am J Respir Crit Care Med 1997; 155: 542–548.

110. Woolley K, Gibson P, Carty K, Wilson A, Twaddell S, Woolley M. Eosinophil apoptosis and the resolution of airway inflammation in asthma. Am J Respir Crit Care Med 1996; 154: 237–243.

111. Gibson PG, Wong BJ, Hepperle MJ, Kline PA, Girgis-Gabardo A, Guyatt G, Dolovich J, Denburg JA, Ramsdale EH, Hargreave FE. A research method to induce and examine a mild exacerbation of asthma by withdrawal of inhaled corticosteroid. Clin Exp Allergy 1992; 22: 525–532.

112. Kraan J, Koeter G, van der Mark T *et al*. Dosage and time effects of inhaled budesonide on bronchial hyperreactivity. Am Rev Respir Dis 1988; 137: 44–48.
113. Wolfe J, Selner J, Mendelson L. Effectiveness of fluticasone propionate in patients with moderate asthma: a dose-ranging study. Clin Ther 1996; 18: 635–646.
114. Juniper E, Kline P, Vanzielegher H, Ramsdale E *et al*. Effect of longterm treatment with a inhaled corticosteroid (budesonide) on airway hyperresponsiveness and clinical asthma in nonsteroid-dependant asthmatics. 1990; 140: 832–836.
115. Brown J, Greville W, Finucane K. Asthma and irreversible airflow obstruction. Thorax 1984; 39: 131–136.
116. Bhagat R, Grunstein M. Effect of corticosteroids on bronchial responsiveness to methacholine in asthmatic children. Am Rev Respir Dis 1985; 131: 902–906.
117. Barnes P. Anti-IgE antibody therapy for asthma. N Engl J Med 1999; 341: 2006–2008.
118. Milgrom H, Fick R, Su J, Reimann J, Bush R, Waltrous M *et al*. Treatment of allergic asthma with monoclonal anti-IgE antibody. N Engl J Med 1999; 341: 1966–1971.
119. Busse W, Lemanske R. Advances in immunology: asthma. N Engl J Med 2001; 344: 350–362.

*R.M. Grounds*

# Reducing mortality and complications in patients undergoing surgery at high risk for postoperative complications and death

Over the last quarter to half century there has been reasonable evidence to suggest that the incidence of death following surgery, which can be directly attributable to anaesthesia, has fallen. Yet on the other hand the overall incidence of death following surgery has remained almost unchanged. In 1954 and 1956 three studies by, Beecher and Todd,[1] Edwards *et al.*,[2] and Dornette and Orth,[3] all suggested that the postoperative mortality solely associated with anaesthesia was approximately 1:2,500 and that anaesthesia was a factor contributory to postoperative death in approximately 1:1,500 cases. By 1987, the contribution of anaesthesia to postoperative death had declined significantly. Buck and Devlin[4] showed that incidence of death solely attributable to the anaesthesia had declined from 1:2,500 to 1:185,000. However, they also showed that anaesthesia was still a contributory factor in approximately 1:1,500 cases. So 30 years had shown a marked decline in the incidence of postoperative death as a direct consequence of the anaesthesia but little or no change in the contribution to the incidence of postoperative death associated with the anaesthetist. Clearly, however, the risk of death in the perioperative period will depend not only on the skills of the surgeon, anaesthetists and their teams but also upon the operation that the patient requires and the preoperative physiological status of the patient. One simple method for assessing the physiological status of the patient prior to surgery

**Table 1** ASA status and mortality rate

| ASA status | Number of cases | Mortality rate (%) |
|------------|-----------------|--------------------|
| I          | 18,320          | 0.06               |
| II         | 10,609          | 0.40               |
| III        | 3,820           | 4.30               |
| IV         | 1,073           | 23.40              |
| V          | 323             | 50.70              |

Modified from Marx, Mateo, and Orkin, 1973.[6]

is the American Society of Anesthesiologists (ASA) classification, a simple but robust classification introduced in 1941 by the ASA (table 1).[5,6] This simple classification has been shown to reflect the increasing surgical and anaesthetic mortality associated with increasing preoperative physiological dysfunction.

For the general surgical population the risk of death within 30 days of an operation is less than 1% and even more complex surgery such as cardiac surgery has an elective surgery mortality of between 2 and 4%. However, when patients with poor preoperative physiology undergo major surgery then the mortality is considerably higher. In a 1 year analysis of all colo-rectal cancer patients undergoing surgical treatment in the Trent Region of the UK, Mella et al.,[7] showed that of 3,520 patients studied, 91.5% under-went surgery and 17% had emergency/urgent surgery. The overall 30-day post surgery mortality was 7.6% but for the emergency surgery group of patients the 30-day mortality was 21%. Furthermore, they were able to categorise their patients into their preoperative ASA groups and show that although the 30-day mortality was 4% for both elective or emergency surgery for ASA I patients the mortality for ASA IV patients was 22% for elective patients and greater than 55% for emergency operations. A number of other sources confirm this high mortality in patients undergoing major surgery who have poor physiological reserve prior to surgery.

In England, Wales and Northern Ireland, there are approximately 2.8 million surgical operations performed every year and in the region of 20,000 deaths within 30 days of operation are reported annually to the National Confidential Enquiry into Post Operative Deaths (NCEPOD). Of these deaths 87% are in patients over 60 years of age and over 75% are in patients over 70 years old. 85% of patients have co-existing medical disorders with 45% having limited cardiovascular reserve and significant cardiovascular disease and 30% having significant reduction in respiratory reserve.[8] Despite this only 32% of these patients are currently admitted to an intensive care unit (ICU) or high dependency unit (HDU).

**Table 2** Summary of mortality data from UK ICU databases

|  | Total number of surgical patients in database | Total surgical mortality (%) | Elective mortality (%) | Emergency mortality (%) |
|---|---|---|---|---|
| SW Thames[a] | 8,718 | 19.3 | 11.5 | 30.2 |
| RIP[b] | 11,960 | 19.9 | 8.4 | 31.5 |
| ICNARC[c] | 26,228 | 24.4 | 10.7 | 36.8 |
| Scottish ICS[d] | 13,711 | 16.6 | 8.7 | 25.0 |

Data from following sources.
[a]South West Thames (Ward watcher) ICU database for 17 ICU with 31,138 admissions from July 1995 to June 1999.
[b]RIP (Riyadh Intensive Care Program) database with 26,000 patients from 1990 to 1999.
[c]Intensive Care National Audit and Research Centre (ICNARC) Case Mix Database of 91 ICU's with 46,587 admissions from December 1995 to March 1999.
[d]Scottish Intensive Care Society (ICS) Audit Group Database of 23 ICU's with 28,097 admissions from January 1995 to December 1998.

This high mortality among a select group of surgical patients was first noted by Shoemaker et al.[9] They noted that there was a difference in the cardio-respiratory responses seen between survivors and non-survivors following major surgery. A year later they defined the physiological endpoints for survival in patients undergoing major surgery.[10] They pointed out that survivors and non-survivors differed in their postoperative cardiovascular responses. Shoemaker et al. showed that patients at high risk could be identified in advance of surgery.[9-11] They examined over 30 physiological variables in several thousand patients and showed that only those variables, which related to blood volume and flow, had significant prognostic value for the patient in terms of mortality and morbidity. They found that the most commonly measured variables in this group of patients (blood pressure, pulse rate, temperature, central venous pressure (CVP) and urine output) conferred little prognostic value for the patient's outcome. The less commonly measured variables relating blood flow, oxygen delivery and oxygen consumption were highly prognostic of postoperative outcome. They were able to demonstrate that the three most prognostic variables of survivors in their data set were, cardiac index, oxygen delivery and oxygen consumption and the median values of survivors were:

| Cardiac index | $4.5\,l^{-1}\,min^{-1}\,m^2$ (body surface area) |
|---|---|
| Tissue oxygen delivery | $600\,ml^{-1}\,min^{-1}\,m^2$ (body surface area) |
| Tissue oxygen consumption | $170\,ml^{-1}\,min^{-1}\,m^2$ (body surface area) |

This concept of limited cardiovascular reserve leading to a poor post-operative outcome had been proposed earlier, Clowes and Del Gurcio[12] in a report on the outcome of thoracic surgery indicating that immediately following surgery 84% of their patients increased their cardiac output. These patients all survived. Whereas, 16% of their patients had not increased their cardiac output in response to major surgery and did not survive. Furthermore, a number of studies have demonstrated that poor cardio-respiratory reserve will lead to a poor postoperative outcome. A history of myocardial infarction or cardiac failure significantly increases perioperative mortality. The risk of perioperative mortality has been studied by Goldman et al.,[13] who published a predictive index of cardiac mortality for patients undergoing non-cardiac surgery. This indicated that patients with a previous history of cardiovascular disease, and in particular previous myocardial infarction, cardiac failure and stroke, were at particularly high risk of perioperative complications and death. Their findings have been confirmed particularly by Mangano et al.[14] These authors followed 474 patients with proven (or at high risk for) coronary artery disease for 2 days prior to their non-cardiac elective surgery until 2 years after their surgery. They found that 18% of these patients had severe postoperative cardiac events including death, myocardial infarction, unstable angina and ventricular tachycardia. Furthermore, 41% of their patients were demonstrated to have perioperative myocardial ischaemia. They postulated that of the 25 million non-cardiac surgery operations performed in the USA annually, 7–8 million of these patients were at risk of perioperative cardiac death and complications.

The suggestion, therefore, from these studies is that there is a group of patients who are at high risk from perioperative complications and death when undergoing major surgery. Intuitively many clinicians would accept that patients with preoperative cardiac disease would probably be at high risk. However, this may hide the extent of the problem. Reports from NCEPOD suggest that the median day of death is not the day of the operation but 6 days postoperatively. Many of these high-risk patients do not die a swift complete death but die from the insidious onset of Multiple Organ Dysfunction Syndrome (MODS)[15] which commences at the time of surgery and gradually causes death over the next 1–4 weeks. A number of factors acting either independently or in combination trigger the onset of MODS.[16] Recent studies suggesting that there is alteration in micro vascular blood flow associated with surgery and injury[17] and the concept of cell death due to inadequate oxygen supply to the tissues at the time of surgery, leading directly to cell hypoxia and tissue damage and eventually death is persuasive.[18]

## Preoperative Selection of the 'High-Risk' Patient

Preoperative identification of high-risk patients will be required to select patients who, by virtue of their preoperative physiological status, are at high risk of perioperative morbidity and mortality. However, this preoperative risk assessment must also take into consideration the type and nature of the surgery to be undertaken. Certain branches of surgery, such as cardiac surgery and thoracic surgery, perceived by the general public and much of the medical profession, as being high risk do in fact have relatively low perioperative mortality. The mortality rate, for example, associated with elective cardiac surgery is between 2 and 4%. Compare this with the mortality of approximately 10% for vascular surgery and over 50%[7] for colo-rectal surgery in an ASA IV patient who requires emergency surgery. Shoemaker et al.,[9–11,19] indicated in a series of studies that they could identify in advance of surgery those patients who were likely to be unable to mount an appropriate physiological response to the proposed surgery and who were thus likely to have postoperative death or complications. They believe that in the patients they have identified as being at high risk the patients will have a 30–40% post surgical 28-day mortality rate.

Other groups have suggested different techniques for identifying the 'at risk' patient. Goldman et al.,[13] identified that the presence of cardiac ischaemia with or without heart (pump) failure was highly predictive of perioperative complications and death. Mangano et al.,[14] have shown that myocardial ischaemia during the first 48 h after surgery confers a three-fold increase in postoperative complications. Recent recommendations for the perioperative investigation of the cardiac patient about to undergo non-cardiac surgery have been published by the American College of Cardiology and American Heart Association.[20] Other methods of assessing cardiac performance prior to surgery have been suggested including dipyridamole ECHO stress testing,[21] or dobutamine stress testing.[22–25] Older et al.,[26] have suggested a system of preoperative cardio-pulmonary exercise testing for identifying these high-risk patients. They have shown that patients with a low anaerobic threshold have a mortality of 18% for their subsequent surgery whereas those patients with a high anaerobic threshold had a mortality of only 0.8%.

Other risk factors must also be considered. Different types of surgery carry different risks of perioperative mortality and morbidity. Interestingly, cardiac surgery, which is perceived as a high-risk surgical speciality, actually has a very low postoperative death rate of only 2–4%. Major vascular surgery carries a postoperative mortality rate of between 7 and 15% for elective surgery and this rises to between 30 and 50% for emergency surgery. Similarly, major colo-rectal surgery carries a risk of death of 8% and a complication rate of 35% but this postoperative death rate is increased to 20–30% if the surgery is performed as an emergency.[7] This increase in mortality associated with emergency surgery is confirmed by other studies. In a study of the outcome of patients over 65 undergoing surgery, Edwards et al.,[27] showed that non-elective admissions had a 30% mortality rate whereas elective admissions had only a 5% mortality rate. They also demonstrated a major difference between ASA status and outcome from surgery, with patients in ASA groups III or IV having a significantly worse outcome. Furthermore, these outcome results for surgery are also complicated by the socio-economic status of the patient and the experience of the surgeon.[28] Some studies relate outcome to the patient's preoperative physiology or pre-existing medical condition. A study by Fowkes et al.,[29] revealed that in 108,878 patient operations between 1972 and 1977 the overall mortality rate was 2.2% but that this rose considerably to 7% for patients with co-existing disease and to nearly 16% for patients with ischaemic heart disease or heart failure. Again as in other studies the mortality rate was increased considerably if the operation was undertaken as an emergency.

Therefore it is possible to identify a group of patients who are at 'High Risk' of postoperative death and complications. This group of patients can be identified without difficulty, prior to surgery by their poor preoperative physiological condition, their age, the type of surgery that is to be undertaken and the seniority and experience of the surgeon who is to perform the surgery. The preoperative high-risk physiological conditions can be identified from the table suggested by Shoemaker (table 3). The highest risks seem

---

**Table 3** Shoemaker et al.,[19] criteria for preoperative identification of patient at high risk of postoperative death and complications following major surgery

- Current or previous severe, cardio-respiratory illness (myocardial infarction, stroke, heart failure, chronic obstructive airways disease, emphysema, severe asthma)
- Acute abdominal catastrophe with haemodynamic instability (pancreatitis, perforated bowel with peritoneal soiling, severe gastrointestinal bleeding)
- Acute renal failure (acute onset renal dysfunction with blood urea >18 mmol$^{-1}$ or blood creatinine >265 mmol$^{-1}$)
- Severe multiple trauma (more than three major organs involved or more than two systems or surgical opening of more than two body cavities)
- Evidence of limited physiological reserve in one or more of the vital organs in elderly patients over 70 years of age
- Shock (mean arterial pressure [MAP] <60 mm Hg, and urine output <0.5 ml kg$^{-1}$ h$^{-1}$)
- Acute respiratory failure (PaO$_2$ < 60 mm Hg with FiO$_2$ >0.4 shunt fraction >30% mechanical ventilation required for more than 48 h)
- Septicaemia, positive blood culture or septic focus with associated haemodynamic instability requiring inotropic support

Shoemaker et al., also suggested another group of patients who would be at high risk. These were those patients who were scheduled to have extensive ablative surgery for carcinoma (oesophagectomy or total gastrectomy). This risk factor seems to have been misinterpreted by some investigators and as a consequence some young patients who clearly have normal physiological reserve have been submitted to unnecessary perioperative invasive intervention.
It is also possible that the risk factors defined by Shoemaker et al. do not all have the same prognostic value or weighting.

**Table 4** Identification of type of surgery and the patients at 'High Risk' from post operative death and complications

- Patients with poor physiological status prior to operation. See list table 3 above. In particular,
  - Elderly patients with poor physiological reserve.
  - Preoperative evidence of heart failure or poor cardiac performance.
- Colo-rectal, vascular, intra-abdominal surgery, trauma surgery involving more than two body cavities or where there is intraperitoneal soiling by bowel contents.
- Patients undergoing prolonged surgery (longer than 1½ h).
- Emergency surgery.
- Inexperienced surgeon or surgeon not regularly specialising in the type of surgery being performed.
- Lack of postoperative intensive care or high dependency facilities.

to be associated with poor preoperative cardiovascular performance and in particular the presence of heart failure at the time of surgery or in the period immediately prior to surgery. The high-risk surgical operations are particularly associated with colo-rectal surgery, abdominal surgery, vascular surgery and trauma surgery (particularly where there is intraperitoneal soiling by bowel contents) (table 4). The risk from surgery is greatly increased if the operation is performed as an emergency or by a surgeon who is not a specialist in that particular type of surgery.[30]

There will be some groups of patients who are clearly at high risk because of other less common causes and they will also benefit from being treated and cared for in the same facilities as these patients. There is some evidence[4,8,31–34] to suggest that as many as 5–7% of all surgical patients fall into this high-risk category and that they have a postoperative mortality of between 20 and 35% and that they represent over 85% of all reported postoperative deaths.

## Perioperative Strategies for Reducing Postoperative Death and Complications

From the early studies[9,12,34] it is apparent that the appropriate reaction to major surgery is to increase cardiac output in response to increased metabolic demand and thus increase tissue oxygen delivery to accommodate a rising tissue oxygen consumption. In 1972, Shoemaker et al.,[9] showed that in major surgery, the median values of the measured physiological parameters of survivors is a cardiac index of $>4.5\,l^{-1}\,min^{-1}\,m^2$ (body surface area), and oxygen delivery of $>600\,ml^{-1}\,min^{-1}\,m^2$ (body surface area) and an oxygen consumption $>170\,ml^{-1}\,min^{-1}\,m^2$ (body surface area). Since then they and a number of other groups[19,35–47] have undertaken studies of early goal directed therapy with a view to improving cardiovascular performance so as to ensure that all patients achieve the same tissue oxygen delivery as those survivors in the earlier observational studies (table 5).

Whilst Shoemaker et al.,[9] suggested that there were three physiological variables (cardiac index, oxygen delivery and oxygen consumption), which were the most predictive determinants of outcome, most groups have taken the more pragmatic view that only two of these were amenable to intervention prior to or during surgery and the perioperative phase, namely increasing cardiac output and increasing oxygen delivery. Using a combination technique of identification of the 'at risk' patient prior to surgery, and then adopting a technique of early goal directed therapy using intravenous fluid and inotropes prior to surgery and in the immediate postoperative period, Shoemaker et al.,[19] demonstrated a reduction in surgical mortality from 33 to 4%. They also demonstrated a reduction in the numbers of postoperative complications (table 6).

**Table 5** Mortality outcome following goal directed studies

| Study | Type of surgery | Mortality control (%) | Mortality treatment (%) |
|---|---|---|---|
| Shultz et al.[36] | Vascular | 29.0 | 2.9 |
| Shoemaker et al.[19] | General | 33.0 | 4.0 |
| Berlauk et al.[43] | Vascular | 9.5 | 1.5 |
| Fleming et al.[38] | Trauma | 44.0 | 24.0 |
| Boyd et al.[44] | General and vascular | 22.2 | 5.7 |
| Bishop et al.[40] | Trauma | 37.0 | 18.0 |
| Sinclair et al.[45] | Hip fracture | 10.0 | 5.0 |
| Zeigler et al.[46] | Peripheral vascular | 9.0 | 5.0 |
| Wilson et al.[41] | Elective general | 17.0 | 3.0 |
| Polonen et al.[47] | Elective cardiac | 3.0 | 1.0 |
| Lobo et al.[42] | General and vascular | 50.0 | 15.7 |

**Table 6** Summary of incidence of postoperative complications (mean number of complications per patient) in studies of goal directed therapy for patients at high risk of post surgical complications

| | Control | Protocol |
|---|---|---|
| Shoemaker 1988[19] | 1.03 CVP 1.3 PA | 0.39 |
| Fleming 1992[32] | 1.79 | 0.79 |
| Boyd 1993[39] | 1.4 | 0.68 |
| Bishop 1995[40] | 1.62 | 0.74 |
| Wilson 1999[41] | 0.6 | 0.52 adrenaline 0.30 dopexamine |
| Lobo 2000[42] | 1.5 | 0.57 |

There have been a number of different methods for enhancing cardio-vascular performance during the perioperative phase. In principle they adopt the technique of maximising intravenous fluid therapy by the use of cardiac flow measuring devices (pulmonary artery catheters or oesophageal Doppler measurements) and then the judicious addition of an inotrope or vasodilator if the goals have not been achieved with this intravenous fluid. One such protocol is outlined in table 7. Most studies have used dobutamine as the inotrope for this cardiovascular improvement but more recently a number of studies[39,41] have suggested that dopexamine may be a more useful agent. One work[42] compared two different inotropic agents (adrenaline and dopexamine) for the protocol group. Although similar results were found between the two agents in terms of mortality, nevertheless the use of dopexamine was associated with fewer postoperative complications in the survivors. It would appear that the choice of flow measurement technique is not critical and new methods of achieving this should be as efficacious. Although some authors have cast doubt on the efficacy of the use of pulmonary artery catheters[48] there is no doubt that the selective use of pulmonary artery catheters for goal directed therapy in this highly selected group of patients has been shown to be consistently effective. Furthermore, it is clear from some of these studies that not all patients will be able to achieve the goals that have been set. In these patients, it is still worth attempting to achieve the optimisation goals since a number of studies[39,41] have shown that merely improving oxygen delivery to that individual patient's maximum will reduce the postoperative mortality and complication rate. These studies have shown that even with patients who failed to achieve the oxygen delivery goal of $>600\,ml^{-1}\,min^{-1}\,m^2$ (body surface area) these patients still attained a better outcome than if their oxygen delivery had not been enhanced from their preoperative baseline.

It is also apparent that oxygen delivery will be improved if the patients' haemoglobin concentration is increased (oxygen delivery depends on cardiac output, haemoglobin concentration, oxygen carrying capacity of that haemo-globin and the oxygen saturation of the blood) but this must not be increased at the expense of a reduction of flow in the tissues due to the increased viscosity of the blood. A compromise haemoglobin concentration that most investigators seem to have adopted has been a target of haemoglobin concen-tration of $10\,g\,dl^{-1}$, although this issue has never been formally studied. It is important during the goals directed therapy that monitoring of the haemo-globin concentration is performed as a significant increase in intravascular fluid volume achieved by the titration of extra crystalloid or colloid solutions may lead to an increase in cardiac output without a similar increase in oxygen delivery due to a dilutional effect that reduces the haemoglobin concentration.

**Table 7** Simplified protocol for performing goal directed cardio-respiratory optimisation for patients undergoing major surgery who are at high risk for postoperative death or complications

*Identify the operation*
- Operations likely to last longer than 1½ h.
- Especially emergency surgery but also colo-rectal surgery, vascular surgery, abdominal surgery, trauma surgery (particularly surgery involving two or more body cavities or faecal soiling of the peritoneal cavity).
- Surgeons who are not experienced at this particular type of surgery (this is more likely in the emergency surgery situations).
- Lack of postoperative critical care facilities.

*Identify the high-risk patient*
- See table 3 above (Shoemaker criteria).
- Particularly identify elderly patients with poor cardio-respiratory reserve, ischaemic heart disease or evidence of current or previous heart failure.

*Perioperative goal directed therapy*
- Assess patients preoperatively: perform cardiovascular measurements to assess cardiac performance. Perform cardiac output and oxygen delivery measurements.
- If cardiac index >4.5 $l^{-1}$ $min^{-1}$ $m^2$ (body surface area) and oxygen delivery >600 ml $^{-1}$ $min^{-1}$ $m^2$ (body surface area). Then no further goal directed therapy will be indicated. Patient can proceed to operation with normal anaesthesia and resuscitation therapy.
- If cardiac index <4.5 $l^{-1}$ $min^{-1}$ $m^2$ (body surface area) and/or oxygen delivery <600 ml $^{-1}$ $min^{-1}$ $m^2$ (body surface area). Then further goal directed therapy is indicated prior to surgery. (If this cannot be performed or has not been performed prior to surgery, then a number of studies have shown that similar results can be obtained if this goal directed therapy is applied immediately on arrival in the ICU at the end of surgery. If goal directed therapy is delayed or not achieved within 1 h after surgery then technique will confer no benefit to the patient's outcome).
- If oxygen delivery <600 ml $^{-1}$ $min^{-1}$ $m^2$ (body surface area).
  - Increase intravenous fluid therapy using flow directed monitoring equipment to improve intravascular filling to pulmonary artery occlusion pressure of 12–16 mm Hg. (or equivalent if using other forms of monitoring not pulmonary artery catheter).
  - Maintain haemoglobin concentration 10 g $dl^{-1}$ by transfusion if necessary.
  - Maintain blood oxygen saturation 95% or greater by use of supplementary oxygen therapy where appropriate.
- If despite these measures oxygen delivery is still <600 ml $^{-1}$ $min^{-1}$ $m^2$ (body surface area).
  - Consider the use of inotrope or inodilator therapy. Although a number of different agents have been used in these studies, the use of dopexamine hydrochloride seems to have achieved the best results.
  - Start dopexamine at 0.5 $\mu$g $kg^{-1}$ $min^{-1}$ and increase incrementally every 15 min by a further 0.5 $\mu$g $kg^{-1}$ $min^{-1}$ until either a target oxygen delivery is achieved or there is an increase in heart rate of 20% over the patients resting rate. (If the patient is very tachycardic prior to starting this goal directed therapy then it is important to recognise this and not to attempt to increase cardiac output at the expense of increasing this already raised heart rate. If the patients' heart rate increases to more than 20% above baseline then the infusion rate of the inotrope should be reduced to the previous dose where the heart rate had not achieved this 20% increase and held at that rate).
  - Maintain intravascular filling pressures (PAOP 12–16 mm Hg), haemoglobin concentration (10 g $dl^{-1}$) and arterial oxygen saturation (>95%) at the figures given above during this period of vasoactive therapy.
- Maintain this goal directed therapy in the immediate postoperative period until there is evidence that the intraoperative oxygen debt has been repaid.
  - Maintain therapy until Base deficit returns to normal (less than your units maximum normal range). Blood lactate concentration (within normal range for your unit/lab). Mixed venous oxygen saturation is above 70%.

A number of other studies have considered the prophylactic use of nitrates, calcium channel blockers or β-blockers for patients who are at risk of perioperative myocardial ischaemia. With the exception of β-blockade there has been no demonstrable improvement in postoperative outcome. Mangano *et al.*,[49] established an improvement in outcome in patients undergoing vascular surgery when they used atenolol prophylactically. They demonstrated that there were no deaths in the 6 months following surgery in those patients who were electively started on prophylactic atenolol compared with their control group who had an 8% mortality over the same period. This study has recently been repeated by Poldermans *et al.*,[50] using the β-blocking agent bisoprolol. They also demonstrated a mortality of 17% in patients who did not receive prophylactic β-blockade against a mortality of only 3.4% in those patients who did. In this study the authors[50] screened 846 patients who seem to have fulfilled the Shoemaker criteria as being 'High Risk' and then dobutamine stress echocardiography tested them and selected those with evidence of myocardial ischaemia for study. This would suggest that approximately 20% of patients being recruited to the major 'optimisation studies' might actually have benefited from β-blockade therapy rather than cardio-respiratory enhancement therapy. At present the total number of patients who have been enrolled in studies involving β-blockade is only 312 patients. Despite the small numbers studied it has been recommended that all patients about to undergo vascular surgery at 'High Risk' should receive prophylactic β-blockade. This may be an over generalisation but some system of preoperative assessment must be developed to determine which patients receive either of the two treatments, as it is possible that the 80% in the Poldermans study who did not receive β-blockade may have benefited from cardiovascular enhancement.

## Outcome of Studies using Goal Directed Therapy for High-Risk Surgical Patients

There have been 14 studies investigating the perioperative use of goal directed therapy in high-risk surgical patients involving a total of 1,132 patients. A number of these have involved patients with a very high post-operative mortality rate (>15%) and a number have had a postoperative mortality which was <15%. The odds ratio for 12 of these studies are shown in figure 1.

From this it can be seen that in those studies where the control mortality is >15% there is no doubt as to the benefit of this form of goal directed therapy for these patients who are at high risk of postoperative death or complications. While the benefit is not so marked in the studies where the control group mortality is <15% nevertheless most studies show a small but

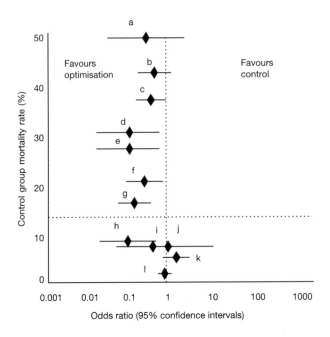

**Figure 1** Graph showing the odds ratio and 95% confidence intervals for 12 studies investigating the effect of goal directed therapy for 'High-Risk' surgical patients. a) Lobo et al. 2000;[42] b) Fleming et al. 1992;[38] c) Bishop et al. 1995;[40] d) Shoemaker et al. 1988;[19] e) Schultz et al. 1985;[36] f) Boyd et al. 1993;[39] g) Wilson et al. 1999;[41] h) Durham et al. 1996;[57] i) Sinclair et al. 1997;[45] j) Berlauk et al. 1991;[43] k) Ziegler et al. 1997;[46] l) Mythen and Webb 1995.[58]

significant improvement in outcome in the patients who have received goal directed therapy.

Critics of this form of therapy often cite a number of studies[51–55] to suggest that this technique of therapy is not effective. However, this argument does stand serious scrutiny. All five of the studies Yu et al., 1993,[51] Hayes et al., 1994,[56] Gattinoni et al., 1995,[53] Yu et al., 1998[55] and Alia et al., 1999[54] studied patients after organ failure had developed. Some studies[51,55] only enrolled postoperative patients who had developed organ failure several days after surgery. These two studies showed that even at this late stage there was still a small improvement in outcome associated with this goal directed therapy. However, the other studies[52–54] examined either post surgical patients or medical patients who had developed sepsis or sepsis syndrome and who were then subsequently admitted to ICU for treatment. Only when in ICU and after organ failure or severe organ dysfunction had set in did the goal directed therapy commence. In the report by Gattinoni et al.,[53] they did not recruit patients and commence therapy until conventional therapy had been administered for 48 h in an ICU and this therapy had failed to improve the patient. Their analysis found no difference in outcome between those patients being treated with goal directed therapy and those patients being treated conventionally. Both the Hayes[52] and the Alia[54] studies recruited medical and surgical patients who had developed sepsis or sepsis syndrome and had been admitted to ICU after demonstrating significant organ dysfunction and at least one organ system failure. Both groups of researchers demonstrated a lack of benefit for patients who had been treated with the Shoemaker variables of goal directed therapy at this late stage. Although frequently cited as showing lack of evidence for goal directed therapy in 'High-Risk' surgical patients these three studies[52–54] should not be included in any meta-analysis of goal directed therapy in this group of patients because they have not studied surgical patients having the goal directed therapy performed at or around the time of surgery.

Shoemaker et al.[31] have suggested that at the time of major surgery there is a development of an oxygen debt. Furthermore, they postulate that if this oxygen debt is repaid within 6–8 h of surgery then the patient will survive and is unlikely to have any major postoperative complications. If the patient is able to repay the oxygen debt within 12–30 h then the patient will survive but will develop varying amounts of postoperative complications depending on the degree of organ dysfunction caused by this prolonged oxygen debt. Finally if the patient does not mount a sufficient increase in cardiovascular response to ever repay this oxygen debt then these are the patients who will subsequently die in the 28-day period following surgery. This may be a rather simplistic overview of what is a very complex process but it helps to give framework on which to build future understanding of the process. It does however, neatly explain why this type of goal directed therapy does not work in the late stages after onset of organ failure, by which time no amount of extra oxygen is going to resuscitate dead tissue or cells. The secret lies in preventing cell death by adequate or increased amounts of oxygen being supplied at the time of development of oxygen debt.

## Conclusion

There is good evidence to suggest that patients with poor cardio-respiratory reserve have a high mortality and complication rate when they undergo major surgery. Many of these patients can be identified by simple clinical methods prior to their surgery. A number of randomised, controlled clinical studies have consistently demonstrated the improvement in outcome that can be achieved for these patients by the use of goal directed therapy aimed at temporarily improving the cardiovascular performance of high-risk patients so that non-survivors have the same cardio-respiratory performance as the survivors. Benefit can be achieved in a wide range of patients and in a wide range surgery including vascular surgery, colo-rectal surgery, trauma, orthopaedic surgery, major cancer surgery and cardiac surgery. The benefit is greatest in any of these types of surgery when the operation is performed as an emergency. Goal directed therapy to achieve a cardiac index of $>4.5 \, l^{-1} min^{-1} m^2$ (body surface area) or an oxygen delivery of $>600 \, ml^{-1} min^{-1} m^2$ (body surface area) should be standard aims and objectives of therapy for any high-risk surgical patient. When implemented early and aggressively this will reduce postoperative deaths and complications.

## References

1. Beecher HK, Todd DP. A study of the deaths associated with anaesthesia and surgery. Ann Surg 1954; 140: 2–5.
2. Edwards G, Morton HJV, Pask EA *et al*. Deaths associated with anaesthesia. Anaesthesia 1956; 11: 194–220.
3. Dornette WHL, Orth OS. Death in the operating room. Anesth and Analg 1956; 3: 545–569.
4. Buck N, Devlin HB, Lunn JN. The Report of a Confidential Enquiry into Perioperative Deaths. London: The Nuffield Provincial Hospitals Trust and the King Edwards Hospital Fund for London. 1987.
5. Saklad M. Grading of patients for surgical procedures. Anesthesiology 1941; 2: 281.
6. Marx GF, Mateo CV, Orkin LR. Computer analysis of postanesthetic deaths. Anesthesiology 1973; 39: 54–58.
7. Mella J, Biffin A, Radcliffe AG, Stamatakis JD, Steele RJ. Population-based audit of colorectal cancer management in two UK health regions. Colorectal Cancer Working Group, Royal College of Surgeons of England Clinical Epidemiology and Audit Unit. Br J Surg 1997; 84: 1731–1736.
8. Sherry KM. Clinical Co-ordinator, NCEPOD. Demographics: National Confidential Enquiry into Perioperative Death (NCEPOD). Clinical Intensive Care 2000; 11: 2–3.
9. Shoemaker WC. Cardiorespiratory patterns of surviving and nonsurviving post-operative patients. Surg Gynecol Obstet 1972; 134: 810–814.
10. Shoemaker WC, Montgomerry ES, Kaplan E, Elwyn DH. Physiologic patterns in surviving and nonsurviving shock patients. Use of sequential cardiorespiratory variables in defining criteria for therapeutic goals and early warning of death. Arch Surg 1973; 106: 630–636.
11. Shoemaker WC, Czer LS. Evaluation of the biologic importance of various hemodynamic and oxygen transport variables: which variables should be monitored in postoperative shock? Crit Care Med 1979; 7: 424–431.
12. Clowes GHAJ, Del Guercio LRM. Circulatory response to trauma of surgical operations. Metabolism 1960; 67–81.
13. Goldman L, Caldera DL, Nussbaum SR *et al*. Multifactorial index of cardiac risk in noncardiac surgical procedures. N Engl J Med 1977; 297: 845–850.
14. Mangano DT, Browner WS, Hollenberg M *et al*. Association of perioperative myocardial ischemia with cardiac morbidity and mortality in men undergoing noncardiac surgery. The Study of Perioperative Ischemia Research Group. N Engl J Med 1990; 323: 1781–1788.

15. Deitch EA. Overview of multiple organ failure, in Critical care: state of the art. Society of Critical Care Medicine: Anaheim, Ca. 1993; 131–168.

16. Livingston DH, Mosenthal AC, Deitch EA. Sepsis and multiple organ dysfunction syndrome: A clinical-mechanistic overview. New Horiz 1995; 3: 257–266.

17. Kirkpatrick CJ, Bittinger F, Klein CL *et al.* The role of the microcirculation in multiple organ dysfunction syndrome (MODS): a review and perspective. Virchows Arch 1996; 427: 461–476.

18. Granger DN. Role of xanthine oxidase and granulocytes in ischemia-reperfusion injury. Am J Physiol 1988; 255: 1269–1275.

19. Shoemaker WC, Appel PL, Kram HB *et al.* Prospective trial of supranormal values of survivors as therapeutic goals in high-risk surgical patients. Chest 1988; 94: 1176–1186.

20. Eagle KA, Brundage BH, Chaitman BR *et al.* Guidelines for perioperative cardio-vascular evaluation for noncardiac surgery. Report of the American College of Cardiology/American Heart Association Task Force on Practice Guidelines. Committee on Perioperative Cardiovascular Evaluation for Noncardiac Surgery. Circulation 1996; 93: 1278–1317.

21. Pasquet VA, D'Hondt AM, Verhelst R *et al.* Comparison of dipyridamole stress echocardiography and perfusion scintgraphy for cardiac risk stratification in vascular surgery patients. Am J Cardiol 1998; 82: 1468–1474.

22. Marcovitz PA. Prognostic issues in stress echocardiography. Prog Cardiovasc Dis 1997; 39: 533–542.

23. Van Damme H, Pierard L, Gillain D *et al.* Cardiac risk assessment before vascular surgery: A prospective study comparing clinical evaluation, dobutamine stress echocardiography, and dobutamine Tc-99 sestamibitomoscintigraphy. Cardiovasc Surg 1997; 5: 54–64.

24. Ryckwaert F, Leclerq F, Colson P. Dobutamine echocardiography for the pre-operative evaluation of patients for surgery of the abdominal aorta. Ann Fr Anesth Reanim 1998; 17: 13–18.

25. Poldermans D, Arnesc M, Fioretti PM *et al.* Sustained prognostic value of dobutamine stress echocardiography for late cardiac events after major noncardiac vascular surgery. Circulation 1997; 95: 53–58.

26. Older P, Smith R, Courtney P, Hone R. Preoperative evaluation of cardiac failure and ischemia in elderly patients by cardiopulmonary exercise testing. Chest 1993; 104: 701–704.

27. Edwards AE, Seymour DG, McCarthy JM, Crumplin MKH. A 5-year survival study of general surgical patients aged 65 and over. Anesthesiology 1996; 51: 3–10.

28. Anderson I. The surgeon. Consensus Meeting: Management of the High Risk Surgical Patient. Clinical Intensive Care 2000; 11: 8–10.

29. Fowkes FGR, Lunn SC, Farrow SC *et al.* Epidemiology in anaesthesia III: Mortality risk in patients with coexisting physical disease. Br J Anaesth 1982; 54: 819–824.

30. Porter GA, Soskolne CL, Yakimets WW, Newman SC. Surgeon-related factors and outcome in rectal cancer. Ann Surg 1998; 227: 157–167.

31. Shoemaker WC, Appel PL, Kram HB. Role of oxygen debt in the development of organ failure sepsis, and death in high-risk surgical patients. Chest 1992; 102: 208–215.

32. Treasure T, Bennett ED. Reducing the risk of major elective surgery. BMJ 1999; 318: 1087–1088.

33. Then and Now: The 2000 report of the NCEPOD. 2000, NCEPOD: London.

34. Clowes Jr GH, Vucinic M, Weidner MG. Circulatory and metabolic alterations associated with survival or death in peritonitis: clinical analysis of 25 cases. Ann Surg 1966; 163: 866–885.

35. Shoemaker WC, Appel PL, Waxman K *et al*. Clinical trial of survivors' cardiorespiratory patterns as therapeutic goals in critically ill postoperative patients. Crit Care Med 1982; 10: 398–403.

36. Schultz RJ, Whitfield GF, LaMura JJ *et al*. The role of physiologic monitoring in patients with fractures of the hip. J Trauma 1985; 25: 309–316.

37. Tuchschmidt J, Fried J, Astiz M, Rackow E. Elevation of cardiac output and oxygen delivery improves outcome in septic shock. Chest 1992; 102: 216–220.

38. Fleming A, Bishop M, Shoemaker WC *et al*. Prospective trial of supranormal values as goals of resuscitation in severe trauma. Arch Surg 1992; 127: 1175–1179.

39. Boyd O, Grounds RM, Bennett ED. A randomized clinical trial of the effect of deliberate perioperative increase of oxygen delivery on mortality in high-risk surgical patients. JAMA 1993; 270: 2699–2707.

40. Bishop MH, Shoemaker WC, Appel PL *et al*. Prospective, randomized trial of survivor values of cardiac index, oxygen delivery, and oxygen consumption as resuscitation endpoints in severe trauma. J Trauma 1995; 38: 780–787.

41. Wilson J, Woods I, Fawcett J *et al*. Reducing the risk of major elective surgery: randomised controlled trial of preoperative optimisation of oxygen delivery. BMJ 1999; 318: 1099–1103.

42. Lobo SM, Salgado PF, Castillo VG *et al*. Effects of maximizing oxygen delivery on morbidity and mortality in high-risk surgical patients. Crit Care Med 2000; 28: 3396–3404.

43. Berlauk JF, Abrams JH, Gilmour IJ *et al*. Preoperative optimization of cardiovascular hemodynamics improves outcome in peripheral vascular surgery. A prospective, randomized clinical trial. Ann Surg 1991; 214: 289–297.

44. Boyd O, Grounds RM, Bennett ED. The use of dopexamine hydrochloride to increase oxygen delivery perioperatively. Anesth Analg 1993; 76: 372–376.

45. Sinclair S, James S, Singer M. Intraoperative intravascular volume optimisation and length of hospital stay after repair of proximal femoral fracture: randomised controlled trial. BMJ 1997; 315: 909–912.

46. Ziegler DW, Wright JG, Choban PS, Flancbaum L. A prospective randomized trial of preoperative 'optimization' of cardiac function in patients undergoing elective peripheral vascular surgery. Surgery 1997; 122: 584–592.

47. Polonen P, Rukonen E, Hippelainen M *et al*. A prospective, randomized study of goal-oriented hemodynamic therapy in cardiac surgical patients. Anesth Analg 2000; 90: 1052–1059.

48. Connors Jr AF, Speroff T, Dawson NV *et al*. The effectiveness of right heart catheterization in the initial care of critically ill patients. SUPPORT Investigators. JAMA 1996; 276: 889–897.

49. Mangano DT, Layag EL, Wallace A, Tateo I. Effect of atenolol on mortality and cardiovascular morbidity after noncardiac surgery. Multicenter Study of Perioperative Ischemia Research Group. N Engl J Med 1996; 335: 1713–1720.

50. Poldermans D, Boersema E, Bax JJ, *et al*. The effect of bisoprolol on perioperative mortality and myocardial infarction in high-risk patients undergoing vascular surgery. Dutch Echocardiographic Cardiac Risk Evaluation Applying Stress Echocardiography Study Group. N Engl J Med 1999; 341: 1789–1794.

51. Yu M, Levy MM, Smith P *et al*. Effect of maximizing oxygen delivery on morbidity and mortality rates in critically ill patients: a prospective, randomized, controlled study. Crit Care Med 1993; 21: 830–838.

52. Hayes MA, Timmins AC, Yau EH *et al*. Elevation of systemic oxygen delivery in the treatment of critically ill patients. N Engl J Med 1994; 330: 1717–1722.

53. Gattinoni L, Brazzi L, Pelosi P *et al*. A trial of goal-oriented hemodynamic therapy in critically ill patients. SvO2 Collaborative Group. N Engl J Med 1995; 333: 1025–1032.

54. Alia I, Esteban A, Gordo F *et al*. A randomized and controlled trial of the effect of treatment aimed at maximising oxygen delivery in patients with severe sepsis or septic shock. Chest 1999; 115: 453–461.

55. Yu M, Burchell S, Hasaniya NW *et al*. Relationship of mortality to increasing oxygen delivery in patients greater than 50 years of age: a prospective, randomized trial. Crit Care Med 1998; 23: 1025–1032.

56. Hayes MA, Yau EH, Timmins AC *et al*. Response of critically ill patients to treatment aimed at achieving supranormal oxygen delivery and consumption. Relationship to outcome. Chest 1993; 103: 886–895.

57. Durham RM, Neunaber K, Mazaski JE *et al*. The use of oxygen consumption and delivery as endpoints for resuscitation in critically ill patients. J Trauma 1996; 41: 32–39.

58. Mythen MG, Webb AR. Perioperative plasma volume expansion reduces the incidence of gut mucosal hypoperfusion during cardiac surgery. Arch Surg 1995; 130: 423–429.

*L. Gattinoni   D. Chiumello   P. Pelosi*

CHAPTER

# 6

# Prone ventilation of the lungs

In the last 15 years, the prone position has been used increasingly in patients with acute lung injury (ALI) or with acute respiratory distress syndrome (ARDS). Its positive benefits on arterial oxygenation are now well established, while its impact on outcome or in the prevention of ventilation-induced lung injury is still under investigation. The prone position has allowed a better understanding of the pathophysiology of ALI-ARDS, which is a fundamental step for tailoring better respiratory support. In this chapter, we will review the pathophysiology related to the prone position, the mechanisms of improving gas exchange and the clinical data obtained by employing the prone position in ALI-ARDS patients, as well as in other clinical scenarios, such as in trauma and brain-injured patients with acute respiratory failure, general anaesthesia and in morbidly obese patients.

## Physiological Effects of Prone Position Ventilation

### Lung volumes

Early studies in ALI-ARDS patients[1] suggested that prone position ventilation allowed an increase in functional residual capacity (FRC). However, when the FRC was actually measured by the Helium dilution technique, no significant increase was found between the supine and the prone position, either in an experimental model[2] or in ALI-ARDS patients.[3] Similar findings were reported by Guerin *et al.*, who found lung recruitment in the prone compared to the supine position but only in a minority of ALI-ARDS patients.[4] When measuring a single computed tomography (CT) scan slice, representative of the entire lung, no difference in the gas volume was observed.[5]

Thus, there is little evidence that changing position in ALI-ARDS patients induces a systematic increase in overall lung volume or in lung recruitment. However, as we discuss later, regional changes in lung volume and in lung recruitment/derecruitment may occur when changing position.

## Respiratory mechanics

The effects of prone position on static respiratory compliance are uncertain: some authors have found an increase[6,7] while others have found[3,4] no difference when changing body position. By partitioning the static respiratory compliance into its chest wall and lung components, the prone position usually decreases chest wall compliance without any change in lung compliance.[3,4] When ALI-ARDS patients return to the supine position, chest wall compliance returns to baseline values while the total respiratory and/or lung compliance can increase.[3,4]

The effects on intra-abdominal pressure are also uncertain, as some authors report a moderate increase[8] while others report no change.[3] These effects are independent of attempts to restrict or enhance movement of the abdominal wall.

## Regional lung inflation

### Regional inflation in the supine position

Regional analysis of lung inflation has been investigated with the radioactive xenon technique or by morphometry.[9] However, computed tomography (CT) scanning offers a better means of analysis and quantification of regional lung inflation.[10]

In healthy subjects, as well as in ALI-ARDS patients who are placed in the supine position, there is a vertical gradient of lung inflation, with the ventral regions, located near the sternum (i.e. non-dependent) being more inflated than the dorsal regions, located near the vertebrae (i.e. dependent).[11] Regional inflation exponentially decreases with the height of the lung and this decay can be defined by a specific constant (Kd). Kd represents the distance from the sternum at which regional inflation decreases to 36%. The lower the value of Kd, the higher the rate of decrease of regional lung inflation. In ALI-ARDS patients, Kd is significantly lower compared with healthy subjects 7.8 ± 0.8 vs 13.9 ± 1.3 cm.

Regional lung inflation depends on the local transpulmonary pressure, defined as the difference between alveolar and pleural pressures.[12] Since pleural pressure is higher and transpulmonary pressure is lower in the dorsal regions compared with the ventral regions, regional lung inflation is lower in the dorsal regions compared to the ventral regions. Normally, the pleural pressure gradient is 0.2–0.3 cmH$_2$O cm$^{-1}$.[13]

Several factors have been postulated to affect the pleural pressure gradient and, consequently, regional lung inflation such as:

- the superimposed pressure on the lung

- cardiac mass

- cephalic displacement of the diaphragm

- lung mass/shape

1. The superimposed pressure on the lung is calculated as the height of the lung times its density.[14] The assumption is that the lung behaves as a fluid and that hydrostatic pressure is transmitted through the lung parenchyma as it is in a liquid. In ALI-ARDS patients, due to the oedema which increases lung weight, 974 $\pm$ 220 g in healthy subjects vs 2590 $\pm$ 1201 g in ALI-ARDS patients,[5] the superimposed pressure on the lung is significantly higher when compared with healthy subjects. The increase in superimposed lung pressure has been found, in an experimental setting, to be the major determinant of the pleural pressure gradient.[15]

2. Cardiac mass (the mass of the heart overlying both lungs) is involved in the genesis of the vertical gradient of pleural pressure.[16] In particular, in ALI-ARDS patients, the cardiac mass is usually heavier (27% more than in the healthy subjects) thus further increasing the pleural pressure gradient when compared with healthy subjects.[17]

3. Cephalic displacement of the dorsal regions of the diaphragm may be induced by sedation and paralysis, which in turn suppresses the muscular tone of the diaphragm[18] and further increases the pleural pressure gradient.[19]

4. Lung mass/shape may also influence regional pleural pressure;[20] however, the importance of this factor in ALI-ARDS patients has yet to be defined.

In summary, in ALI-ARDS patients in the supine position, regional lung inflation is greater in the ventral (non-dependent) regions compared with the dorsal (dependent) regions. Increases in lung weight and cardiac mass, loss of muscular tone, cephalic displacement of the diaphragm, change in thoracic-lung shape may all affect the pleural pressure gradient and regional lung inflation.

## Regional inflation in the prone position

When ALI-ARDS patients are turned from the supine to the prone position, the distribution of regional lung inflation changes. It increases in the dorsal regions and decreases in the ventral regions; the Kd is higher, compared with the supine position, and the changes in regional inflation are paralleled by an opposing redistribution of densities (from dorsal to ventral regions).[5] The prone position, by reducing the pleural pressure gradient,[21] also causes a more homogeneous distribution of transpulmonary pressures and of regional lung inflation.[5]

Modifications of superimposed pressure on the lung could explain, in part, the redistribution of regional lung inflation. In the supine position, the superimposed pressure on the lung causes a collapse in the dorsal regions (i.e. dependent zone), while in the prone position, the dependent zones (with the higher superimposed pressure on the lung) are the ventral regions, which collapse. Moreover, in the prone position, the cardiac mass lies on the sternum without acting as a compressive force on the lungs. In the presence of abdominal distension, the decrease in abdominal pressure in the prone position, by unloading the weight of the abdominal content against the diaphragm, may reduce the cephalic displacement of the diaphragm and change its motion.[22] Modifications of the thoracic-lung shape and the regional mechanical properties of the lungs and of the chest wall may also redistribute the forces acting on the pleural pressure gradient.

In summary, in ARDS patients, the prone position, by reversing the pleural pressure gradient, prevents compression from the weight of the cardiac mass and possibly reduces the cephalic displacement of the diaphragm, resulting in a more homogeneous regional lung inflation.

## Alveolar ventilation

### Distribution of alveolar ventilation in the supine position

For a number of years, using different techniques such as chest radiography and single photon emission CT, it has been known that the supine position in ventilated, sedated and paralyzed subjects is associated with preferential distribution of alveolar ventilation towards non-dependent regions.[23] CT scanning has confirmed these results when end-expiratory pressure is equal to zero. However, it was shown that by increasing end expiratory positive pressure (PEEP), alveolar ventilation-distribution becomes more homogeneous (i.e. the ratio of non-dependent and dependent regions of alveolar ventilation is 1:1).[24] This probably results from a combination of two effects: maintenance of lung opening in dependent regions by PEEP and stretching of non-dependent regions, which are more inflated but less ventilated. A more homogeneous distribution of alveolar ventilation is usually associated with better oxygenation.

## Distribution of alveolar ventilation in the prone position

Albert *et al*. provided evidence of improvement in alveolar ventilation-distribution in dorsal regions during prone position ventilation in an experimental setting.[2] Unfortunately, direct data of alveolar ventilation-distribution in human beings are lacking. Nevertheless, one may speculate that alveolar ventilation-distribution improves in the dorsal regions during prone position ventilation based on the findings of a more homogeneous lung inflation, a decreased transpulmonary pressure gradient and changes in chest wall compliance (see below). All of these findings indirectly suggest a more homogeneous alveolar ventilatory distribution in the prone compared with the supine position.

## Pulmonary perfusion

### Distribution of perfusion in the supine position

The most popular model to explain pulmonary perfusion is the gravitational one, in which gravity is the principal determinant of regional lung perfusion.[25] This model assumes that pulmonary blood flow is regulated by pulmonary arterial (Pa), venous (Pv) and alveolar (PA) pressures modeled as a Starling resistor. According to this gravitational model, perfusion should progressively increase from the non-dependent regions to the dependent regions.

However, several studies have noted a paradoxical decrease in pulmonary perfusion along the ventral axis despite increasing hydrostatic pressure in the most dependent regions,[26,27] suggesting that the pulmonary vessels system is not a passive one comprising infinitely compliant vessels.

In ALI-ARDS patients, several factors are known to influence the gravitational distribution of perfusion: for example, hypoxic vasoconstriction,[28] vessel obliteration and extrinsic vessel compression.[29] Hypoxic pulmonary vasoconstriction in the dependent regions can reverse blood flow toward the non-dependent regions, due to low alveolar ventilation.[28] Besides macro-microthrombi, extrinsic vessel compression due to higher superimposed pressure on the lung, or a reduction in extra-alveolar vessel calibre due to low lung volume can affect pulmonary perfusion. Hypoxic vasoconstriction and external or internal obstruction of pulmonary vessels, present mainly in the dependent regions, should reverse blood flow toward the non-dependent regions, so 'protecting' against hypoxaemia. However there is strong indirect pathophysiological evidence indicating that regional perfusion in ALI-ARDS is not gravity dependent and not homogeneously distributed. In fact, considering that some parts of the lung may be airless (up to 60–70%) and that these regions are located in the dependent portions of the lung, if perfusion were to be homogeneously distributed, the resulting shunt would lead to a degree of hypoxaemia incompatible with life.[30]

### Distribution of perfusion in the prone position

Most of the data concerning lung perfusion in the prone position arise from experimental work. Direct evidence on ALI-ARDS patients is lacking. The experimental data suggest that the gravitational model does not apply in the prone position. Glenny *et al.* showed that in the prone position, the gravitational gradient is reduced with a more homogeneous distribution of blood flow, i.e. similar blood flow in dependent and non-dependent lung regions.[31] Thus, in ALI-ARDS patients, prone position ventilation may cause a more homogeneous distribution of perfusion that is relatively unaffected by gravity.

In summary, the available evidence suggests that perfusion is not dramatically changed by body position.[32]

## Mechanisms Improving the Arterial Oxygenation in the Prone Position

By definition, hypoxaemia is due to an alteration of the ventilation-perfusion ratio (i.e. 'true shunt' V/Q < 0.01 and 'low V/Q' of 0.05–0.1). Lung regions characterized by a V/Q ratio of 0–0.1 contribute to arterial hypoxaemia.[33] Pappert *et al.* using the inert gas technique to quantify the V/Q impairment, found that, in ALI-ARDS patients ventilated in the supine position, an overall decrease of V/Q ratio due to 'true shunt' and 'low V/Q' while V/Q ratio improved when changing to prone position ventilation, particularly its 'true shunt'.[34] Unfortunately, the inert gas technique used in this study does not allow an anatomical regional description of the V/Q ratio distribution.

We will now discuss the factors leading to this improvement in the alveolar ventilation, bearing in mind that these different factors may operate at different degrees in different patients, depending on underlying pathophysiology, ARDS aetiology and the time course of the disease.

The main factors known to lead to possible improvements of V/Q may be grouped as followed:

• more homogeneous distribution of alveolar ventilation

• lung mass/shape

• changes in chest wall compliance.

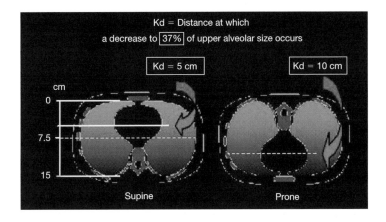

**Figure 1** Constant deflation decay (Kd) in the supine and prone positions.

## More homogeneous distribution of alveolar ventilation

As previously discussed, the prone position *per se* induces a more homogeneous distribution of regional lung inflation and by inference a more homogeneous alveolar ventilation-distribution. In fact, quantifying the homogeneity of the regional lung inflation by Kd, we found that arterial oxygenation improved when Kd increased from supine to prone, did not change when Kd was unmodified, and decreased when Kd was lower in prone compared with the supine position (fig. 1). This suggests that the rate of response in arterial oxygenation is associated with the rate of change in regional lung inflation.

## Lung mass/shape

Lung superimposed pressure is greatly increased in patients with ALI-ARDS. It is important to remember that lung superimposed pressure is a function of the density and the height of the lung. As shown in figure 2, the shape of the lung in general is such that the dependent lung mass is greater in the supine than in the prone position. For example, if the patient is ventilated in the supine position and the alveoli start to collapse at 50% of lung height, then 58% of the total lung mass would collapse. However, in the prone position, if collapse started to occur at the same lung height, only 38% of the lung mass would be dependent and would collapse. This means that part of the effect of the prone position is due to the lung mass undergoing collapse and the extent of this collapse may be different in different ALI-ARDS patients according to their individual lung shape. We found that the greater the mass of the lung in the upper lung in the prone position, the greater the improvement in arterial oxygenation.

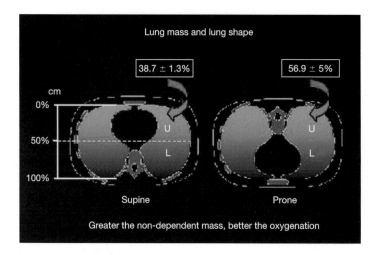

**Figure 2** Different lung mass/shape in the supine and prone positions.

## Changes in chest wall compliance

Changes in total respiratory compliance are unpredictable. While there is sufficient evidence to state that chest wall compliance decreases in the prone position, it is important to realize that chest wall compliance is the sum of the ventral chest wall, dorsal chest wall and diaphragm compliances. The dorsal chest wall, for anatomical reasons, is stiffer than the ventral chest wall and it is likely that diaphragmatic compliance does not change from the supine to the prone position. Thus the reduction in chest wall compliance in the prone position is most probably due to a reduction in ventral chest wall compliance, i.e. the ventral chest wall is stiffer in prone ventilation due to its limited range of movement, lying against the mattress surface.[3]

We have found that the greater the reduction of chest wall compliance, the greater the improvement in arterial oxygenation. A possible explanation is that a decrease in chest wall compliance may lead to a redistribution of alveolar ventilation towards the ventral and abdominal compartments, making alveolar ventilation-distribution more homogeneous.[3] However, further data are needed to confirm this hypothesis, since Geurin *et al.* did not find any correlation between the decrease in chest wall compliance and the increase in arterial oxygenation.[4]

Indeed, all three factors may contribute to improve the V/Q ratio. The more homogeneous distribution of alveolar ventilation, the more chest wall compliance changes may act on intra-tidal gas distribution while the change in the lung mass/shape may promote regional lung recruitment.

In addition, the prone position offers good secretion removal, which can be difficult to obtain using normal tracheal suctioning in the supine position, so contributing to improved distribution of alveolar ventilation.[35]

## Respiratory Factors Influencing the Different Responses of Respiratory Function in the Prone Position

The majority of studies have found a systematic improvement in arterial oxygenation when the body position is changed from supine to prone position. The improvement seen in responders (responders being defined as patients who show an increase in the arterial oxygenation of at least 1.3 kPa) is large, ranging from 57 to 100% (table 1). Several factors have been suggested to influence the rate of the response, according to a variety of inclusion criteria ALI, ARDS, aetiology, different duration and timing of pronation, different modes of mechanical ventilation.

### Pathogenic pathways

Since its original description, it has been recognized that ARDS may derive from a pulmonary (i.e. primary ARDS) or an extrapulmonary insult (i.e. secondary ARDS). This distinction was thought to be irrelevant in clinical practice. However, recently we have described differences in mechanical behaviour[49] and in lung morphology between primary and secondary ARDS.[50] Primary ARDS is characterized predominantly by consolidation and appears to be less responsive to the application of PEEP and recruitment manoeuvres. In contrast, secondary ARDS is characterized predominantly by atelectasis and is more responsive to the application of PEEP and recruitment manoeuvres.

We speculate that the main mechanism explaining the improvement of arterial oxygenation in prone position ventilation in secondary ARDS is regional recruitment due to the lung mass/shape. Secondary ARDS in the early stage fits the 'sponge lung model' with an homogeneous involvement of all parenchyma exposed via the bloodstream to the mediators originating in the extrapulmonary foci with consequent prevalent interstitial oedema, an increase in lung superimposed pressure and lung collapse.

Indeed, the amount of collapse/decollapse in the prone position may represent the main mechanism effecting the improvement in arterial oxygenation in prone position ventilation in secondary (extrinsic) ARDS.

In contrast, in primary ARDS, the amount of oedema and the potential for recruitment is lower. We may speculate that the main mechanism operating

**Table 1** Rate of responders, $PaO_2/FiO_2$ during supine, prone, return to supine position and time spent in prone position

| Study | No. of patients (absolute) | No. of responders absolute (%) | $PaO_2/FiO_2S$ (kPa) | $PaO_2/FiO_2P$ (kPa) | $PaO_2/FiO_2S^1$ (kPa) | T (h) |
|---|---|---|---|---|---|---|
| Phiel[36] | 5 | 5 (100) | 12.40 ± 1.33 | 18.80 ± 3.33 | – | – |
| Douglas[1] | 6 | 5 (83) | 11.87 ± 7.33 | 21.87 ± 9.73 | – | 4 |
| Langer[35] | 13 | 8 (61) | 13.33 ± 3.33 | 18.40 ± 2.67 | 17.07 ± 2 | 2 |
| Pappert[34] | 12 | 8 (66) | 14.53 ± 7.60 | 25.33 ± 13.73 | 16.40 ± 11.87 | 2 |
| Fridrich[37] | 20 | 20 (100) | 16.80 ± 1.07 | 32.93 ± 2.40 | 21.60 ± 1.87 | 20 |
| Stocker[38] | 16 | 16 (100) | 9.87 ± 3.47 | 30 ± 7.60 | – | * |
| Servillo[7] | 12 | 10 (83) | 16.53 ± 3.07 | 20.40 ± 2.27 | 18.80 ± 2.67 | 0.15 |
| Chatte[39] | 32 | 25 (78) | 13.33 ± 4 | 20 ± 8 | 17.33 ± 6.67 | 4 |
| Blanch[6] | 23 | 16 (70) | 10.40 ± 4.93 | 15.33 ± 6.80 | – | 1.5 |
| Papazian[40] | 14 | 9 (64) | 17.06 ± 5.87 | 25.73 ± 11.06 | – | 5 |
| Pelosi[3] | 16 | 12 (75) | 20.13 ± 4.67 | 25.47 ± 6.40 | 23.07 ± 10.67 | 2 |
| Jolliet[41] | 19 | 11 (57) | 9.07 ± 0.93 | 13.87 ± 2.40 | 12.93 ± 1.33 | 12 |
| Martinez[42] | 14 | 10 (71) | 14.67 ± 7.33 | 21.47 ± 11.87 | – | 2 |
| Guerin[4] | 12 | 10 (83) | 18.13 ± 2.27 | 27.20 ± 3.20 | 20.93 ± 2.80 | 1 |
| Voggenreiter[43] | 22 | 20 (90) | 28 ± 1.87 | 49.47 ± 3.47 | – | 8 |
| Dupont[44] | 27 | 16 (59) | 12.93 ± 6.13 | 22.53 ± 10.13 | – | 4 |
| Nakos[45] | 15 | 12 (80) | 11.07 ± 2.13 | 18 ± 3.73 | 17.87 ± 3.60 | 6 |
| Gattinoni[46] | 152 | 110 (73) | 17.33 ± 1.33 | 27.33 ± 2 | 20.67 ± 1.33 | 7 |
| Rialp[47] | 15 | 12 (80) | 14.13 ± 8 | 24.53 ± 8.93 | – | 0.5 |
| Venet[48] | 25 | 22 (90) | 18.93 ± 1.33 | 27.73 ± 1.33 | 22 ± 1.33 | 2 |

*The positioning procedures were continued until gas exchange remained stable at $PaO_2/FiO_2 > 20$ kPa.

in this situation is due to a more homogeneous intra-tidal gas distribution. Interestingly, the relationship that we described between the decrease in chest wall compliance and increase in arterial oxygenation was found in 16 patients, 13 of whom presented with primary ARDS.[3] It is important to stress that at present, these findings are mainly speculative and further studies are needed to confirm this hypothesis.

## Stage of disease

Most current studies on the prone position are limited to the early phase of ARDS, which is usually defined as being limited to the first week. In addition, the distinction between primary and secondary ARDS makes sense only in the early phase of the disease. In fact, in the late phase, the lung undergoes deep remodelling with structural changes, i.e. fibrosis, bullous emphysema-like lesions.[51]

In most studies, non-responders endured more days of mechanical ventilation than responders since the initial diagnosis of ARDS (11.8 $\pm$ 16 vs 32.78 $\pm$ 42 days).[6,39,41] Similarly, patients in the early phase of ARDS (i.e. with more pronounced pulmonary oedema) exhibited a greater improvement in arterial oxygenation compared with patients in the late phase of ARDS (i.e. with more pulmonary fibrosis), who usually did not respond.[45] However, it is important to note that even in late ARDS, some patients may respond to prone position ventilation with an improvement in arterial oxygenation. The main mechanism operating in this phase is likely to be one related to intra-tidal gas distribution, as the potential for recruitment is likely to be marginal at best.

## Ventilation-Induced Lung Injury and the Prone Position

Ventilation-induced lung injury is now widely recognized as a major problem in the management of acute respiratory failure.[52] The use of high transpulmonary pressures (i.e. ventilation with high tidal volumes or high pressures) which overstretches the alveoli can cause epithelial and endothelial disruption and induce lung oedema. Furthermore, failure to apply adequate PEEP levels can further increase the shear forces resulting from repeated air space opening and closing. When ALI-ARDS patients are in the supine position, with air spaces opening and closing, the largest alveolar volume excursion and the smallest end-expiratory alveolar volumes are preferentially distributed in the dorsal regions due to the more positive pleural pressure and the lower regional FRC. The prone position, by reducing the gravitational gradient of pleural pressure, can increase transpulmonary pressure and regional FRC. Moreover, prone position ventilation, can limit the shear forces and alveolar volume excursions in the dorsal regions. Similarly, prone position ventilation causes more homogeneous pulmonary blood flow distribution and may limit the capillary stress and reduce lung oedema.

Recent animal data showed that in the prone position, either in a healthy or a lung injury model, lung oedema and the severity of histological abnormalities were less severe in the prone compared with the supine position.[53,54] In the supine position, the distribution of lung oedema and histological abnormalities was higher in the dorsal regions, while in the prone position they were more uniform between the dorsal and the ventral regions. Furthermore, it has been shown that prone position ventilation may also reduce the incidence of pneumothorax.[55]

In summary, the use of the prone position, besides improving gas exchange, may also limit ventilation-induced lung injury.[56]

## Clinical Use of Prone Position Ventilation

### In acute respiratory failure

Although prone position ventilation has been shown to be effective in improving arterial oxygenation, its effects on patient outcome are still under investigation. So far, most studies are too limited in size to detect effects of outcome, and only one large randomized trial has been completed to date.[46] In a multicenter trial, 305 ALI-ARDS patients were randomized to be kept prone for at least 6 h per day for a period of 10 days. 152 patients were assigned to a prone group and 152 to a supine (control) group. Mortality did not differ significantly between the prone and the supine groups at the end of the 10-day study period (21 vs 25%), at the time of discharge from intensive care (50 vs 48%) or at 6 months (62 vs 59%). In a *posthoc* analysis, it was found that there was a significantly lower 10-day mortality rate in the prone group than in the supine group in those patients with the lowest PaO$_2$/FiO$_2$ ratio (<11.7 kPa), with the highest Simplified Acute Physiologic Score (>49) and the highest tidal volume (>12 ml/kg).

These negative results could be explained by a true lack of effect of the prone position on outcome or alternatively by an inadequate statistical power, the short duration of the prone position (an average of only 7 h per day, meaning that patients were supine for more than 70% for each day) or the limitation of the prone position to only 10 days.

Considering these potential limitations, we believe that, at present, prone position ventilation using this protocol should not be adopted in all

ALI-ARDS patients but limited to the most severe cases of respiratory failure.[57]

### When should the prone position be initiated?

We do not know at present when ALI-ARDS patients should be turned prone.[58] We suggest turning ALI-ARDS patients prone from the earliest phase of the disease and simultaneously to try to recruit the lung maximally using manoeuvres such as sighs or sustained inflations. This use of prone position ventilation in the early phase may maximize the effectiveness of the manoeuvre due to the predominant position of oedema and atelectasis (i.e. increased amount of recruitable tissue).

### Length of time spent for each prone position

There are no guidelines to suggest how long the prone position should be maintained in order to obtain the maximal beneficial effect on respiratory function. The literature suggests that most of the improvement occurs rapidly, within a few minutes of turning prone. However, a continuous increase in arterial oxygenation can be obtained even after 6 h in the prone position.[46]

In some responders, the improvement in arterial oxygenation is partially maintained when they are returned supine (i.e. persistent responders), while other responders rapidly lose this gain when returned supine (non-persistent responders).[39] A possible explanation for this is that, in the persistent responders, the recruited lung volume from prone ventilation is better maintained when returned to supine. So, in the persistent responders, a strategy of repeated supine-prone cycles could be useful, avoiding the complications of a prolonged time in the prone position. On the contrary, in non-persistent responders, we suggest increasing the duration of prone position ventilation, in order to decrease the risk of severe hypoxaemia when returning supine. In our clinical practice we continue to use prone position ventilation until an arterial oxygenation of at least 13.3 kPa is reached with a PEEP of 10 cm H$_2$O and FiO$_2$ of 40%. Then, we return to supine ventilation and begin an assisted mode of ventilation plus weaning procedures.

### Recruitment manoeuvre: PEEP during prone position

CT scan studies in supine ALI-ARDS patients have shown that the presence of lung collapse was not only along a vertical gradient (i.e. ventral to dorsal) but also along a cephalo- to caudal axis. Recruitment manoeuvres are recommended as a useful tool to re-open these collapsed lung regions and to improve arterial oxygenation. However, recruitment manoeuvres in the supine position, besides reopening the dorsal regions (i.e. collapsed ones) will also overdistend the already maximally open alveoli. Prone position ventilation, by reducing the pleural pressure gradient, can increase the transpulmonary pressure in the dorsal regions. This property of prone position ventilation causes a greater lung recruitment in the dorsal regions and enhanced arterial oxygenation improvement when the recruitment manoeuvres are applied in the prone compared with the supine position. This has been shown both in an experimental setting and in ALI-ARDS patients.[59,60]

PEEP is one of the most important treatment modalities used to improve arterial oxygenation in severe respiratory failure. PEEP, by opposing the critical closing pressure (i.e. superimposed pressure), can maintain alveoli open at end-expiration. Data from animal studies suggest that PEEP in the prone position will cause a more homogeneous distribution of pulmonary blood flow compared with the supine position.[61] Due to the lower closing pressures and more favourable pulmonary blood distribution in the prone position, lower PEEP levels are likely to result in the same increase in arterial oxygenation compared with supine.[59,62]

CT scanning has shown that the ventral regions remained aerated at lower PEEP levels in the prone position, while the previously collapsed dorsal regions in the supine position became aerated. For the same dorsal regions to remain aerated in supine positions, higher levels of PEEP are needed and this can cause an overdistension of the ventral regions. Thus, the prone position compared with the supine position, can enhance the beneficial effect of a recruitment manoeuvre to increase arterial oxygenation and requires lower PEEP levels to maintain this increase.

### Nitric oxide and the prone position

Nitric oxide (NO) is a vasodilator that, when inhaled by ALI-ARDS patients, causes a dilatation of the pulmonary vessels supplying the ventilated alveolar regions, thus improving blood flow to ventilated areas of lung. It has been shown to be beneficial by increasing arterial oxygenation in ALI-ARDS patients.[40,47,63]

When NO is inhaled by a patient undergoing prone position ventilation, it causes a greater improvement in arterial oxygenation than either treatment used alone. This improvement in arterial oxygenation allows a faster reduction of the inspired oxygen fraction. Furthermore, the combination of prone position ventilation and inhaled NO may lead to a decrease in the required dose of NO, thus reducing the accumulation of toxic pro-inflammatory degradation products such as nitrogen dioxide ($NO_2$).

The effects of NO may be different in primary and secondary ARDS. Rialp *et al.*[47] found an improvement with NO and prone positioning only in primary ARDS. However, all studies so far have addressed only the short term effects of inhaled NO combined with prone positioning, and further studies are necessary to evaluate the real benefits of this fascinating dual therapy to outcome in ALI-ARDS patients.

Another potentially beneficial strategy may be to combine inhaled NO with almitrine bysmesylate to enhance the beneficial effects of prone positioning on arterial oxygenation. Almitrine bysmesylate increases hypoxic vasoconstriction, so redirecting pulmonary blood flow to the well-ventilated regions of the lung. Combining inhaled NO and almitrine bysmesylate in prone position ventilation may enhance arterial oxygenation when compared with inhaled NO in this situation.[64] However, almitrine bysmesylate may also increase mean pulmonary arterial pressure and right ventricular workload, although this may be attenuated by the addition of inhaled NO. Nevertheless, particular caution will be necessary in case this therapy causes severe pulmonary hypertension or right ventricular failure. One suggested approach would be to start with inhaled NO and then later add almitrine bysmesylate in an increasing but low dose (i.e. <1 mg/kg/h).[64]

### In trauma induced acute respiratory failure

Several studies have shown the usefulness of prone positioning in improving arterial oxygenation in trauma patients with severe respiratory failure. In these studies, different types of trauma patients were enrolled (e.g. multiple trauma, blunt chest trauma, abdominal trauma and patients with multiple fractures). The use of prone positioning was safe and caused only minor complications such as swelling and oedema of the face and pressures sores. In one study by Fridrich *et al.*[37] trauma patients with ARDS were treated for at least 20 consecutive hours per day in the prone position (mean $8 \pm 4$ days) without any significant side-effects.[37] They did, however, exclude patients with raised intracranial pressure (ICP) >3.3 kPa, or unstable cervical spine fractures.

### Brain-injured patients with acute respiratory failure

Brain-injured patients have an increased risk of extracerebral organ dysfunction, mainly pulmonary.[65] Patients with brain injury are characterized by an increased risk of developing ventilator-associated pneumonia (30–50% compared to 20% of the normal ICU population).[66,67] Studies have indicated that pulmonary dysfunction after brain injury may significantly increase the length of stay in intensive care and mortality and worsen the neurological outcome.[68]

The use of prone positioning in patients with brain injury has not usually been considered due to two possible negative effects on brain perfusion and ICP.

For this reason, strict exclusion criteria must be adopted when the prone position is used in this group of patients:

- presence of unstable clinical situation (unstable ICP, and/or ICP higher than 2.7–3.3 kPa despite adequate treatment).

- evidence of ischaemia, as indicated by a low jugular venous oxygen tension ($SjO_2$ below 7.3–8 kPa). Furthermore, in this particular patient group, it is necessary to consider the following: the adequacy of the level of sedation; careful positioning of the patient in the reverse Trendelenburg position (head and trunk at 20°) with a good alignment of the cervical with the thoracic spine; in more severe brain-injured patients, monitoring of ICP and $SjO_2$ may be required; careful clinical monitoring of the central nervous system (in particular, pupillary diameter in the acute phases of positioning and overall neurological status and daily clinical assessments).

We recently investigated the effect of a short period of prone positioning, in a randomized controlled study, in severe brain-injured patients sedated and paralyzed with acute respiratory failure due to ventilator-associated pneumonia.[69] During prone position ventilation in these patients, arterial oxygenation markedly improved within 4 h and this improvement was maintained 24 h later when returned to the supine position. No significant increase in ICP was found in the prone position and no patients experienced an increase in ICP >3.3 kPa. Although these are only preliminary data, obtained in a small study population, they suggest that, over a short time period, the prone position in brain-injured patients is safe to use, may improve oxygenation and that the improvement may be maintained for at least 24 h when the patient is returned to the supine position. If carefully performed for a moderate period of time and carefully monitored, the prone position does not negatively affect brain perfusion and ICP.

## General anaesthesia

The prone position is frequently used during general anaesthesia for specific neurosurgical (spinal cord, occipital lobe, craniosynostosis and posterior fossa) procedures, orthopaedic or recto-perineal procedures.[70] The main focus of attention during general anaesthesia has been on the positioning procedure and pressure injuries.

Data concerning the physiological effects of the prone position on respiratory function in spontaneously breathing or mechanically ventilated normal subjects are scanty. Lynch *et al.* were the first to report that anaesthetized subjects, when breathing spontaneously in the prone position, were unable to maintain an adequate tidal volume and showed a concomitant decrease in arterial oxygenation.[71] Similarly, Safar *et al.* reported a reduction of 20–30% in the compliance of the respiratory system using the prone position.[72] Overall these data suggest that the prone position can be associated with adverse effects on pulmonary function during anaesthesia, hence it should be applied with caution in healthy subjects. Nevertheless, Lumb *et al.* reported that the prone position did not affect respiratory function in conscious healthy male volunteers, possibly increasing the FRC.[73]

We studied a group of normal subjects receiving general anaesthesia for elective surgery requiring the prone position.[74] The prone position did not significantly affect the respiratory system, lung or chest wall compliance. Both FRC and arterial oxygenation markedly increased from supine to prone (53% and 24% respectively).

It is worth noting that, in contrast to previous studies,[71,72] we positioned our patients as described by Smith *et al.*[75] ensuring free abdominal movements by the use of upper chest and pelvic supports, with less constriction of the chest wall movements. This suggests that this kind of prone positioning can affect respiratory function differently.

## Obese patients

In obese patients, general anaesthesia is known to negatively affect respiratory mechanics and arterial oxygenation more than in normal subjects.[76] In particular, the increased intra-abdominal pressure which characterizes obese patients can lead to a more obvious cranial shift of the diaphragm, i.e. producing a marked reduction in lung volume and reduction of the movement of the dependent part of the diaphragm. Both of these phenomena predispose the patient to the formation of more overt atelectasis with a marked deterioration in oxygenation, and respiratory mechanics.

The beneficial effects of the prone position may be greater in obese patients compared with normal subjects, due to a greater reduction in intra-abdominal pressure and in the abdominal-to-diaphragmatic load leading to a greater improvement in lung volume, oxygenation and respiratory mechanics.

We studied a group of obese patients receiving general anaesthesia for elective surgery requiring the prone position.[77] We found that lung compliance increased while chest wall compliance decreased, but that the total compliance of the whole respiratory system was essentially unchanged. Improvements in FRC and lung compliance were paralleled by an increase in oxygenation in all patients when their position was changed from supine to the prone position. Overall, the differences in arterial oxygenation from supine and prone position were not significantly related to the differences in FRC. The relative improvement in oxygenation in FRC and arterial oxygenation between supine and prone positions was significantly greater in obese patients compared with normal subjects ($0.89 \pm 0.33$ vs $1.98 \pm 0.85\,L$ and $130 \pm 30$ vs $180 \pm 28\,mm\,Hg$ in obese patients and $1.93 \pm 0.57$ vs $2.92 \pm 0.68$ and $160 \pm 37$ vs $199 \pm 16\,mm\,Hg$ in normal subjects). This demonstrates that the most probable effect of prone position is to unload the abdominal pressure pushing on the diaphragm, allowing an increase in FRC with consequent beneficial effects on respiratory mechanics and oxygenation. In our study, most of the changes in respiratory function observed in supine obese patients were, at least in part, reversed by prone positioning. Hence, the use of the prone position only in these patients does not seem to have any adverse effects on pulmonary function but may actually improve FRC, lung compliance and arterial oxygenation.

## How to Perform the Prone Manoeuvre

There are no published guidelines for the optimal turning and positioning of patients. We describe here how we perform the prone positioning manoeuvre in our clinical practice. Before starting the turning sequence, an adequate level of sedation (which may also require neuromuscular blockades) must be achieved to maximize patient compliance with the ventilator. Tracheal suctioning is performed before turning, to prevent mobilization of airway secretions during the manoeuvre. All patients, during the turning and once in prone position, should be monitored with an electrocardiogram, pulse oximetry and invasive arterial pressure. At least five attendants (one doctor and four nurses) are required to perform the manoeuvre. The doctor usually places themself at the patient's head and is responsible for the endotracheal or tracheostomy tube and the breathing system connections. The four nurses, two for each side, turn the patient first to the lateral position, and sequentially to the prone position. When the patient is in the lateral position, two thick pillows are put under the shoulder and under the bony pelvis respectively. This allows free abdominal wall motion and tension-free positioning of the head. The arms can lie parallel to the body with the head turned either to the right or left, avoiding extreme cervical rotation. Alternatively, one arm can lie parallel to the body and the other arm can lie above the head and the head turned towards the same side. The cervical spine should not be in excessive extension and a thin pillow should be placed under the patient's face. When the patient is in the prone position, maximal consideration must be applied to ensuring that the patient is in a position which places no tension on the neck or arms, so as to avoid peripheral nerve injury. However, if this

**Table 2** Contraindications to the prone position

*Absolute*
Haemodynamic instability
Increased ICP (>25 mm Hg)
Unstable spinal and pelvic fractures

*Relative*
Face injury
Uncontrolled dysrhythmias
Acute bleeding
Recent tracheostomy or rachis, abdominal surgery
Broncho-pleural fistula
Haemodialysis

positioning is maintained for a long time, it could become dangerous; we recommend regularly alternating the position, changing the orientation of the head and the arms.

Pressure on the eyes must be avoided to eliminate the possibility of blindness. The frequency of tracheal suctioning will need to be increased to prevent secretions being mobilized from dorsal regions and subsequently aspirated into ventral regions. Absolute and relative contraindications to turning patients into the prone position are detailed in table 2.

## Complications and Technical Aspects of the Prone Manoeuvre

Use of the prone position is not without risk, firstly due to complications associated with turning the patient prone and secondly with the maintenance of the prone position. The frequency of complications in a large multicentre trial associated with prone and supine positioning involving more than 300 ALI-ARDS patients are reported in table 3.[46] At enrollment, the number of patients with pressure sores and the number of pressure sores per patient were similar between the two groups.

The study showed that the number of new pressure sores per patient was significantly higher in the prone group than in the supine group. The weight-bearing sites in the prone position (thorax, cheekbone, iliac crest, breast and knee) were more likely to be significantly affected in the prone group (70 of 158 sores were at these sites, compared with 12 of 102 sores in the supine group). The percentages of patients with accidental displacement of the endotracheal or thoractomy tube or loss of venous access were low and similar in the two groups. The most frequent acute complications during the prone position

**Table 3** Incidence of acute complications

| Complications related to manoeuvre | Supine group (n = 152) | Prone group (n = 152) | P |
|---|---|---|---|
| Pressure sores at entry (% of patients) | 22.5 | 24.0 | 0.78 |
| No. of pressure sores/patient at entry | 1.6 ± 0.9 | 1.9 ± 2.4 | 0.23 |
| No. of new or worsening pressure sores/patient | 1.9 ± 1.3 | 2.7 ± 1.7 | 0.04 |
| Displacement of thoracotomy tube (% of patient) | 0.7 | 3.9 | 0.12 |
| Loss of venous access (% of patient) | 9.2 | 5.3 | 0.27 |
| Displacement of tracheal tube (% of patient) | 9.9 | 7.9 | 0.68 |
| | | | |
| Complications related to prone (% of patient) | Prone group | | |
| Need for increased sedation | 55.2 | | |
| Need for increased muscle relaxants | 27.7 | | |
| Airway obstruction | 39.3 | | |
| Transient desaturation | 18.7 | | |
| Hypotension | 12.3 | | |
| Vomiting | 7.6 | | |
| Displacement of thoracotomy tube | 0.5 | | |
| Accidental extubation | 0.5 | | |
| Facial oedema | 29.8 | | |

From Gattinoni L et al;[46] Multicenter study 300 patients.

were the need for increased sedation, muscle relaxants, immediate tracheal suctioning and facial oedema. However, despite these reservations, the prone position appears to be a safe manoeuvre if performed carefully.

Besides these acute complications, chronic complications such as contractures, calcifications of shoulder and hip joints[78] and nerve lesions may also occur as a direct result of the use of the prone position, particularly if it is used on a long-term basis. These chronic complications may be very severe and will also have a negative impact on the course and the recovery of the patients.

## References

1. Douglas WW, Rehder K, Beynen FM, Sessler AD, Marsh H. Improved oxygenation in patients with acute respiratory failure: the prone position. Am Rev Respir Dis 1977; 115: 559–566.
2. Albert RK, Leasa D, Sanderson M, Robertson TH, Hlastala MP. The prone position improves arterial oxygenation and reduces shunt in oleic acid induced acute lung injury. Am Rev Respir Dis 1987; 135: 628–633.
3. Pelosi P, Tubiolo D, Mascheroni D, Vicardi P, Crotti S, Valenza F, Gattinoni L. Effects of the prone position on respiratory mechanics and gas exchange during acute lung injury. Am J Respir Crit Care Med 1998; 157: 1–7.

4. Guerin C, Badet M, Rosselli S *et al*. Effects of prone position on alveolar recruitment and oxygenation in acute lung injury. Intensive Care Med 1999; 25: 1222–1230.
5. Gattinoni L, Pelosi P, Vitale G, Pesenti A, D'Andrea L, Mascheroni D. Body position changes redistribute lung computed tomographic density in patients with acute respiratory failure. Anesthesiology 1991; 74: 15–23.
6. Blanch L, Mancebo J, Perez M *et al*. Short term effects of prone position incritically ill patients with acute respiratory distress syndrome. Intensive Care Med 1997; 23: 1033–1039.
7. Servillo G, Roupie E, De Robertis E *et al*. Effects of ventilation in ventral decubitus position on respiratory mechanics in adult respiratory distress syndrome. Intensive Care Med 1997; 23: 1219–1224.
8. Hering R, Wrigge H, Vorwerk R, Brensing K *et al*. The effect of prone position on intraabdominal pressure and cardiovascular and renal function in patients with acute lung injury. Anest Analg 2001; 92: 1226–1231.
9. Milic Emili J. Radioactive Xenon in the evaluation of regional lung function. Semin Nucl Med 1971; 2: 246–262.
10. Gattinoni L, Pesenti A, Bombino M *et al*. Relationship between lung computed tomographic density gas exchange and PEEP in acute respiratory failure. Anesthesiology 1988; 69: 824–832.
11. Pelosi P, D'Andrea L, Vitale G, Pesenti A, Gattinoni L. Vertical gradient of regional lung inflation in adult respiratory distress syndrome. Am J Respir Crit Care Med 1994; 149: 8–13.
12. In: Macklem PT, Mead J. (eds) Handbook of Physiology. American Physiological Society, Bethesda 1986; Vol. 3, 561–574.
13. In: Macklem PT, Mead J. (eds) Handbook of Physiology. American Physiological Society, Bethesda 1986; Vol. 3, 531–559.
14. Krueger JJ, Boin T, Patterson L. Elevation gradient of intrathoracic pressure. J Appl Physiol 1961; 16: 465–468.
15. Pelosi P, Golmer M, McKibben A *et al*. Recruitment and derecruitment during acute respiratory failure: an experimental study. Am J Respir Crit Care Med 2001; 164: 122–130.
16. Albert RK, Hubmayr R. The prone position eliminates compression of lungs by the heart. Am J Respir Crit Care Med 2000; 16: 1660–1665.
17. Malbuisson LM, Bush L, Puybasset L, Lu Q, Cluzel P, Rouby JJ. Role of the heart in the loss of aeration characterizing lower lobes in acute respiratory distress syndrome. Am J Respir Crit Care Med 2000: 161: 2005–2012.
18. Frose AB, Bryan AC. Effects of anesthesia and paralysis on diaphragmatic mechanics in man. Anesthesiology 1974; 4: 242–254.
19. Warner DO, Warner MA, Ritman EL. Human chest wall function while awake and during anesthesia: I Quiet breathing. Anesthesiology 1995; 82: 6–19.
20. Margulies SS, Rodarte JR. Shape of the chest wall in the prone and supine anesthetised dogs. J Appl Physiol 1990; 68: 1970–1978.
21. Muthot T, Guest RJ, Lamm WJE, Albert RK. Prone position alters the effect of volume overload or regional pleural pressures and improves hypoxemia in pigs in vivo. Am Rev Respir Dis 1992; 146: 300–306.
22. Mure M, Glemmy Rw, Domino KB, Hlastalo MP. Pulmonary gas exchange improves in the prone position with abdominal distension. Am J Respir Crit Care Med 1998; 157: 1785–1790.
23. Tokics L, Hedenstierna G, Svensson L, Brismar B, Cederlund T, Lundquist H. V/D distribution and correlation to atelectasis in anesthetized paralyzed humans. J Appl Physiol 1996; 4: 1822–1833.

24. Gattinoni L, Pelosi P, Crotti S, Valenza F. Effects of positive end expiratory pressure on regional distribution of tidal volume and recruitment in adult respiratory distress syndrome. Am J Respir Crit Care Med 1995; 151: 1807–1815.
25. West JB, Dolley CT, Noimark A. Distribution of blood flow in isolated lungs: relation to vascular and alveolar pressures. J Appl Physiol 1964; 19: 713–724.
26. Hughes JMB, Glazier JB, Maloney JE, West JB. Effect of lung volume on the distribution of pulmonary blood flow in man. Respir Physiol 1968; 4: 58–72.
27. Prefaut C, Engel LA. Vertical distribution of perfusion and inspired gas in supine man. Respir Physiol 1981; 43: 209–219.
28. Arborelius M, Lunding G, Suanberg L, Defares JG. Influence of unilateral hypoxia on blood flow through the lungs in man in lateral position. J Appl Physiol 1960; 15: 595–597.
29. Vesconi S, Rossi GP, Pesenti A, Fumagalli R, Gattinoni L. Pulmonary microthrombosis in severe adult respiratory distress syndrome. Crit Care Med 1988; 16: 111–113.
30. Gattinoni L, Pelosi P, Pesenti A et al. CT scan in ARDS: clinical and physiopathological insights. Acta Anaesthesiol Scand 1991; 35: 87–96.
31. Glenny RW, Lamm WJE, Albert RK, Robertson HT. Gravity is a minor determinant of pulmonary blood flow distribution. J Appl Physiol 1991; 71: 620–629.
32. Lamm WJE, Graham MM, Albert RK. Mechanism by which the prone position improves oxygenation in acute lung injury. Am J Respir Crit Care 1994; 150: 184–193.
33. Tokics L, Hedenstierna G, Strandberg A, Brismar B, Lundquist H. Lung collapse and gas exchange during general anesthesia: effects of spontaneous breathing, muscle paralysis, and positive end-expiratory pressure. Anesthesiology 1987; 66: 157–167.
34. Pappert D, Rossaint R, Slama K, Gruning T, Falke K. Influence of positioning on ventilation perfusion relationships in severe adult respiratory distress syndrome. Chest 1994; 106: 1511–1516.
35. Langer M, Mascheroni D, Marcolin R, Gattinoni L. The prone position in ARDS patients. A clinical study. Chest 1988; 94: 103–107.
36. Piehl MA, Brown RS. Use of extreme position changes in acute respiratory failure. Crit Care Med 1976; 4: 13–14.
37. Fridrich P, Krafft P, Hochleuthner H, Mauritz W. The effects of long term prone positioning in patients with trauma induced adult respiratory distress syndrome. Anesth Analg 1996; 83: 1206–1211.
38. Stocker R, Neff T, Stein S, Ecknauer E, Trentz O, Russi E. Prone positioning and low volume pressure limited ventilation improve survival in patients with severe ARDS. Chest 1997; 111: 1008–1017.
39. Chatte G, Sab JM, Dubois JM, Sirodot M, Gaussorgues P, Robert D. Prone position in mechanically ventilated patients with severe acute respiratory failure. Am J Respir Crit Care Med 1997; 155: 473–478.
40. Papazian L, Bregeon F, Caillot F et al. Respective and combined effects of prone position and inhaled nitric oxide in patients with acute respiratory distress syndrome. Am J Respir Crit Care Med 1998; 157: 580–585.
41. Jolliet P, Bulpa P, Chevrolet JC. Effects of the prone position on gas exchange and hemodynamics in severe acute respiratory distress syndrome. Crit Care Med 1998; 26: 1977–1985.
42. Martinez M, Diaz E, Joseph D, Villagrà A, Mas A, Fernandez R, Blanch L. Improvement in oxygenation by prone position and nitric oxide in patients with acute respiratory distress syndrome. Intensive Care Med 1999; 25: 29–36.

43. Voggenreiter G, Neudeck F, Aufmkock M *et al.* Intermittent prone positioning in the treatment of severe and moderate posttraumatic lung injury. Crit Care Med 1999; 27: 2375–2382.

44. Dupont H, Mentec H, Cheval C, Moine P, Fierobe L, Timsit JF. Short term effect of inhaled nitric oxide and prone positioning on gas exchange in patients with severe acute respiratory distress syndrome. Crit Care Med 2000; 28: 304–308.

45. Nakos G, Tsangaris I, Kostanti E *et al.* Effect of the prone position on patients with hydrostatic pulmonary edema compared with patients with acute respiratory distress syndrome and pulmonary fibrosis. Am J Respir Crit Care Med 2000; 161: 360–368.

46. Gattinoni L, Tognoni G, Pesenti A *et al.* Effect of prone position on the survival of patients with acute respiratory failure. N Engl J M 2001; 345: 568–573.

47. Rialp G, Betbese AJ, Marquez MP, Mancebo J. Short term effects of inhaled nitric oxide and prone position in pulmonary and extrapulmonary acute respiratory distress syndrome. Am J Respir Crit Care Med 2001; 164: 243–249.

48. Venet C, Guyomarc'h S, Migeot C *et al.* The oxygenation variations related to prone positioning during mechanical ventilation: a clinical comparison between ARDS and non ARDS hypoxemic patients. Intensive Care Med 2001; 27: 1352–1359.

49. Gattinoni L, Pelosi P, Suter PM, Pedoto A, Vercesi P, Lissoni A. Acute respiratory distress syndrome caused by pulmonary and extrapulmonary disease: different syndromes? Am J Respir Crit Care Med 1998; 158: 3–11.

50. Gattinoni L, Caironi P, Pelosi P, Goodman LR. What the computed tomography taught us about the acute respiratory distress syndrome. Am J Respir Crit Care Med 2001; 164: 1701–1711.

51. Gattinoni L, Bombino M, Pelosi P, Lissoni A, Pesenti A, Fumagalli R, Tagliabue M. Lung structure and function in different stages of severe adult respiratory distress syndrome. JAMA 1994; 271: 1772–1779.

52. Gillette MA, Hess DR. Ventilator induced lung injury and the evolution of lung protective strategies in acute respiratory distress syndrome. Respir Care 2001; 46: 130–148.

53. Broccard A, Shapiro RS, Schmitz LL, Adams AB, Nahum A, Marini JJ. Prone position attenuates and redistributes ventilator induced lung injury in dogs. Crit Care Med 2000; 28: 295–303.

54. Broccard A, Shapiro RS, Schmitz LL, Ravenscraft SA, Marini JJ. Influence of prone position on the extent and distribution of lung injury in a high tidal volume oleic acid model of acute respiratory distress syndrome. Crit Care Med 1997; 25: 16–27.

55. Yamado HDL, Orii R, Suzuki S, Sawamura S, Suwa K, Hanaoka K. Beneficial effects of the prone position on the incidence of barotrauma in oleic acid induced lung injury under continuous positive pressure ventilation. Acta Anaesthesiologica Scandinavica 1997; 4: 701–707.

56. Albert RK. Prone position in ARDS: What do we know and What do we need to know. Crit Care Med 1999; 11: 2574–2575.

57. Slutsky AS. The acute respiratory distress syndrome, mechanical ventilation and the prone position. N Engl J Med 2001; 345: 610–611.

58. Albert RK. The prone position in acute respiratory distress syndrome: where we are, and where do we go from here. Crit Care Med 1997; 25: 1453–1454.

59. Cakar N, Van der Kloot T, Youngblood M, Adams A, Nahum A. Oxygenation response to a recruitment maneuver during supine and prone positions in an oleic acid induced lung injury model. Am J Respir Crit Care Med 2000; 161: 1946–1956.

60. Pelosi P, Bottino N, Caironi P, Panigada M, Eccher G, Mondino M, Gattinoni L. Sigh in acute respiratory distress syndrome: effects in supine and in prone position. Intensive Care Med 2000; 26: s263.

61. Walther SM, Domino KB, Glenny RW, Hlastala MP. Positive end-expiratory pressure redistributes perfusion to dependent lung regions in supine but not in prone lambs. Crit Care Med 1999; 27: 37–45.

62. Lim CM, Koh Y, Chin JY et al. Respiratory and haemodynamic effects of the prone position at two different levels of PEEP in a canine acute lung injury model. Eur Respir J 1999; 13: 163–168.

63. Borrelli M, Lampati L, Vascotto E, Fumgalli R, Pesenti A. Hemodynamic and gas exchange response to inhaled nitric oxide and prone positioning in acute respiratory distress syndrome patients. Crit Care Med 2000; 28: 2707–2712.

64. Jolliet P, Bulpe P, Ritz M, Ricon B, Lopez J, Chevrolet JC. Additive beneficial effects of the prone position nitric oxide and almitrine bysmesylate on gas exchange and oxygen transport in acute respiratory distress syndrome. Crit Care Med 1997; 25: 786–794.

65. Mascia L, Andreus PJ. Acute lung injury in head trauma patients. Intensive Care Med 1988; 24: 1115–1116.

66. Rello J, Ausina V, Ricart M et al. Nosocomial pneumonia in critically ill comatose patients: need for a differential therapeutic approach. Eur Respir J 1992; 5: 1249–1253.

67. Ewig S, Torres A, El-Ebiary M et al. Bacterial colonization patterns in mechanically ventilated patients with traumatic and medical head injury. Incidence, risk factors and association with ventilator associated pneumonia. Am J Respir Crit Care Med 1999; 159: 188–198.

68. Gruber A, Reinprect A. Pulmonary function and radiographic abnormalities related to neurological outcome after aneurismal subaracnoid hemorrhage. J Neurosurg 1998; 88: 28–37.

69. Pelosi P, Colombo G, Gamberoni C, Mascheroni C, Aspesi M, Severgnini P. Acute respiratory failure in brain injured patients. Recent Res Devel Resp Critical Care Med 2001; 1: 19–37.

70. Smith RH. The prone position. In: Martin JT. (ed) Positioning in anesthesia and surgery. Philadelphia: 1978; 32–43.

71. Lynch S, Brand L, Levy A. Changes in lung thorax compliance during orthopedic surgery. Anesthesiology 1959; 20: 278–282.

72. Safar P, Agusto-Escarraga L. Compliance in apneic anesthetized adults. Anesthesiology 1959; 20: 283–289.

73. Lumb AB, Nunn JF. Respiratory function and rib cage contribution to ventilation in body positions commonly used during anesthesia. Anesth Anal 1991; 73: 422–426.

74. Pelosi P, Croci M, Calappi E et al. The prone position during general anesthesia minimally affects respiratory mechanics while improving functional residual capacity and increasing oxygenation. Anesth Anal 1995; 80: 955–960.

75. Smith RH. One solution to the problem of the prone position for surigal procedures. Anesth Anal 1974; 53: 211–224.

76. Hedenstierna G, Santesson J. Breathing mechanics, dead space and gas exchange in extremely obese breathing spontaneously and during anesthesia with intermittent positive pressure ventilation. Acta Anaesthesiol 1976; 20: 248–254.

77. Pelosi P, Croci M, Calappi E, Mulazzi D et al. Prone positioning improves pulmonary function in obese patients during general anesthesia. Anesth Anal 1996; 83: 578–583.

78. Willems MCM, Voets AJ, Welten RJTJ. Two unusual complications of prone dependency in severe ARDS. Intensive Care Med 1998; 24: 276–281.

*J. Chastre   J.-L. Trouillet*

CHAPTER

# 7

# Antibiotics and nosocomial infection in the ICU

Over the past decade, resistance patterns of bacteria to antimicrobial agents have changed substantially in intensive care units (ICUs).[1-5] The unique nature of the ICU environment makes this part of the hospital a focus for the emergence and spread of many antibiotic-resistant pathogens. There are ample opportunities for the cross-transmission of resistant bacteria from patient to patient, and patients are commonly exposed to broad-spectrum antimicrobial agents. Therefore, rates of antibiotic resistance have increased for most bacteria associated with nosocomial infections among ICU patients, and rates are almost invariably higher among ICU patients compared with non-ICU patients.[2-5]

Infections caused by antibiotic-resistant organisms are more likely to prolong hospitalization, to increase the risk of death, and to require treatment with more toxic or more expensive antibiotics.[6] Inappropriate therapy, including therapy to which a pathogen is resistant, has been identified as an independent risk factor for increased mortality in patients with Gram-negative bacteraemia or nosocomial pneumonia, and estimates of the excess hospital costs due to antibiotic resistance range from $100 million to $30 billion annually in hospitals in the USA.[6-9] Such bacterial resistance limits the available treatment options. Clinicians feel impelled to use antibiotic regimens combining several broad-spectrum drugs in ICU patients with a clinical suspicion of infection, even if the pretest probability of the disease is low, as initial inappropriate antimicrobial therapy can be associated with poor prognosis.[10-12]

Besides its economic impact, this practice increasingly leads to the unnecessary administration of antibiotics in many ICU patients with no infection.
Paradoxically this results in the emergence of infections caused by more
antibiotic-resistant bacteria, and this in turn is associated with increased
rates of patient mortality and morbidity.

This account summarizes rates of resistance of the most common pathogens
associated with nosocomial infections among ICU patients. It reviews important aspects of antimicrobial therapy that contribute to the spread of multiresistant microorganisms in this setting, and provides recommendations for
avoiding and, when necessary, controlling antibiotic problems in ICUs.

## Rates of Antimicrobial Resistance in ICUs

Bacteria possess a remarkable number of genetic mechanisms for resistance
to antimicrobials. They can:

• undergo chromosomal mutations,

• express a latent chromosomal resistance gene,

• acquire new genetic resistance material through direct exchange of DNA
  (by conjugation), through a bacteriophage (transduction),

• acquire new genetic extrachromosomal plasmid DNA (by conjugation), or

• acquire new genetic material by acquisition of DNA via transformation.

The information encoded in this genetic material enables a bacterium to
develop resistance through three major mechanisms:

• production of an enzyme that will inactivate or destroy the antibiotic;

•  alteration of the antibiotic target site to evade action of the antibiotic; or

• prevention of antibiotic access to the target site. Importantly, it is not
  unusual for a single bacterial strain found in a hospital to possess several
  of these resistance mechanisms simultaneously.[13]

Although it has often been stated that antibiotic-resistant bacteria tend to be
less virulent than their susceptible parents, this is not always true, and even
these less virulent bacteria can be dangerous pathogens for some immunocompromised patients. Many resistant pathogens are just as virulent as the
susceptible parents in animal models and in patients. For example this was
perfectly demonstrated by Harbarth *et al.*, for methicillin-resistant *S. aureus*.[14]

The most representative data on nosocomial infection rates have been provided
by the National Nosocomial Infections Surveillance (NNIS) system in the
USA.[15,16] Table 1 shows the eight most common pathogens associated with
nosocomial infections among ICU patients from January 1989 until June 1998.

**Table 1** Eight most common pathogens associated with nosocomial infections in ICU patients, National Nosocomial Infections Surveillance System, January 1989–June 1998 (adapted from ref. 16)

| Pathogen | Relative percentage by site of infection | | | | | |
| --- | --- | --- | --- | --- | --- | --- |
| | All sites n = 235,758 | BSI n = 50,091 | PNEU n = 64,056 | UTI n = 47,502 | SSI n = 22,043 | Others n = 52,066 |
| Coagulase-negative staphylococci | 14.3 | 39.3 | 2.5 | 3.1 | 13.5 | 15.4 |
| Staphylococcus aureus | 11.4 | 10.7 | 16.8 | 1.6 | 12.3 | 13.7 |
| Pseudomonas aeruginosa | 9.9 | 3.0 | 16.1 | 10.6 | 9.2 | 8.7 |
| Enterococci spp. | 8.1 | 10.3 | 1.9 | 13.8 | 14.5 | 5.9 |
| Enterobacter spp. | 7.3 | 4.2 | 10.7 | 5.7 | 8.8 | 6.8 |
| Escherichia coli | 7.0 | 2.9 | 4.4 | 18.2 | 7.1 | 4.0 |
| Candida albicans | 6.6 | 4.9 | 4.0 | 15.3 | 4.8 | 4.3 |
| Klebsiella pneumoniae | 4.7 | 2.9 | 6.5 | 6.1 | 3.5 | 3.5 |
| Others | 30.7 | 21.8 | 37.1 | 25.6 | 26 | 37.7 |
| Total | 100 | 100 | 100 | 100 | 100 | 100 |

BSI = laboratory confirmed (primary) bloodstream infection; PNEU = pneumonia; UTI = urinary tract infection; SSI = surgical site infection.

Each of the pathogens listed has demonstrated antimicrobial resistance to at least one, if not several, of the antimicrobial agents commonly used to treat infections caused by them. During the past decade Gram-positive bacteria have gradually emerged as the most frequent cause of nosocomial disease. Methicillin-resistant strains now make up 60–90% of all isolates of coagulase-negative staphylococci; the most frequent cause of infection is related to intravascular catheters and prosthetic devices. In large teaching hospitals, the proportion of methicillin-resistant *Staphylococcus aureus* among nosocomial staphylococcal isolates increased from 8% in 1986 to 40% in 1992.[17] *S. aureus* is the most frequent cause of skin and wound infections and bacteraemia and the second most frequent cause of lower respiratory tract nosocomial infections. Strains of methicillin-resistant *S. aureus*, formerly confined to large teaching hospitals, spread by the early 1990s into smaller hospital units and into the nursing homes. The majority of methicillin-resistant *S. aureus* isolates are also resistant to most other antibiotics, necessitating the use of the glycopeptide antibiotic vancomycin for treatment.[5,18]

In response to the increasing numbers of infections with methicillin-resistant *S. aureus*, which requires treatment with vancomycin, there has also been a dramatic rise in the percentage of enterococcal isolates resistant to vancomycin – from 0.5% in 1989 to 22% in 1997 among ICU patients with nosocomial infections reported to National Nosocomial Infections Surveillance.[18] Nearly 90% of these isolates are also resistant to β-lactam antibiotics, aminoglycosides, fluoroquinolones, tetracyclines, and teicoplanin. Mortality among patients with bacteraemia and vancomycin-resistant isolates has been reported as 36.3%, compared to 16.4% among patients who have infections with vancomycin-susceptible isolates.[17]

Multiresistant Gram-negative bacilli are also increasingly associated with nosocomial infections in ICU patients, particularly ventilator-associated pneumonia and urinary catheter-associated infections. Evaluation of data from National Nosocomial Infections Surveillance hospitals shows an increase in the proportion of *Klebsiella pneumoniae* resistant to cefotaxime or ceftazidime over the past decade.[2,16,19] Other common antibiotic-resistant pathogens encountered among ICU patients include *Pseudomonas aeruginosa* resistant to imipenem and *P. aeruginosa* or *Enterobacter* spp. resistant to third-generation cephalosporins, such as cefotaxime, ceftriaxone, or ceftazidime, even if the rates of resistance among these pathogens have been relatively stable over the past decade.[2]

Several other studies conducted outside North America have confirmed these results. For example, in a study of 9,166 aerobic Gram-negative bacilli isolated from consecutive patients in 118 ICUs in five European countries, the most frequently isolated organisms were Enterobacteriaceae (59%) followed by *P. aeruginosa* (24%). A high incidence of antibiotic resistance was seen in all microorganisms but particularly among *P. aeruginosa* (up to 37% resistant to ciprofloxacin in Portuguese ICUs and 46% resistant to gentamicin in French ICUs), *Enterobacter* spp., *Acinetobacter* spp., and *Stenotrophomonas maltophilia*, also have a high resistance in Portugal as does *Klebsiella* spp. in France (figs 1–4).[20] Jarlier *et al.*, reported that susceptibility against *Klebsiella pneumoniae* in French ICUs was 36% in 1991.[21] In the United States, resistance to ceftazidime among *K. pneumoniae* in ICU isolates increased from 3.6% in 1990 to 14.4% in 1993.[22]

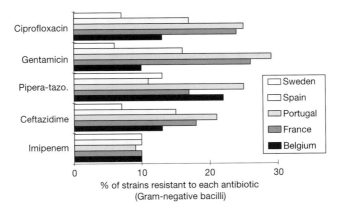

**Figure 1** Decreased antibiotic susceptibility among 9,166 aerobic Gram-negative bacilli in 118 ICUs in five European countries (adapted from ref. 20).

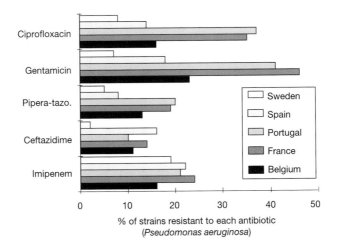

**Figure 2** Decreased antibiotic susceptibility among 2,200 *P. aeruginosa* in 118 ICUs in five European countries (adapted from ref. 20).

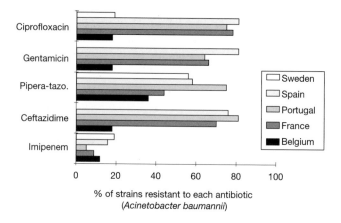

Figure 3 Decreased antibiotic susceptibility among 642 *A. baumannii* in 118 ICUs in five European countries (adapted from ref. 20).

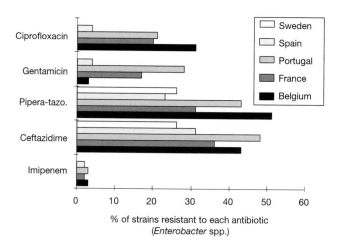

Figure 4 Decreased antibiotic susceptibility among 1,054 *Enterobacter* spp. in 118 ICUs in five European countries (adapted from ref. 20).

*Acinetobacter* spp. and *Stenotrophomonas maltophilia* have developed most resistance to all investigated drugs. Although Acinetobacter is not a very virulent Gram-negative pathogen, Acinetobacter is an increasingly infectious threat, especially for patients receiving broad-spectrum antimicrobiotic therapy. A Spanish study has shown that *Acinetobacter* spp. isolates, often acquired in burns and ICU, are multiresistant and may cause severe infections associated with a high mortality.[23] Riley *et al.*, have recently described the failure to prevent the spread of gentamicin-resistant *Acinetobacter baumannii* in an Australian ICU despite measures to control infection.[24]

Resistance of aerobic Gram-negative bacilli to third-generation cephalosporins was also found to be an emerging problem in 396 ICUs in North America between 1990 and 1993.[22] Amikacin and imipenem were the most active agents against the 33,869 nonduplicate isolates (those recovered only once) tested, with an overall antimicrobial susceptibility rate of 92% and 91%, respectively. However, from 1990 to 1993 increases in rates of resistance to ceftazidime among isolates of *K. pneumoniae* (from 3.6% to 14.4%; $P < 0.01$) and *Enterobacter* species (from 30.8% to 38.3%; $P = 0.0004$) were noted (fig. 5). Ceftazidime-resistant bacteria were also frequently cross-resistant to other antimicrobial classes (figs 6–8). Finally, many factors correlated with the

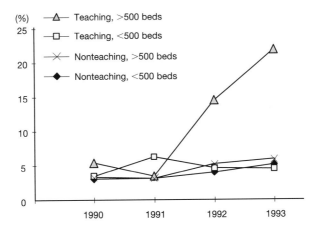

**Figure 5** Ceftazidime-resistance rates by hospital type and year for *K. pneumoniae* (adapted from ref. 22).

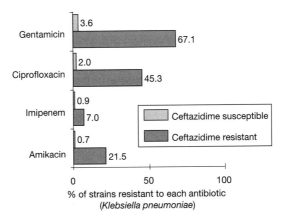

**Figure 6** Cross-resistance rates to other antimicrobial classes of ceftazidime-resistant and ceftazidime-susceptible *K. pneumoniae* (adapted from ref. 22).

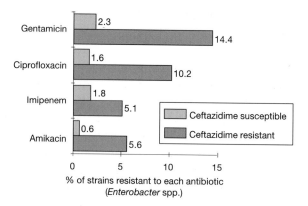

**Figure 7** Cross-resistance rates to other antimicrobial classes of ceftazidime-resistant and ceftazidime-susceptible *Enterobacter* species (adapted from ref. 22).

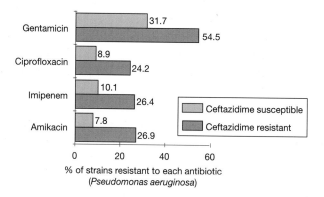

**Figure 8** Cross-resistance rates to other antimicrobial classes of ceftazidime-resistant and ceftazidime-susceptible *Pseudomonas aeruginosa* (adapted from ref. 22).

recovery of antibiotic-resistant bacteria, including the number of beds in the hospital, the teaching status of the hospital, prior exposure to antimicrobials, and specific body sites from which the isolates were recovered.

## Antimicrobial Therapy as a Factor Promoting Antimicrobial Resistance in the ICU

The most important factor in the development of bacterial resistance is the use of antimicrobial agents. Meyer *et al.*, reported the largest outbreak of ceftazidime-resistant Klebsiella infections yet to occur in a general hospital in North America.[25] This outbreak coincided with increasing use of ceftazidime and declined after restricting the use of this antimicrobial agent, implying a causal relationship.

Other studies have confirmed that nosocomial infections in ICU patients presumably occur as a consequence of selection of more resistant bacterial pathogens such as *Acinetobacter* or *Pseudomonas* spp. during treatment with antibiotics. Fagon *et al.*, conducted a study of 567 consecutive patients receiving mechanical ventilation. Eighty-nine percent of patients who developed pneumonia due to *Pseudomonas* or *Acinetobacter* species had been receiving antimicrobial therapy prior to the onset of pneumonia. Of the patients who developed pneumonia who had not been receiving antibiotics only 17% had pneumonia due to multiresistant *Pseudomonas* or *Acinetobacter* spp. ($P < 0.02$).[26] Rello *et al.*, also evaluated the impact of recent antibiotics on the aetiology of nosocomial pneumonia in a large series of patients who developed ventilator-associated pneumonia.[27] The most striking finding was that the incidence of pneumonia caused by *P. aeruginosa* was significantly higher in patients who had received prior antibiotic treatment. The incidence of pneumonia caused by Gram-positive cocci or *H. influenzae* was significantly lower. Stepwise logistic regression analysis could only identify prior antibiotic use as a significant factor increasing the risk of death from pneumonia (Odds ratio = 9.2).

Our own experience is based on a prospective study.[28] In 135 consecutive ventilator-associated pneumonia in our ICU we documented the responsible bacteria specimens. The distribution of infecting pathogens was influenced by previous duration of mechanical ventilation and prior antibiotic use (table 2).[28] Early-onset pneumonias in patients who had not already received antibiotic treatment were mainly caused by sensitive Enterobacteriaceae, *Haemophilus* species, methicillin-sensitive *S. aureus* and *Streptococcus pneumoniae*. However early-onset pneumonias in patients who had already received antibiotics were commonly caused by nonfermenting Gram-negative bacilli such as *P. aeruginosa*, in addition to streptococci and *Haemophilus* spp. Late-onset pneumonias which occurred in those who had not received antibiotics in the 15 days before the onset of infection were caused by streptococci, methicillin-sensitive *S. aureus*, and Enterobacteriaceae (some of them being, however, multiresistant). Late-onset pneumonias in patients having received prior antibiotic treatment were commonly caused by multiresistant pathogens, such as *P. aeruginosa*, *A. baumannii* and methicillin-resistant *S. aureus*. When all these variables were entered into a logistic regression model, recent prior use of antibiotics was identified as the prime variable that was associated with the occurrence of ventilator-associated pneumonia, with an OR = 13.5 (95% CI: 3.3–55.0).

**Table 2** Bacteriology of 135 ventilator-associated pneumonia according to duration of mechanical ventilation and prior antimicrobial therapy (adapted from ref. 28)

| Microorganisms | Percentage of infection caused by each organism | | | |
|---|---|---|---|---|
| | MV < 7 d ABs = no | MV < 7 d ABs = yes | MV ≥ 7 d Abs = no | MV ≥ 7 d ABs = yes |
| **Multiresistant bacteria** | | | | |
| P. aeruginosa | 0 | 20 | 6 | 22 |
| A. baumannii | 0 | 5 | 3 | 13 |
| Stenotrophomonas maltophilia | 0 | 0 | 0 | 4 |
| MRSA | 0 | 5 | 3 | 20 |
| **Other bacteria** | | | | |
| Enterobacteriaceae | 24 | 20 | 22 | 15 |
| Haemophilus | 19 | 10 | 3 | 3 |
| MSSA | 15 | 0 | 22 | 5 |
| Streptococcus pneumoniae | 7 | 0 | 0 | 0 |
| Other streptococci | 17 | 25 | 22 | 9 |
| Neisseria spp. | 12 | 10 | 12 | 2 |
| Other pathogens | 5 | 5 | 6 | 8 |

MRSA = methicillin-resistant S. aureus; MSSA = methicillin-sensitive S. aureus

## Optimizing Use of Antimicrobial Agents

As already indicated patients infected with resistant strains of bacteria are more likely than control patients to have previously received prior antimicrobials. Hospital areas that have the highest prevalence of resistance also have the highest rates of antibiotic use.[3] For these reasons, programs to prevent or control the development of resistant organisms should focus on the overuse or inappropriate use of antibiotics. Surprisingly, only about 30% of all antibiotics in hospitals are used in a situation where a positive bacterial culture has been established and the appropriate antibiotic selectivity is known.[29,30]

The objective is that only those patients who have developed infection, should be treated with the most effective, least toxic, and least costly antibiotic. Five possible strategies to optimize the use of antimicrobial agents in the ICU are possible:

- development of guidelines and treatment algorithms, designed to permit optimal use;
- selective removal or control of use of specific antibiotics or classes of antibiotics;
- rotational or cyclic antibiotic use;
- use of combination antimicrobial therapy to reduce the emergence of resistance;
- shortening the duration of antimicrobial therapy.

## Development of guidelines and treatment algorithms designed to permit optimal use

Using such a strategy, prescribers are encouraged to follow strict guidelines when confronted with an infectious disease or even its suspicion and to seek guidance from specialists. So far, such programs have not been particularly successful, however, modern electronic communications assist physician-pharmacy interactions. Evans *et al.*, have developed a computerized decision-support program linked to computer-based patient records. These assist physicians in the use of anti-infective agents and thus improve the quality of care.[31] This program presents epidemiological information, together with detailed antibiotic therapy recommendations and warnings. In a before-and-after study, all 545 patients admitted during the intervention period were cared for with the aid of the antiinfectives-management program. Historical control outcomes from these patients were compared with 1,136 patients who had been admitted to the same unit in the 2 years before the intervention period. The use of the programme led to significant reductions in adverse drug reactions, total hospital cost and length of stay.[31]

Another example of the benefits associated with the use of a specific algorithm for managing ICU patients with a clinical suspicion of infection is the study by Fagon *et al.*[32] In their randomized study, two diagnostic strategies were compared prospectively in 413 patients who were suspected of having ventilator-associated pneumonia. In a non-invasive group (n = 209), antibiotic therapy was on the basis of the presence of bacteria in the Gramstain from endotracheal aspirates. Therapy was adjusted or discontinued according to the results of semiquantitative cultures. In cases of severe sepsis, therapy was started without the laboratory result. This resembles clinical practice in most ICUs, 91% of patients received empirical therapy for suspected ventilator-associated pneumonia and only 7% did not. In the invasively investigated group, bronchiolar lavage was performed with direct microscopic examination of the fluid and cells recovered. Therapy was then commenced if the results were positive. A definitive diagnosis based on quantitative, culture results of the specimens obtained using this technique was awaited before starting, adjusting, or discontinuing therapy. In contrast to the empirical approach using this strategy 44% of patients (90/204) did not receive antibiotics. Furthermore, compared with patients who received clinical management, there was a reduction in mortality at day 14 (16% and 25%; $P = 0.022$), a reduction in mean Sepsis-related Organ Failure Assessment scores at day 3 and day 7 ($P = 0.03$), and an increase in the number of antibiotic-free days, $5 \pm 5$ and $2 \pm 3$; $P < 0.001$. These differences were maintained at 28 days ($11 \pm 9$ compared with $7 \pm 7$; $P < 0.001$).

Thus, use of bronchoscopic techniques for the diagnosis of ventilator-associated pneumonia reduces antibiotic use and improves outcome. Pertinently, in that study, invasive-group patients had 22 infections at other sites that required specific therapeutic measures versus only 5 in the clinical group. This difference suggests that reliance on non-invasive techniques and the consequent overestimation of VAP may mean that diagnoses of non-pulmonary infections are missed. Many hospitalized patients with negative bronchoscopic specimen cultures have other potential sites of infection that can more readily be identified in the absence of antibiotic interference.[33] Delaying diagnosis or definitive treatment of the true infection site may lead to prolonged antibiotic therapy, more antibiotic-associated complications and induction of additional organ dysfunctions.[34]

## Selective removal or control of use of specific antimicrobial agents

The second method of antimicrobial control, selective removal or control of use of specific agents or classes of agents, has been employed in many studies.[13] Most have shown significant reductions in antibiotic resistance, but a return of resistance when restriction is lifted. For example, decreased use of broad-spectrum cephalosporins has been associated with decreased antibiotic resistance among Gram-negative bacilli. Decreased use of third-generation cephalosporins and vancomycin has been associated with a decreased incidence of vancomycin-resistant enterococcus VRE.[13] White *et al.*, evaluated the policy that required prior authorization for selected parenteral antibiotics.[35] Total parenteral antibiotic expenditures decreased by 32%. Sensitivities to all β-lactam and quinolone antibiotics increased, particularly sensitivities in the isolates recovered in ICUs and in other inpatient sites, with little change in sensitivities to isolates recovered from outpatient sites. For patients with bacteraemia caused by Gram-negative bacilli, the restrictions did not change overall survival, time from positive blood culture to the prescription of an appropriate antibiotic or time to discharge from hospital.[35]

In a recent study in two identical neonatal ICUs, De Man *et al.*, showed that by modifying the antibiotic therapy in septicaemic patients to penicillin and tobramycin and by not using broad-spectrum betalactam antibiotics (amoxycillin and cefotaxime) they were able to reduce the relative risk for colonization with strains of bacteria that were resistant to the empirical therapy per 1,000 at risk patient days by 18 times.[36]

Therefore, policies regarding the empirical use of antibiotics can have an effect on control of antimicrobial resistance. The indiscriminate use of antimicrobial agents in ICU patients may have immediate as well as long-term consequences, which contribute to the emergence of multiresistant pathogens and increasing the risk of severe superinfections. This risk is not limited to an individual patient but may raise the risk of multidrug-resistance to patients throughout the entire hospital.[30,37]

## Cyclic use of antibiotics

Rotating antibiotic therapy might reduce the emergence of resistance and the associated morbidity. However, to date this has not been fully tested in ICU patients.[38] In one study during which ciprofloxacin was used in place of ceftazidime for the empirical treatment of suspected Gram-negative bacilli infections, ventilator-associated pneumonia occurred significantly less frequently during the period after compared with the period before (7 vs. 12%; $P = 0.03$) but there were no outcome differences noted between the two groups of patients.[39]

A similar reduction in the rates of infection caused by multiple classes of resistant bacteria was recently demonstrated by Raymond *et al.*, when they tested antibiotic rotation in 1,456 consecutive admissions to the ICU.[40] Furthermore, outcome analysis revealed a significant reduction of the mortality associated with infection (2.9 deaths/100 admissions vs. 9.6 deaths/100 admissions, $P < 0.0001$) during antibiotic rotation. Further studies in this area are necessary to understand these effects more fully. Whether antibiotic rotation can maintain lower levels of antimicrobial resistance and mortality over time remains to be seen.

## Use of combination antimicrobial therapy

Use of combination antimicrobial therapy to reduce emergence of resistance is theoretically attractive and is the basis for current treatment of tuberculosis. However, in studies conducted in the ICU, there is no benefit to be gained by combination therapy.[34]

β-lactam-aminoglycoside combinations have been reassessed in the treatment of infections. A prospective, randomized, controlled study compared imipenem alone to imipenem plus netilmicin as the empirical regimen for nosocomial pneumonia and other severe infections in non-neutropenic patients.[41] Two hundred and eighty patients enrolled in the study. Forty eight percent had pneumonia and required mechanical ventilation. The addition of an aminoglycoside to imipenem did not significantly improve the outcome. This combination therapy was unable to prevent the colonization of resistant strains *P. aeruginosa* or prevent the emergence of resistant strains. Moreover the addition of the aminoglycoside increased the incidence of nephrotoxicity.

Such results have been seen in another study using cephalosporins alone or in combination with amikacin.[42]

Further trials are needed to clarify all these uncertainties because those studies included non-homogeneous populations of patients with different types of infections. In the meantime, it is probably safer to use a β-lactam antibiotic in combination with an aminoglycoside or a quinolone for patients with severe nosocomial infection, at least for the first days of therapy, while culture results are pending. Possibly monodrug therapies for nosocomial infection are best reserved for infections in which *P. aeruginosa* or other multiresistant microorganisms, such as *Klebsiella, Enterobacter, Citrobacter, Serratia* or *Acinetobacter* spp. have been excluded as the etiologic agents.

### Duration of therapy

As already mentioned, there is a relationship between the use of antibiotic (and also its duration) and the emergence of resistant bacteria. In a recent study in which a total of 102 consecutive patients with ventilator-associated pneumonia were prospectively evaluated before and after the application of a clinical guideline which restricted the total duration of antimicrobial therapy to 7 days, no statistically significant differences in hospital mortality and hospital lengths of stay were found between the two study groups. However, patients in the before group for whom the mean duration of treatment was 14.8 days – were more likely to develop a second episode of ventilator-associated pneumonia compared with those in the group in which antibiotics were restricted to 7 days.[43]

Nevertheless, a regimen of insufficient duration can be the source of therapeutic failure or relapse defined as the reappearance of signs of infection and isolation of the same pathogen(s) whether or not they have acquired resistance. The risk is probably small for bacteria considered susceptible but might be high for certain strains, especially *P. aeruginosa* and methicillin-resistant *S. aureus*, which are particularly difficult to eradicate. This situation is further aggravated in immunocompromised patients. Thus, at present, a short-term regimen is rarely prescribed, despite the major advantages it might have in terms of bacterial ecology, the prevention of the emergence of multiresistant bacteria and, lower costs. Lowering the quantity of antibiotics administered to ICU patients is a primary objective of every strategy aimed to prevent the emergence and dissemination of such bacteria.

### Conclusion

The rapid emergence and dissemination of antimicrobial-resistant microorganisms in hospitals is a major worldwide problem. The root causes of this problem are multifactorial, but the core issues are clear. The emergence of antimicrobiotic resistance is highly correlated with selective pressures that results from inappropriate use of antimicrobiotics. Despite the emergence of control strategies, interventions are unlikely to be successful unless strategic objectives are formulated to control the resistant organisms. The appropriate use of antimicrobiotic includes not only the limitation of use of inappropriate agents but also the appropriate selection, dosing, and duration of antimicrobial therapy to achieve optimal efficacy in managing infections.

## *References*

1. Jarvis WR. Preventing the emergence of multidrug-resistant microorganisms through antimicrobial use controls: the complexity of the problem. Infect Control Hosp Epidemiol 1996; 17: 490–495.
2. Fridkin SK, Gaynes RP. Antimicrobial resistance in intensive care units. Clin Chest Med 1999; 20: 303–316, viii.
3. Fridkin SK, Steward CD, Edwards JR, Pryor ER, McGowan Jr JE, Archibald LK, Gaynes RP, Tenover FC. Surveillance of antimicrobial use and antimicrobial resistance in United States hospitals: project ICARE phase 2. Project Intensive Care Antimicrobial Resistance Epidemiology (ICARE) hospitals. Clin Infect Dis 1999; 29: 245–252.
4. Weber DJ, Raasch R, Rutala WA. Nosocomial infections in the ICU: the growing importance of antibiotic-resistant pathogens. Chest 1999; 115: 34S–41S.
5. Flaherty JP, Weinstein RA. Nosocomial infection caused by antibiotic-resistant organisms in the intensive-care unit. Infect Control Hosp Epidemiol 1996; 17: 236–248.
6. Holmberg SD, Solomon SL, Blake PA. Health and economic impacts of antimicrobial resistance. Rev Infect Dis 1987; 9: 1065–1078.
7. Bisbe J, Gatell JM, Puig J, Mallolas J, Martinez JA, Jimenez de Anta MT, Soriano E. Pseudomonas aeruginosa bacteremia: univariate and multivariate analyses of factors influencing the prognosis in 133 episodes. Rev Infect Dis 1988; 10: 629–635.
8. Saito H, Elting L, Bodey GP, Berkey P. Serratia bacteremia: review of 118 cases. Rev Infect Dis 1989; 11: 912–920.
9. Torres A, Aznar R, Gatell JM, Jimenez P, Gonzalez J, Ferrer A, Celis R, Rodriguez-Roisin R. Incidence, risk, and prognosis factors of nosocomial pneumonia in mechanically ventilated patients. Am Rev Respir Dis 1990; 142: 523–528.
10. Alvarez-Lerma F. Modification of empiric antibiotic treatment in patients with pneumonia acquired in the intensive care unit. ICU-acquired pneumonia study group. Intensive Care Med 1996; 22: 387–394.
11. Kollef MH, Ward S. The influence of mini-BAL cultures on patient outcomes: implications for the antibiotic management of ventilator-associated pneumonia. Chest 1998; 113: 412–420.
12. Rello J, Gallego M, Mariscal D, Sonora R, Valles J. The value of routine microbial investigation in ventilator-associated pneumonia. Am J Respir Crit Care Med 1997; 156: 196–200.
13. Shlaes DM, Gerding DN, John Jr JF, Craig WA, Bornstein DL, Duncan RA, Eckman MR, Farrer WE, Greene WH, Lorian V *et al*. Society for healthcare

epidemiology of America and infectious diseases society of America joint committee on the prevention of antimicrobial resistance: guidelines for the prevention of antimicrobial resistance in hospitals. Clin Infect Dis 1997; 25: 584–599.

14. Harbarth S, Rutschmann O, Sudre P, Pittet D. Impact of methicillin resistance on the outcome of patients with bacteremia caused by Staphylococcus aureus. Arch Intern Med 1998; 158: 182–189.

15. Richards MJ, Edwards JR, Culver DH, Gaynes RP. Nosocomial infections in medical intensive care units in the United States. National Nosocomial Infections Surveillance System. Crit Care Med 1999; 27: 887–892.

16. National Nosocomial Infections Surveillance (NNIS) System report, data summary from January 1990–May 1999, issued June 1999. Am J Infect Control 1999; 27: 520–532.

17. Emori TG, Gaynes RP. An overview of nosocomial infections, including the role of the microbiology laboratory. Clin Microbiol Rev 1993; 6: 428–442.

18. Fridkin SK. Increasing prevalence of antimicrobial resistance in intensive care units. Crit Care Med 2001; 29: N64–N68.

19. Richards MJ, Edwards JR, Culver DH, Gaynes RP. Nosocomial infections in medical intensive care units in the United States. National nosocomial infections surveillance system. Crit Care Med 1999; 27: 887–892.

20. Hanberger H, Garcia-Rodriguez JA, Gobernado M, Goossens H, Nilsson LE, Struelens MJ. Antibiotic susceptibility among aerobic gram-negative bacilli in intensive care units in 5 European countries. Jama 1999; 281: 67–71.

21. Jarlier V, Fosse T, Philippon A. Antibiotic susceptibility in aerobic gram-negative bacilli isolated in intensive care units in 39 French teaching hospitals. Intensive Care Med 1996; 22: 1057–1065.

22. Itokazu GS, Quinn JP, Bell-Dixon C, Kahan FM, Weinstein RA. Antimicrobial resistance rates among aerobic gram-negative bacilli recovered from patients in intensive care units: evaluation of a national postmarketing surveillance program. Clin Infect Dis 1996; 23: 779–784.

23. Cisneros JM, Reyes MJ, Pachon J, Becerril B, Caballero FJ, Garcia-Garmendia JL, Ortiz C, Cobacho AR. Bacteremia due to Acinetobacter baumannii: epidemiology, clinical findings, and prognostic features. Clin Infect Dis 1996; 22: 1026–1032.

24. Riley TV, Webb SA, Cadwallader H, Briggs BD, Christiansen L, Bowman RA. Outbreak of gentamicin-resistant Acinetobacter baumannii in an intensive care unit: clinical, epidemiological and microbiological features. Pathology 1996; 28: 359–363.

25. Meyer KS, Urban C, Eagan JA, Berger BJ, Rahal JJ. Nosocomial outbreak of Klebsiella infection resistant to late-generation cephalosporins. Ann Intern Med 1993; 119: 353–358.

26. Fagon JY, Chastre J, Domart Y, Trouillet JL, Pierre J, Darne C, Gibert C. Nosocomial pneumonia in patients receiving continuous mechanical ventilation. Prospective analysis of 52 episodes with use of a protected specimen brush and quantitative culture techniques. Am Rev Respir Dis 1989; 139: 877–884.

27. Rello J, Ausina V, Ricart M, Castella J, Prats G. Impact of previous antimicrobial therapy on the etiology and outcome of ventilator-associated pneumonia. Chest 1993; 104: 1230–1235.

28. Trouillet JL, Chastre J, Vuagnat A, Joly-Guillou ML, Combaux D, Dombret MC, Gibert C. Ventilator-associated pneumonia caused by potentially drug-resistant bacteria. Am J Respir Crit Care Med 1998; 157: 531–539.

29. Bergmans DC, Bonten MJ, Gaillard CA, van Tiel FH, van der Geest S, de Leeuw PW, Stobberingh EE. Indications for antibiotic use in ICU patients: a one-year prospective surveillance. J Antimicrob Chemother 1997; 39: 527–535.

30. Kollef MH, Fraser VJ. Antibiotic resistance in the intensive care unit. Ann Intern Med 2001; 134: 298–314.

31. Evans RS, Pestotnik SL, Classen DC, Clemmer TP, Weaver LK, Orme Jr JF, Lloyd JF, Burke JP. A computer-assisted management program for antibiotics and other antiinfective agents. N Engl J Med 1998; 338: 232–238.

32. Fagon JY, Chastre J, Wolff M, Gervais C, Parer-Aubas S, Stephan F, Similowski T, Mercat A, Diehl JL, Sollet JP *et al.* Invasive and noninvasive strategies for management of suspected ventilator-associated pneumonia. A randomized trial. Ann Intern Med 2000; 132: 621–630.

33. Meduri GU, Mauldin GL, Wunderink RG, Leeper Jr KV, Jones CB, Tolley E, Mayhall G. Causes of fever and pulmonary densities in patients with clinical manifestations of ventilator-associated pneumonia. Chest 1994; 106: 221–235.

34. Chastre J, Fagon JY. Pneumonia in the ventilator-dependent patient. In: Tobin MJ. (ed) Principles and Practice of Mechanical Ventilation. New York: McGraw-Hill, 1994; 857–890.

35. White Jr AC, Atmar RL, Wilson J, Cate TR, Stager CE, Greenberg SB. Effects of requiring prior authorization for selected antimicrobials: expenditures, susceptibilities, and clinical outcomes. Clin Infect Dis 1997; 25: 230–239.

36. de Man P, Verhoeven BA, Verbrugh HA, Vos MC, van den Anker JN. An antibiotic policy to prevent emergence of resistant bacilli. Lancet 2000; 355: 973–978.

37. Neu HC. The crisis in antibiotic resistance. Science 1992; 257: 1064–1073.

38. Gruson D, Hilbert G, Vargas F, Valentino R, Bebear C, Allery A, Gbikpi-Benissan G, Cardinaud JP. Rotation and restricted use of antibiotics in a medical intensive care unit. Impact on the incidence of ventilator-associated pneumonia caused by antibiotic-resistant gram-negative bacteria. Am J Respir Crit Care Med 2000; 162: 837–843.

39. Kollef MH, Vlasnik J, Sharpless L, Pasque C, Murphy D, Fraser V. Scheduled change of antibiotic classes: a strategy to decrease the incidence of ventilator-associated pneumonia. Am J Respir Crit Care Med 1997; 156: 1040–1048.

40. Raymond DP, Pelletier SJ, Crabtree TD, Gleason TG, Hamm LL, Pruett TL, Sawyer RG. Impact of a rotating empiric antibiotic schedule on infectious mortality in an intensive care unit. Crit Care Med 2001; 29: 1101–1108.

41. Cometta A, Baumgartner JD, Lew D, Zimmerli W, Pittet D, Chopart P, Schaad U, Herter C, Eggimann P, Huber O *et al.* Prospective randomized comparison of imipenem monotherapy with imipenem plus netilmicin for treatment of severe infections in nonneutropenic patients. Antimicrob Agents Chemother 1994; 38: 1309–1313.

42. Solberg CO, Sjursen H. Safety and efficacy of meropenem in patients with septicaemia: a randomised comparison with ceftazidime, alone or combined with amikacin. J Antimicrob Chemother 1995;36 Suppl A:157–166.

43. Ibrahim EH, Ward S, Sherman G, Schaiff R, Fraser VJ, Kollef MH. Experience with a clinical guideline for the treatment of ventilator-associated pneumonia. Crit Care Med 2001; 29: 1109–1115.

*A.B. Petrenko   T. Yamakura*
*H. Baba   K. Shimoji*

# Neuropathic pain

According to the International Association for the Study of Pain (IASP) pain terminology, neuropathic pain is defined as pain initiated or caused by a primary lesion or dysfunction in the nervous system.[1] This includes pain associated with damage to peripheral nerves (peripheral neuropathic pain), spinal roots (radiculopathic pain) and to the central nervous system (CNS) (central pain). Examples of lesions that affect the nervous system at each level of neural axis are shown in table 1. Neuropathic pain is a complex entity; it is a formidable syndrome that complicates a variety of disease states. Amputation, cancer, diabetes, metabolic disorders, infection and stroke may all result in neuropathic pain. Such pain is often severe, delayed in onset after the noxious event, can be shooting, lancinating, or burning in quality, and manifests even in the absence of an ongoing primary source for the pain. An area of sensory loss, either partial or complete, is an essential component of neuropathic pain; it can involve all sensory modalities, but damage to the classical thermonociceptive pathways, such as peripheral small diameter sensory fibers and the spinothalamic tract anywhere along its course from the dorsal horn to cerebral cortex, is prerequisite for neuropathic pain to be manifest clinically. Most neuropathic pain conditions involve the peripheral nervous system (PNS), at least in the early stages. Thus, peripheral neuropathic pain is the primary focus of attention of this chapter. Central pain arising from the damage to the CNS is less common and is not discussed here. Neuropathic pain responds poorly to traditional therapeutic approaches and represents an area of an unmet clinical need. It can persist for years and is lifelong in some patients. This often results in physical, occupational and social disability, psychological distress/depression and increased use of healthcare resources.

**Table 1** Causes of neuropathic pain according to disease and location of the lesion

| Peripheral nerve | Spinal cord | Brain |
|---|---|---|
| Neuropathies | Traumatic injury | Stroke |
| Amputations | Vascular lesions | Multiple sclerosis |
| Traumatic injury | Multiple sclerosis | Syringobulbia |
| Entrapments | Avulsion injuries | Parkinson's disease |
| Herpes zoster | Syringomyelia | Epilepsy |
| Neoplastic invasion | Prolapsed disk | Tumours |
| Nerve root disorders | Arachnoiditis Tumours | Abscesses |

Why can treatment of neuropathic pain be so frustrating? According to the 'failsafe' theory,[2] any insult to the nervous system, be it physical injury or any disorder, initiates adaptive responses that ensure adequacy of neurotransmission, regardless of whether such transmission ultimately evokes normal or abnormal sensations. Such adaptive responses will act to oppose and surmount any pharmacological intervention aimed to diminish pain through attenuation of signal conduction.

Why should a damaged sensory nerve cause pain? Intuitively nerve injury should deaden or dull sensation, not amplify it! Basic research with animal and human models of neuropathic pain has begun to provide some clues to the problem. To date, a number of distinct phenotypic and related functional changes have been documented to take place in the nervous system as a result of an insult. For example, axotomy-induced changes have been reported for essentially all of the functional classes of molecules known to be involved in pain processing: neurotransmitters, receptors, structural and regulatory proteins, ion channels etc. These changes are not necessarily unidirectional; in some cases gene expression in the associated dorsal root ganglia is increased (up-regulated), in others decreased (down-regulated). Moreover, occasionally these changes occur in some neuronal types in the dorsal root ganglia, but not in the others. Not surprisingly, almost any consistent axotomy-induced change in a molecule, a structure, or a neurophysiological process anywhere in the pain-relaying system can form a rational basis for a pain theory. However, it is very unlikely that all of these theories will prove to describe processes that have significant impact on neuropathic pain. The 'ectopic pacemaker' theory[3] might offer a cogent explanation for the paradox of neuropathic pain. It states that electrical hyperexcitability of primary afferent neurons following axonal injury and demyelination is an essential substrate of neuropathic pain. If we accept this theory, many of the apparent differences between neuropathic syndromes will turn out to reflect subtleties of the ectopic firing process. For example, sympathetic related pain conditions may be distinguished by excess ectopic adrenosensitivity, while trigeminal neuralgia is distinguished by excess ectopic cross-excitation.

Neuropathic pain is thought to result when sensory neurons generate impulses at abnormal (ectopic) locations, for example at sites of nerve injury or demyelination. In the PNS, in addition to firing spontaneously, these ectopic pacemaker sites are often excited by mechanical forces applied to them during movement. The result is spontaneous and movement-evoked pain. Damage to the CNS, such as stroke or trauma, may cause ectopic firing of central origin, or render brain circuits hyperexcitable, abnormally amplifying input from the periphery. In the light of the ectopic pacemaker theory, ectopic afferent firing is a primary source of spontaneous pain; it initiates and sustains central sensitization that manifests clinically as neuropathic hypersensitivity. This has important implications for therapy and, thus, motivates further research into the underlying mechanisms.

In summary, today it is clear that numerous changes, both central and peripheral, occur following nerve injury. The most important pathophysiological mechanisms known to play a role in neuropathic pain are summarized in table 2. It is beyond the scope of this review to give a detailed description of all of them. However, two functionally important and interrelated phenomena – ectopic hyperexcitability and central sensitization – and their cellular and molecular mechanisms will be briefly discussed here. The relationship between sympathetic activity and the pain is increasingly uncertain[4] and is presented in the section on the complex regional pain syndrome (CRPS). The diagrammatic representation in figure 1 sets out some components of neuropathic pain, which are currently thought to be of importance in pathogenesis.

**Table 2** Mechanisms of neuropathic pain

| Peripheral | Spinal | Brain |
|---|---|---|
| Sensitization and collateral sprouting of spared afferents in partially denervated skin | Central sensitization Increased activity of excitatory systems | Neuronal hyperexcitability in pain-relaying structures Abnormal pain modulation |
| Abnormal electrogenesis in damaged nerves | Reduced segmental inhibition | • Increased facilitation |
| • Spontaneous ectopic firing | Structural reorganization | • Reduced inhibition |
| • Ectopic hyperexcitability | | Structural reorganization |
| Ephaptic cross-talk | | |
| Abnormal adrenosensitivity | | |
| • Up-regulation of adrenoreceptors | | |
| • Sympathetic-sensory coupling | | |

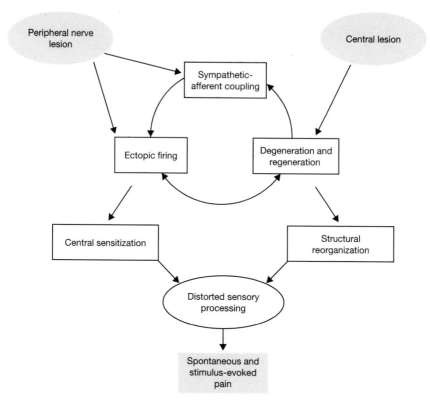

**Figure 1** Simplified diagram illustrating pathogenesis of neuropathic pain. Neuronal injury switches on a survival program that sustains nociceptive transmission and renders neuropathic pain so difficult to treat. Note the vicious circle. The ectopic hyperexcitability is an important component of this circle.

## Pathophysiology

### Ectopic hyperexcitability and abnormal sodium channels

Spontaneous and evoked hyperexcitability of the peripheral nerve after injury is considered to be a principal feature of the underlying pathophysiology associated with neuropathic pain syndromes. Voltage-gated sodium channels, which produce the inward membrane current necessary for regenerative action potential production within the mammalian nervous system, are expressed in primary sensory neurons and have emerged as important targets in the study of the molecular pathophysiology of sensory neuron hyperexcitability producing pain.[5]

It is now clear that nearly a dozen molecularly distinct voltage-gated sodium channels are encoded within mammals by different genes. Dorsal root ganglion neurons, which are known to display two main types of sodium currents – termed tetrodotoxin-sensitive and tetrodotoxin-resistant and identified on the basis of their kinetics and sensitivity to the neurotoxin, tetrodotoxin – express several sodium channel transcripts.[6]

In addition to α-I and Na6 channels, also expressed at high levels by other neuronal cell types within the CNS, dorsal root ganglion neurons are unique in expressing at least three sodium channel transcripts that are not expressed at significant levels in other neuronal cell types:

- PN1/hNE, which is present in virtually all dorsal root ganglion neurons, encodes a tetrodotoxin-sensitive channel;

- SNS/PN3, expressed preferentially in small dorsal root ganglion and trigeminal neurons, produces a sodium current that is relatively resistant to tetrodotoxin;

- NaN, expressed preferentially in small and trigeminal neurons, encodes a tetrodotoxin-resistant sodium channel.

Early studies demonstrated that, after injury to their axons, sensory neurons display changes in excitability, suggesting increased sodium channel expression over the cell body and the dendrites.[7] Abnormal sodium channel accumulation in neuroma endings also has been observed,[8–10] and both electrophysiological and computer simulation studies have suggested that abnormal increases in sodium conductance can lead to inappropriate, repetitive firing.[11–13] There is substantial evidence indicating that the abnormal excitability of dorsal root ganglion neurons, after axonal injury, is associated with an increased density of sodium channels.[13,14] Subsequent observations revealed that, in addition to production of excess channels, there is a switch in the type of channels produced after axonal injury,[15] resulting in a significant up-regulation of expression of the previously silent α-III sodium channel gene in dorsal root ganglion neurons after axotomy. This finding was followed by demonstration of down-regulation of the SNS/PN3 gene expression, which can persist as long as 210 days after axotomy,[16] and of down-regulation of the NaN gene.[17]

In line with this – as demonstrated in patch-clamp studies – there is a loss of tetrodotoxin-resistant sodium currents in dorsal root ganglion neurons after axonal transection.[18] In addition, there is a switch in the properties of the tetrodotoxin-sensitive sodium currents in these cells after axotomy, with the emergence of a rapidly repriming current (i.e. a current that recovers rapidly from inactivation).[19] It has been suggested that the expression of α-III sodium channel underlies the emergence of the rapidly repriming sodium current.[19] Notably, abnormal accumulations of type III sodium channel protein can be detected close to the tips of injured axons within the experimental neuromas,[20] a site where aberrant hyperexcitability has been demonstrated.

Similar, though less extensive, changes occur in sodium channel gene expression in the chronic constriction injury model of neuropathic pain.[21] As would be expected in view of the changes in sodium channel mRNA, tetrodotoxin-resistant sodium currents are attenuated and there is more rapid repriming of tetrodotoxin-sensitive currents in dorsal root ganglion neurons in the chronic constriction injury model.[21]

Increased membrane density of sodium channels and resultant lowered threshold for action potential generation, coexpression of abnormal combinations of several types of channels with overlapping steady-state activation and inactivation curves and their resultant cross-activation, together with the emergence of a rapidly repriming tetrodotoxin-sensitive sodium current confer instability on the neuronal membrane, and, consequently, precipitate ectopic impulse generation.[22]

Delineation of the precise role(s) of each sodium channel subtype in the pathophysiology of pain is currently underway. For example, a potentially specialized, pathophysiological role for tetrodotoxin-resistant SNS/PN3 has been supported by alterations in channel distribution observed in rats with spinal nerve (L5/L6) ligation.[23] The increased number of large-diameter cells expressing PN3 protein after SNL may account, in part, for the observed tactile allodynia. Indeed, evidence shows that spinal administration of an antisense oligodeoxynucleotide to a unique sequence of SNS/PN3 produces a selective and reversible block of channel protein expression and prevents the behavioural thermal hyperalgesia and tactile allodynia evoked by this type of injury. In contrast, NaN/SNS2, another tetrodotoxin-resistant sodium channel recently cloned from rat dorsal root ganglion,[17,24] does not appear to contribute to the maintenance of nerve injury-induced changes in nociceptive thresholds.[23]

These observations suggest that the primary symptoms of neuropathic pain may be significantly attenuated by interfering with the expression and function of PN3. However, the utility of selective blockade of other channel subtypes as an approach to the treatment of pain will require further careful study. Nonetheless, it is quite likely that sodium channel blockade will emerge as a viable strategy for pharmacologic treatment of pain.

## Central Sensitization and N-methyl-D-aspartate (NMDA) Receptor Activation

As already stated, following nerve injury, damaged primary afferent neurons become spontaneously active and generate ectopic action potentials, which create a constant drive of input to the spinal cord. This initiates and maintains a hyperexcitable state of the spinal cord dorsal horn, termed *'central sensitization'*.

The changes that occur in the periphery following trauma lead to the phenomenon of 'peripheral sensitization' and primary hyperalgesia. The sensitization that occurs, however, can only be partly explained by the changes in the periphery, indicating that the hyperalgesia and allodynia after injury has a central component. This is the phenomenon of central sensitization.

Several changes have been noted to occur in the dorsal horn with central sensitization:

- a lowering of activation threshold of spinal neurons;

- an expansion in receptive field size;

- 'wind-up', which manifests as a progressive increase in the magnitude and duration of the response to repetitive painful stimuli;

- a strengthening of the efficacy of synaptic transmission or long-term potentiation.

These changes indicate that, in the presence of injurious stimuli, the sensory response generated by the CNS is not fixed, but dynamic or plastic, and for any pain therapy to be maximally effective we must take into account these changes.

The dorsal horn is the site of termination of primary afferents and there is a complex interaction among afferent fibers, local intrinsic spinal neurons and the endings of descending fibers from the brain. Primary afferent nociceptors terminate preferentially in laminae I, II and V and release the excitatory amino acids glutamate and aspartate upon activation. Nerve injury-induced barrage of nociceptive input leads to the release of glutamate and aspartate from nociceptor central terminals and causes activation of ionotropic α-amino-3-hydroxy-5-methyl-4-isoxazole propionic acid (AMPA) receptors and rapid depolarization of the postsynaptic membrane, and if the threshold is reached, action potential is generated. Another ionotropic glutamate receptor, NMDA receptor, is blocked at resting membrane potentials, because a magnesium ion plugs the channel pore, and, as a consequence, no current is produced when glutamate binds to the receptor. However, this block is voltage-dependent, and membrane depolarization due to sodium influx at the AMPA receptor removes the magnesium block and causes this channel to open. A number of neuropeptides, such as substance P, neurokinin A and calcitonin gene-related peptide (CGRP), are released with glutamate and act on neurokinin 1 (NK-1) receptors, leading to a progressively more depolarized membrane and the loss of the magnesium block of the NMDA receptors. This enables gluta-mate released from primary afferents to generate an inward current upon binding the receptors; calcium enters into the cell and activates protein kinase C (PKC) and protein tyrosine kinases (PTKs), which mediate the phosphory-lation of the NMDA receptor on its serine/threonine and tyrosine residues, respectively. Phosphorylation of NMDA receptors on its serine/threonine residues via PKC decreases the magnesium block at resting membrane poten-tials and produces long-lasting increases in synaptic efficacy.[25] Inhibitors of PKC have been shown to reduce central sensitization of spinothalamic neurons and reduce hyperalgesia,[26] and mutant mice deficient in PKCγ, a PKC isoenzyme with the spinal cord distribution highly restricted to lamina II (substantia gelatinosa), do not develop neuropathic pain-related behaviour after nerve injury.[27] Phosphorylation of the NMDA receptor on its tyrosine residues via the activation of tyrosine kinases also increases excitability by increasing the probability of channel opening.[28] Attention recently has focused on PTK Src, one of the best studied of PTKs that may be important in patho-physiological enhancement of excitatory transmission in the dorsal horn of the spinal cord. The coincidence of Src activation and a rise in the intracel-lular concentration of sodium – a situation known to occur during high levels of firing activity – may be important for boosting NMDA receptor function and inducing persistent alterations in synaptic function.[29]

In the normal state, only C-fiber input can reliably trigger central sensitiza-tion, but the situation changes following nerve injury because some A-fibres switch chemical phenotype and begin to express substance P and other modulators, including BDNF, such that low-intensity stimulation begins to induce central sensitization, which never normally occurs in the naïve animal. In addition, nociceptor input arising from ectopic locations in the damaged nerve maintains central sensitization, which manifests behaviourally as allodynia and hyperalgesia.

It is clear that activation of the NMDA receptor is critical for the initiation and maintenance of the enhanced responsiveness of dorsal horn nociceptive neurons that occurs in the chronic pain setting. Animal studies have demon-strated that NMDA receptor or neurokinin antagonists prevent the estab-lishment of central sensitization, but only NMDA antagonists reverse established central sensitization.[30–32]

Accumulating evidence suggests that NMDA receptor antagonists may have a role in attenuating features of neuropathic pain. For example, as demonstrated in the chronic constriction injury model, preemptive administration of the NMDA receptor antagonist MK-801 can prevent the onset of hyperalgesia,[33,34] or, if given after injury, can significantly reduce pain-related behaviour.[35–37]

Similar results were obtained with other neuropathic pain models, indicating the involvement of NMDA receptors in a number of phenomena associated with neuropathic pain. *In vivo* electrophysiological studies also show that NMDA receptor antagonists significantly reduce the exaggerated responsiveness of dorsal horn sensory neurons after nerve injury.[38,39] It is noteworthy that MK-801 has no effect on the frequency of ectopic baseline firing, suggesting that, in contrast to stimulus-evoked pain, spontaneous pain is not mediated through spinal NMDA receptors.[38]

These observations argue for the role for NMDA antagonists in the treatment of neuropathic pain. Unfortunately, antagonists that completely block NMDA receptors have numerous side effects such as memory impairment, psychotomimetic effects, ataxia and motor incoordination, limiting their use in clinical situation. Nevertheless, there still remains a potential for the development of clinically suitable NMDA receptor antagonists that prevent the pathological activation of NMDA receptors, but do not interfere with their physiological function.[40] Functional inhibition of NMDA receptor can be achieved through actions at different modulation sites located on its NR1 ($\zeta$1) and one of four NR2 (NR2A-B, $\epsilon$1–4) subunits.[41] For example, CP-101,606, an NR2B subunit-selective NMDA receptor antagonist has been found to suppress hyperalgesia in neuropathic rats at doses devoid of negative side effects.[42] It is of note that, in contrast to NR2A subunit widely distributed in the spinal cord except for lamina II, NR2B subunit has a restricted distribution in laminae I, II of the dorsal horn, a region strongly involved in nociception.[42,43] This observation, and the results from our study, in which we were not able to demonstrate antinociceptive effect of the targeted deletion of NMDA receptor $\epsilon$1 (NR2A) subunit on neuropathic pain-related behaviour in mice (unpublished observations), form the basis for the expectation that selective inhibition of NMDA receptor NR2B subunit might offer effective pain relief without a significant incidence of side effects.

The increase in excitability of spinal neurons after peripheral injury, termed central sensitization, has been extensively studied. Although the focus of investigation still remains the spinal cord, and the importance of the spinal NMDA receptor to the induction and maintenance of central sensitization has been documented. There is conclusive evidence suggesting that peripheral injury and persistent input engage spinobulbospinal mechanisms that may be the important contributors to central sensitization and development of secondary hyperalgesia.[44]

A contribution of supraspinal sites to neuropathic pain after spinal nerve ligation was first reported in the rat.[45] The tactile allodynia that develops after unilateral ligation of the $L_5$ and $L_6$ spinal nerves was found to be attenuated by inactivation of the rostral ventromedial medulla (RVM) by lidocaine injection. The lidocaine effect was determined to be localized within the RVM and independent of an opioid mechanism, suggesting an inactivation of a descending facilitatory influence from the RVM. These results were supported in subsequent studies.[46,47] Thus, neuropathic pain after peripheral nerve injury appears to involve, at least in part, activation of descending facilitatory influences from supraspinal sites, including the RVM.

In summary, central sensitization, a state of excessive sensitivity triggered by the nociceptor afferent input due to tissue damage and peripheral inflammation, can potentially help to protect injured body parts from further injury while recuperation or healing occurs. However, the survival advantage of the activity-dependent facilitation of the nociceptive system is lost in patients with neuropathic pain, which can persist indefinitely past the stage of healing of the primary injury.

## Clinical Presentation and Treatment of Neuropathic Pain

Dramatic differences among the various neuropathic pain states have long been recognized. Few conditions can match neuropathic pain for the differences in etiology, clinical features and response to treatment. It might be argued that conditions such as postherpetic neuralgia, intercostal neuralgia and trigeminal neuralgia are fundamentally different diseases. However, as it has been already discussed in the introduction, from the point of view of underlying mechanism the neuropathic pain syndromes have much in common; the apparent differences merely reflect the peculiarities of the ectopic firing process.

The natural course of neuropathic pain varies depending on its etiology. It may begin immediately or, more often, its onset is delayed for many weeks after neural trauma and healing of the primary injury. In some patients pain may begin acutely and acquire other delayed features such as those found in CRPS. In spite of the diverse aetiology and location of neuropathic pain, the clinical picture is in many cases surprisingly similar, suggesting that pain in these disorders shares common mechanisms. The typical patient with neuropathic pain presents to the clinician with a combination of three types of pain. The first type of neuropathic pain is spontaneous constant pain, which fluctuates in intensity and can change in character over time. The second type of pain comprises variable paroxysmal spontaneous attacks or exacerbations of pain, which are frequently very disturbing to a patient. These two types of pain are termed stimulus-independent and are usually described as shooting, stabbing, or electrical. The third type includes stimulus-dependent pains,

**Table 3** Clinical findings in neuropathic pain

| Symptoms | Characteristics |
|---|---|
| Sensory changes | Raised thresholds or total loss of sensibility in the painful area |
| Anaesthesia dolorosa | Pain referred to anesthetic region |
| Hyperaesthesia | Increase sensation to a stimulus |
| • Allodynia | • Pain elicited by non-noxious stimuli |
| • Hyperalgesia | • Increased sensitivity to noxious stimuli |
| Hyperpathia | Abnormal spatial and temporal characteristics of pain |
| • Radiation | • Spread of pain outside the site of stimulation |
| • After sensations | • Persistence of pain after termination of stimulus |
| • Prolonged response latency | • Delay in sensation after a stimulus |
| • Summation | • Progressive worsening of pain on repeated stimulation |
| Paroxysms | Attacks of pain of various severity, duration and periodicity |
| Pareasthesias | Abnormal sensations other than pain ('pins and needles') |
| Dysaesthesias | Abnormal unpleasant sensations, spontaneous and evoked, which may be painful |
| Borderline zone pain | Pain in area adjacent to denervated skin |
| Variability of pain severity | Pain aggravation with anxiety/emotional stress |
| Associated psychological changes | Anxiety, depression, insomnia |

reflecting the hypersensitivity of the nervous system to many external stimuli, such as touch, blunt pressure, hot or cold temperatures, and even internal stimuli such as anxiety or excitement. A summary of various neuropathic pain symptoms is given in table 3. Treating neuropathic pain is no easy task and can be very frustrating. Fortunately, results from clinical trials have led to the improvements in the medical management of neuropathic pain, and a number of treatments are now available (fig. 2). What follows is a brief refresher looking at several peripheral neuropathic pain syndromes, their pathogenesis, clinical picture and therapeutic aspects.

## Phantom Pain

### Clinical features

One type of pain is experienced by virtually all amputees – stump pain. Stump pain is universally seen after a limb amputation, and, quite naturally, it subsides with recuperation. In those few patients who continue to complain of the pain in the stump careful examination usually reveals pathological findings, such as infection, bone spurs, poorly fitted prostheses, neuromas, myofascial trigger points, etc. In general, this type of pain is rare in perfectly healed stumps. It has recently become accepted, however, that in up to 80% of amputees the missing extremity becomes a site of severe and excruciating pain – defined as phantom pain – presenting a serious

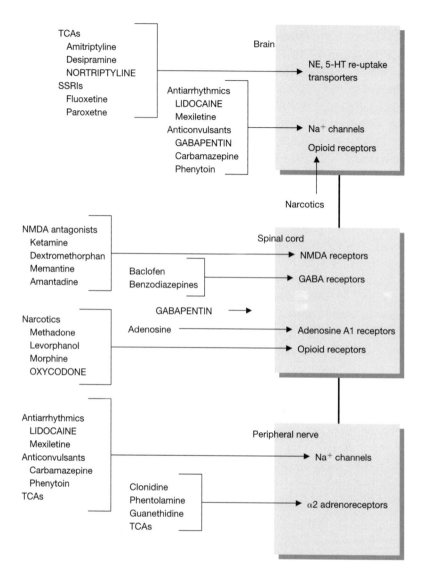

**Figure 2** Pharmacological treatments of neuropathic pain with respect to a class of drugs and site of action. The first-line drugs are capitalized. GABA = γ-aminobutyric acid; 5-HT = 5-hydroxytryptamine (serotonin); NE = norepinephrine; NMDA = N-methyl-D-aspartate; SSRIs = serotonin selective re-uptake inhibitors; TCAs = tricyclic antidepressants.

therapeutic problem. Phantom pain should be distinguished from phantom limb sensation – any non-painful sensation of the absent limb – which is more frequent than phantom pain. Phantom pain is usually intermittent; it is described as shooting or squeezing but may also be described as electric-like and is preferentially experienced in the distal parts of the phantom limb.

## Pathogenesis

The pathophysiology is complex and not completely understood, although it is likely that peripheral factors, such as ectopic discharge from the stump neuromas and sensitization of nociceptors in the pathological stump, contribute to abnormal firing of spinal pain transmission neurons, which, in turn, may generate dysfunction in more rostral CNS centres. Results to date suggest that long-lasting noxious input may trigger and perpetuate long-term changes at all levels of the neuraxis. A reorganization of cerebral cortex and thalamus, when adjacent areas invade the representation zone of the deafferented body part, has been documented in both monkeys and humans following limb amputation and deafferentiation.[48–50] This reorganization was found to be highly correlated with phantom pain and unrelated to the infrequent topographic referred sensations.[51] It should be noted that in contrast to patients with phantom limb pain who showed massive reorganization of primary somatosensory cortex, neuromagnetic source imaging revealed only minimal cortical reorganization in congenital amputees and traumatic amputees without phantom pain.[52] Also, axonal sprouting, which is known to occur in the spinal cord dorsal horn after nerve axotomy, has been recently described in the reorganized cortex of amputated monkeys.[53]

## Treatment

Treatment is difficult. In general, it should be based on non-invasive procedures because surgical treatment can cause further deafferentiation resulting in aggravation of pain. Early reports suggested that perioperative epidural blockade may prevent phantom pain and many anesthesiologists started to offer preoperative epidural catheter to patients scheduled for amputation. However, some of the clinical suggestions of these reports is questionable given the number of methodological problems relative to the study design. Recent evidence now suggests that it may not be possible to prevent phantom pain by using a preemptive approach.[54] Medical treatment is the mainstay of therapy but has variable benefits if symptoms last longer than one year. Tricyclic antidepressants (TCAs), sodium channel blockers, anticonvulsants, NMDA receptor antagonists and calcitonin may be effective in phantom pain. Several authors have described the analgesic effect of oral and intrathecal opioids in phantom pain, but control studies proving their beneficial effect are still lacking.

As already mentioned, intracortical changes may be important in maintaining phantom limb pain. Intensive use of a myoelectric prosthesis or sensory discrimination training, another form of behaviourally relevant stimulation, may lead to significant improvements in phantom limb pain along with a significant reduction of cortical reorganization.[55] This stimulation-based approach may benefit patients who suffer from centrally mediated phantom limb pain, but may be insufficient for those in whom peripheral factors dominate the problem. In the latter case, biofeedback may be more effective.

Spinal cord stimulation (SCS) can relieve both phantom and stump pain in many, but not all, amputees. One half of our patients with phantom limb obtained greater than 50% pain reduction with spinal cord stimulation (table 4).[56] Unfortunately, the effect of spinal cord stimulation appears to wane with time more than in some other conditions. Relief of phantom pain may sometimes be secondary to relief of the exacerbating stump pain. The question of whether pre-emptive spinal cord stimulation influences the development of phantom limb or stump pain remains unresolved.

## Avulsion of the Brachial Plexus

### Clinical features

Avulsion injury to the brachial plexus represents a special type of pain typically seen in patients who have been involved in motorcycle accidents. This injury usually occurs in an abducted and hyperextended position of the arm. Parry found that of 108 cases of brachial plexus avulsion injury, 98 suffered significant pain.[57] Brachial plexus avulsions present as severe burning, crushing, or paroxysmal shooting pain, which is almost invariably felt in the dermatome of the avulsed root. Many patients have a feeling that the hand is on fire or that boiling water is being poured over it. Sudden paroxysms come unpredictably and are sometimes of unbearable intensity. Paresthesias are also common and almost all of the patients complain of tingling, 'pins and needles' or feelings of electricity. Nearly all are aware of a phantom limb with sensations of movement when effort is made to use paralyzed muscles. Spontaneous remission is very rare and may be delayed for a number of years. The pain is usually lifelong and is very difficult to manage.

### Pathogenesis

The pain is thought to result from aberrant and spontaneous firing of deafferented neurons in the spinal cord dorsal horn at the level of the injury. Subsequently, an abnormality in spinal cord neurons generate an abnormality in the responsiveness of thalamic neurons, which, in turn, may generate dysfunction in the cerebral cortex. The lines of evidence suggest that with time, these high-level abnormalities within the pain pathways may become independent of the lower-level abnormalities that generated them.[58]

**Table 4** Relationship between diseases (presented by sex, age, and pain site) and pain relief >50% by epidural spinal cord stimulation [Reproduced with permission from Shimoji K, Hokari T, Kano T et al. Management of intractable pain with percutaneous epidural spinal cord stimulation: differences in pain-relieving effects among diseases and sites of pain. Anesth Analg 1993; 77: 110–116. Lippincott, Williams and Wilkins.]

| Disease | Sex | | Age (yr) (mean ± SE) | Subjective pain relief >50% | | | | | |
| | M | F | | Site of pain[a] | | | | Total | (%) |
| | | | | H-F | N-UE | Tr | L-E | | |
|---|---|---|---|---|---|---|---|---|---|
| Carcinoma/sarcoma | 29/34[b] | 16/18 | 62 ± 2 | 1/1 | 2/3 | 40/43 | 2/5[c] | 45/52[d] | (86.5) |
| Postherpetic neuralgia | 17/72 | 18/54 | 59 ± 4 | 5/13 | 6/11 | 22/88 | 2/14 | 35/126[e] | (27.8) |
| Causalgia | 68/101 | 71/88 | 51 ± 7 | 5/6 | 32/34 | 87/98 | 15/51[f] | 139/189[d] | (73.5) |
| Spinal trauma | 4/11 | 1/1 | 51 ± 8 | 0 | 0 | 0 | 5/12 | 5/12 | (41.7) |
| SMON | 1/3 | 3/6 | 63 ± 2 | 0 | 0/1 | 2/3 | 2/5 | 4/9 | (44.4) |
| Phantom limb | 3/7 | 1/1 | 49 ± 5 | 0 | 4/6 | 0 | 0/2 | 4/8 | (50.0) |
| TAO/ASO | 1/14 | 0 | 67 ± 4 | 0 | 0 | 0 | 1/14 | 1/14[e] | (7.1) |
| Thalamic syndrome | 3/8 | 0/1 | 71 ± 5 | 0 | 3/8 | 0 | 0/1 | 3/9 | (33.3) |
| Tabes dorsalis | 3/3 | 0 | 70 ± 2 | 0 | 0 | 3/3 | 0 | 3/3 | (100.0) |
| Others | 8/14 | 6/18[h] | 58 ± 4 | 4/5 | 1/3 | 7/9 | 2/15[g] | 14/32 | (43.8) |
| | 137/267 | 116/187[h] | 56 ± 2 | 15/25 | 48/66 | 161/244 | 29/199[i] | 253/454 | (55.7) |

[a]When the sites of pain were distributed to more than one region, the most painful site was represented. M, male; F, female; H-F, head and/or face; N-UE, neck and/or upper extremities; Tr, trunk; L-E, lower extremities; SMON, subacute myelo-optico-neuropathy; TAO/ASO, thromboangitis obliterans/arterial sclerosis obliterans.

[b]A numerator and denominator in the sex as well as pain relief columns represent number of patients with pain relief >50% and number of patients treated, respectively. Numbers in parentheses indicate percentage of the patients who showed pain relief >50%. $\chi^2$ test was conducted for evaluation of a significant difference in occurrence.

[c]Significantly lower than Tr ($P < 0.01$) in the same disease.

[d]Significantly higher ($P < 0.01$) than the overall effect (253/454; 55.7%).

[e]Significantly lower ($P < 0.01$) than the overall effect.

[f]Significantly lower than H-F ($P < 0.05$), N-UE ($P < 0.01$), and Tr ($P < 0.01$).

[g]Significantly lower than H-F ($P < 0.05$) and Tr ($P < 0.01$).

[h]Significantly higher ($P < 0.05$) than male patients.

[i]Significantly lower than H-F ($P < 0.01$), N-UE ($P < 0.01$), and Tr ($P < 0.01$).

## Treatment

Pharmacotherapy is usually of limited benefit. Good results of dorsal root entry zone lesions (DREZLs) have been reported in numerous studies and the overall success rate is in the region of 60% with follow-ups for about 10 years. The dorsal root entry zone lesion procedure involves laminectomy and electrocoagulation of the dorsal root entry zone lesion of the avulsed roots. We have had experience with this procedure in our patients with intractable pain who failed all conservative measures.[59,60] Our results with dorsal root entry zone lesion in brachial plexus avulsion have demonstrated that the procedure is efficacious and that complications such as sensory decrease or motor weakness are not a major concern in these patients with a paralyzed arm and an aggressive approach may be taken (fig. 3). Although pain following complete root avulsion is unlikely to respond to spinal cord stimulation, which depends upon intact ascending afferent collaterals, many patients have a mixture of root avulsion and partial damage and are likely to respond to spinal cord stimulation to some extent. In selected patients who showed partial improvement during trial stimulation prior to surgery we used to implant cervical epidural electrodes with a subcutaneous receiver during dorsal root entry zone lesion. However we have been unable to demonstrate better outcomes with this manipulation. Furthermore, spinal cord stimulation is only partially effective against a new type of pain that can appear in some patients as a complication of dorsal root entry zone lesion.

## Complex Regional Pain Syndrome (CRPS)

### Clinical features

CRPS, types I and II, is the name now given to a group of conditions formerly described as reflex sympathetic dystrophy (RSD) and causalgia. CRPS I or RSD includes patients whose pain and associated features follow a variety of insults, most commonly relatively minor, and fully recoverable injuries. CRPS II (causalgia) is in all respects similar to CRPS I except the additional condition that it follows a nerve injury.

The pain is usually present immediately or relatively soon after the injury and is disproportionate to the initiating cause in distribution, severity and duration. Although the injury is sometimes easily defined, such as in direct nerve damage or a fracture, other times it is not easily traceable to a specific event. The symptoms most frequently mentioned by patients are spontaneous burning and stinging pain. In CRPS II patients may often complain of symptoms related to the neuropathy, such as brief electrical sensations or shooting

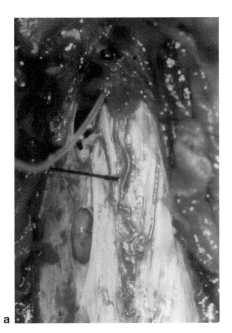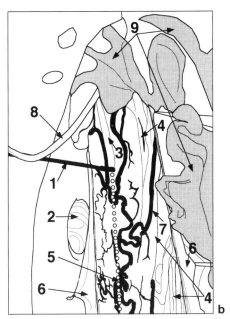

**Figure 3 a** Surgical view of the dorsal root entry zone (DREZ) procedure in a 43 year-old patient with phantom pain caused by left brachial plexus avulsion. **b** A simplified schematic drawing of the same photograph. The DREZ lesion was carried out along the intermediolateral sulcus through $C_4$ to $T_1$ (dotted line). (1) Coagulation electrode inserted into the DREZ; (2) The root sleeve emptied after brachial plexus avulsion on the injury side; (3) A rootlet left at the $C_3$ level on the injury side; (4) Dorsal rootlets on the intact side; (5) DREZ area is highly vascularized due to the traumatic avulsion making it difficult to reach with a coagulation electrode; (6) Dura mater; (7) Posterior spinal artery; (8) Suction catheter; (9) Sponge gauze.

pain. The pain is constant and is often severe so that any contact with the affected part and active or passive movement may be extremely painful, leading to protection of the limb and frequently severe loss of function. In general, there is a marked variation in symptoms present in patients with CRPS. Table 5 lists clinical features of CRPS. Significant findings include muscle wasting and, thinned, cool skin with hyperhidrosis, sensory, motor and autonomic abnormalities. Oedema is often present as an early sign. Muscle wasting and joint stiffness are frequent compounding factors in CRPS.

## Pathogenesis

The primary pathophysiology of CRPS is still poorly understood. Although chronic inflammatory changes in the periphery and altered central processing

**Table 5** Clinical findings in CRPS

History
   Trauma, nerve injury
   Early onset
Sensory changes
   Spontaneous pain
   Evoked pain (allodynia, hyperalgesia)
Musculoskeletal changes
   Decreased range of motion
   Muscle weakness/wasting
   Dystonia
   Tremor
   Joint stiffness/contracture
   Osteoporosis
Autonomic changes
   Vasomotor (temperature/colour abnormalities)
   Sudomotor (hyperhidrosis/sweating asymmetry)
Dystrophic changes/oedema
Loss of function
Psychological changes
   Anxiety/fear/depression

are clearly important, only the role of the sympathetic nervous system in the mechanisms of pain and other clinical features of CRPS will be briefly outlined below.

Sympathetically maintained pain is the component of a patient's pain, which is maintained by efferent noradrenergic sympathetic activity and circulating catecholamines. A number of neuropathic pain states may be partly, if only temporarily, dependent on sympathetic activity.[61] SMP as assessed clinically by the effect of sympathetic blockade is a very variable component of pain in CRPS, not only between individuals but also in the same individual at different times. Therefore, sympathetically maintained pain is correctly not included in the diagnostic criteria for either type of CRPS.[1]

Normally, sympathetic postganglionic neurons do not communicate with afferent neurons in the periphery and the sympathetic nervous system is not involved in the generation of pain. However, there is substantial experimental and clinical evidence in favour of the existence of a sympathetic influence on pain in CRPS and other pain states. Following peripheral nerve injury, sympathetic noradrenergic neurons may influence afferent neurons in several ways. Three sites of sympathetic-sensory interaction after nerve injury have been identified; the region of the nerve damage itself, undamaged fibers distal to the nerve lesion and the dorsal root ganglion.

Activity in sympathetic neurons at physiological frequencies is able to elicit impulses in C-fibre afferents. The sympathetically induced discharges can be mimicked by epinephrine and are blocked by the α-adrenoreceptor antagonist phentolamine.[62] Whether sympathetic-afferent coupling occurs in the nerve proximal to the lesion and whether this coupling is mediated directly by norepinephrine and/or via the blood flow is not known.

Following peripheral nerve lesion, perivascular sympathetic axons start to invade the dorsal root ganglions, which contain axotomized neurons, and form abnormal sympathetic terminal arborizations or 'baskets' around some dorsal root ganglion neurons. This novel sprouting increases with time and, depending on the type of injury, days to weeks after the nerve lesion, some dorsal root ganglion neurons are partially or almost completely surrounded by varicose catecholaminergic terminals. The catecholaminergic varicose terminals surround preferentially large-diameter neurons, which have been lesioned but probably also unlesioned ones.[63]

Nerve injury-induced sprouting of sympathetic fibres is expected to increase the amount of sympathetically released noradrenaline, and to enhance its access to hypersensitive afferent neurons and their axonal endings, even if the sympathetic efferent barrage remains unchanged. The use of receptor-selective pharmacological agents has shown that sympathetic-sensory coupling is mediated primarily by adrenoreceptors of the α2 type, with a minor role played by α1 adrenoreceptors.[64] It should be pointed out that receptor up-regulation occurs following peripheral nerve injury,[65] but at this stage, the relationship of the increased α-adrenoreceptor presence to neuropathic states is a matter of conjecture. Rather, α-adrenoreceptors normally expressed by dorsal root ganglion neurons might yield suprathreshold responses following nerve injury simply due to the electrical hyperexcitability of axotomized sensory neurons.

## Treatment

There are many treatment modalities and drugs that have been suggested in CRPS – a sure indication that no single treatment is superior to others and that nothing is consistently successful – but few have been tested in double-blind, randomized, controlled trials. This is not surprising in a condition, which has proved so difficult to define, and whose limits are still uncertain. Also, many treatments suggested have previously been based on ideas and speculation rather than fact.

Patients with established CRPS should always be referred to a center where a multidisciplinary program for pain management is available. It is always gratifying both to patient and clinician, to obtain analgesia by whatever means, but pain relief alone is insufficient and every period of even partial analgesia should be utilized to begin mobilization and rehabilitation. All treatments should be focused primarily on functional restoration; the use of more aggressive blocks, pharmacotherapy and psychotherapy is reserved for patients failing to progress in 2–4 weeks with physical therapy.[66] The principle of functional restoration is based on steady progression from very gentle movements on an active basis to gentle weight-bearing, such as carrying light bags in upper extremity syndromes or putting partial weight on the lower extremity in gait training. Gradual desensitization to increasing sensory stimuli goes along with increased function. This could include such strategies as progressive stimulation with silk, progressing to cloths of other textures, such as towelling, or contrast baths that progressively broaden the temperature difference between the two baths.

Another basic principle of functional restoration is that if a patient does not progress in a reasonable time, then other interventions, for example, a sympathetic and/or somatic block, will be added progressively to give the patient greater comfort or confidence so that they may proceed to the next level. It is important to manage oedema, optimize the range of motion and encourage general aerobic activity throughout. Interdisciplinary pain management techniques emphasizing functional restoration are thought to be the most effective therapy; they may work to reset altered central processing and/or normalizing the distal environment.

Pharmacotherapy should basically include prophylactic drugs used daily for pain relief and drugs employed for crisis management. Tricyclic anti-depressants are traditional in neuropathic conditions and seem to be partially effective in CRPS, especially in patients with anxiety, fear and depression. Of the anticonvulsant drugs, attention has been recently drawn to gabapentin, which is reported to help in CRPS, but controlled trials are awaited. Membrane-stabilizing anticonvulsants such as phenytoin may be useful, particularly when nerve damage is present or pain is thought to originate from ectopic site, but again randomized controlled trials are lacking.

Many patients report analgesic effects from simple analgesics, codeine and non-steroidal anti-inflammatory drugs, and continue to take these drugs in the absence of more effective treatment. Corticosteroids can be particularly useful in the early/acute phases of CRPS, particularly in cases where there is considerable inflammation. Opioids may be effectively employed in the early stages of CRPS and in crisis management. Although NMDA receptor antagonists have been considered for management of allodynia and/or hyper-pathia, numerous side effects limit their clinical use. The challenge therefore is to develop subunit- and site-specific NMDA receptor antagonists that do not interfere with the physiological function of NMDA receptors, but prevent their pathological activation.[40,41] Meanwhile, low-dose subcutaneous ketamine may have a role in the management of CRPS.

While a variety of block therapies have been the traditional first line of treatment in CRPS, there is very little scientific evidence to support their use. Blocks should be primarily viewed as providing a pain-free period so that patient may progress with the functional restoration. Many blocks have been examined, and the most frequently used are paravertebral sympathetic blocks and epidural blocks.[67] Intravenous phentolamine is widely used in many centres to identify those likely to respond to more prolonged local sympathetic blockade. Intravenous regional sympathetic blockade using guanethidine or bretylium seems to be effective. Sympathectomy has some theoretical support, but the decision to proceed to sympathectomy should be made with care. Some patients do very well in the short term after the procedure, but long-term pain relief is poor. Others present with postsympathectomy pain, which may take months to resolve. This procedure is almost abandoned now.

Although recent randomized controlled trial has shown that spinal cord stimulation can reduce pain and improve the health-related quality of life in CRPS I, more recent results are disappointing.[68] We have reported good outcomes with spinal cord stimulation in CRPS type II.[56] The stimulus frequencies we used were relatively low (1.6–8.0 Hz) compared to those of other investigators. Among 189 patients with causalgia treated in this study, 139 (73.5%) reported greater than 50% pain reduction (table 4). In general, stimulation-produced analgesia tends to decrease during the course of treatment. However, our results demonstrated that the effects of low-frequency spinal cord stimulation did not wane in the long term. It is recognized that the higher the frequency of stimulation, the more rapidly the evoked activities are attenuated. The stimulus frequency of our method was relatively low compared to that used by other investigators, and the duration of stimulation was limited to 30 min. at a time. It is likely that our method of low-frequency and short period stimulation prevents attenuation of the analgesic effect of spinal cord stimulation.

## Diabetic Neuropathy

### Clinical features

Peripheral neuropathy is a very common complication of diabetes. This is a heterogeneous group of disorders that are classified according to nervous system involvement: autonomic neuropathy, distal symmetric polyneuropathy, proximal motor neuropathy, which is also referred to as diabetic amyotrophy, and mononeuropathy. Mononeuropathies occur more frequently in diabetic patients than in the general population, affecting particularly the motor nerves to the extraocular muscles but also single peripheral nerves, preferentially at common sites of nerve entrapment or compression, such as carpal tunnel (median nerve), tarsal tunnel (posterior tibial), and elbow (ulnar nerve). Involvement of small-fibre sensory neurons may result in loss of normal pain and temperature sensation, which can predispose the patient to injury, ulceration, and chronic infection. These patients may experience neuropathic pain manifesting itself as a burning sensation, sharp lancinating pains, dull aches, hyperesthesia and allodynia. Most of these symptoms are often reported to be worse at night. Such patients may cry out when their feet contact a blanket; they often have a poor sleep.

## Pathogenesis

The mechanisms that contribute to the pathogenesis of diabetic neuropathy are still not fully understood. They may include direct metabolic compromise, reduced endoneural blood flow and nerve ischaemia, oxidative stress, and reduced availability of neurotrophic factors. Morphological studies show axonal degeneration and segmental demyelination. Both small- and large-diameter nerve fibres are involved, although initially there is an altered fibre size population with a shift toward larger nerve fiber diameter. The combination of axonal degeneration, spontaneous discharges from both large myelinated and small unmyelinated nerve fibres, hyperglycaemia, and possibly microangiopathic changes and ischaemia contributes to this painful syndrome.

## Treatment

Treatment relies, to a great extent, on measures that can reduce the risk of developing diabetic neuropathy, prevent secondary complications and attenuate symptoms. Strict control of hyperglycaemia may dramatically reduce the risk of developing diabetic neuropathy. Because the most severe complications involve the diabetic foot, patients must be educated in the importance of routine foot care. Pharmacological approach is used to treat diabetic neuropathic pain. It is similar to the medical management of other neuropathic pain syndromes, with some disorders responding variably to different agents. Tricyclic antidepressants and gabapentin are first-line therapy. Alternative treatments include other anticonvulsants, mexiletine and tramadol. Treatment with opioids should be reserved for patients in whom other treatment modalities fail. Spinal cord stimulation has been found to work well in painful diabetic neuropathy and should be considered in patients who do not respond to conventional treatment.[69]

## Postherpetic Neuralgia

### Clinical features

Postherpetic neuralgia, a chronic pain syndrome experienced by some patients after the complete healing of acute herpes zoster lesions, is often refractory to treatment and can persist for years. Although there is no generally agreed definition of postherpetic neuralgia, many investigators consider postherpetic neuralgia as pain that persists longer than one month after the onset of the rash. The incidence of postherpetic neuralgia in patients who have contracted herpes zoster infection is approximately 10%. Age is the greatest risk factor; the elderly are more susceptible to postherpetic neuralgia than are younger individuals. The commonest sites for postherpetic neuralgia are the mid-thoracic dermatomes and the ophthalmic division of the trigeminal nerve, but pain may occur in any dermatome. Postherpetic neuralgia exhibits the cardinal clinical features of neuropathic pain, namely altered sensation, stimulus-independent (ongoing) pain, and allodynic pain after light touch.[70] The cause of postherpetic neuralgia is well-defined; skin changes point at the affected nerve. Unaffected dermatomes provide within-subject control sites, and patients whose herpetic neuralgia does not persist past the stage of healing of the acute eruption provide a control population. Thus, postherpetic neuralgia presents a useful 'human model' for the research into pain mechanisms.[71]

### Pathogenesis

A number of skin biopsy studies of patients with painful neuropathies have shown a loss of epidermal innervation. Almost all epidermal neurites are capsaicin-sensitive nociceptors that signal acute pain. Patients with postherpetic neuralgia have fewer remaining nerve endings in the affected skin than those without postherpetic neuralgia.[72] Because varicella-zoster virus destroys the entire primary afferent neuron including the central axon, the density of neural innervation in the skin reflects the density of the central projection from primary afferent neurons onto second-order sensory neurons within the CNS. Recent study provides new insights into the relationship between neuronal loss and the presence of neuropathic pain.[71] A threshold relationship between the density of remaining epidermal neurites in skin previously affected by herpes zoster and the development of neuropathic pain has been described. It is suggested that the absence of postherpetic neuralgia may require the preservation of a minimum density of primary nociceptive neurons, and that the density of epidermal innervation may provide an object-ive correlate for the presence or absence of neuropathic pain. The phenom-enon of 'minimum residual structure'[73] may apply to the development of postherpetic neuralgia. The minimum residual structure hypothesis states that near-normal function can be preserved after neural injury as long as a certain minimum number of neurons survive. However, abnormal function ensues abruptly if neuronal densities drop slightly below the minimum residual structure value. Minimum residual structure helps maintain function after mild injury.

Why should a neuronal loss cause postherpetic neuralgia pain? A possible explanation is that dorsal horn projection neurons become hyperexcitable after loss of input from peripheral neurons. Additionally, spared nociceptors in postherpetic neuralgia-affected skin may generate ectopic impulses – the irritable nociceptor hypothesis[74] – contributing to ongoing and allodynic pain. Furthermore, damage to primary afferents can cause electrical hyper-activity within the brain. If enough sensory innervation is lost, structural abnormalities similar to those seen in somatosensory cortex and thalamic regions after limb amputation may develop and contribute to the pain in postherpetic neuralgia. Thus, postherpetic neuralgia may be a 'phantom-skin' pain associated with loss of nociceptors.[71]

## Treatment

Antiviral therapy is not helpful in classic postherpetic neuralgia, although it might be effective in patients with continuing low-grade infection manifesting as gradually worsening pain. The important issue of prevention of posther-petic neuralgia has received considerable attention. Use of antiviral therapy (aciclovir, famciclovir or valaciclovir) for acute herpes zoster reduces the risk of developing postherpetic neuralgia and the overall duration of pain.

Postherpetic neuralgia is one of the commonest intractable conditions seen in pain clinics. Initiating treatment as soon as possible after onset of rash may be a key in prevention of postherpetic neuralgia.[75] All the same treatments used in acute herpes zoster have been used in postherpetic neuralgia, although with considerably less success. The mainstay of therapy is often the use of tricyclic antidepressants. Tricyclic antidepressants have an analgesic effect in neuropathic pain that is independent of their antidepressant activity. Since there is often associated depression they represent a logical choice in this clinical setting. Tricyclic antidepressants have significant side effects such as orthostatic hypotension, pronounced sedation and anticholinergic actions. Nortriptyline is now preferred to amitriptyline on the basis of its equivalent efficacy and better tolerability.[75] Topical lidocaine has a good anti-allodynic effect on postherpetic neuralgia skin with minimal systemic absorption and no need for dose titration.[76] Treatment with gabapentin – the only drug indicated for the treatment of all neuropathic pain – has been reported to significantly reduce average pain ratings and improve quality of life in patients with postherpetic neuralgia.[77] The most frequently documented adverse effects of gabapentin include somnolence, dizziness, ataxia, fatigue, but it is generally well tolerated in comparison with other anticonvulsants. In addition to tricyclic antidepressants, topical lidocaine patches and gabapentin, sustained-release oxycodone has also been identified as an effective analgesic for postherpetic neuralgia.[78]

Alternative treatment approaches should be tried in cases where nothing else is helping. They include tramadol, selective serotonin reuptake inhibitors, other anticonvulsants, transcutaneous electrical nerve stimulation (TENS), topical capsaicin, lidocaine infusion followed by oral mexiletine if the patient gets a good response, and nerve blocks.[75] The outcome with spinal cord stimulation is less predictable, some finding spinal cord stimulation effective and others not. We have found it useful in approximately 30% of patients with postherpetic neuralgia.[56] Such heterogeneous results may reflect the variable natural history of the condition.

## Key points for clinical practice

- Neuropathic pain results from injuries and disease that affect the nervous system directly. It is a pathological pain that has no survival advantage and causes suffering and distress.

- Both peripheral and CNS processes play a role in its pathophysiological mechanisms. Increased electrical excitability of sensory neurons following injury and disease, and particularly the emergence of ectopic firing, represent a fundamental substrate of neuropathic pain. Increased nociceptor drive triggers and maintains central sensitization and causes structural reorganization within the CNS. Finally, sensory processing is irreversibly changed.

- The treatment of patients with neuropathic pain is a complex and challenging task. The 'ideal analgesic' for neuropathic pain is most unlikely to be found because of the complexity of pathophysiological and biochemical changes underlying this condition.

- Effective pain therapy requires an understanding of the mechanisms involved; it needs to be more than symptom management. A better understanding of the particular mechanisms responsible for pain in an individual will substantially improve the management of neuropathic pain.

- The treatment is still largely empirical and often unsatisfactory. Tricyclic antidepressants and gabapentin are currently the best-documented therapy for neuropathic pain. Although the use of narcotic analgesics is highly controversial in this setting, they can be very useful and should be tried before invasive therapies are instituted. Alternative treatments include other anticonvulsants, mexiletine, tramadol and topical agents (e.g. capsaicin, lidocaine).

- General treatment principles are the individualization of therapy and the titration of the dose. It should be remembered that the mean dose required for pain reduction with antidepressant is usually lower than doses necessary to treat depression, and that the dosages of anticonvulsants used as analgesics are usually in the anticonvulsant range. Once the decision is made to use these medications, it is advisable to start with low doses and to increase the dose gradually until either pain relief is obtained or side effects are noted.

- A rational polypharmacy is often employed. A combination of drugs targeted at different mechanisms represents a logical choice.

- Clinically available substances with NMDA receptor blocking properties have been shown to reduce spontaneous pain and hyperalgesia, but have a narrow therapeutic window. Given the pivotal role of the NMDA receptors in central sensitization and the strong evidence implicating this phenomenon in neuropathic pain, newer and safer subunit-selective and site-selective drugs having an antagonist action at the NMDA receptor offer a very attractive approach for the management of neuropathic pain.

- Neurosurgical treatment of neuropathic pain should always follow a reasonable trial of conservative therapy and should be undertaken only if the patient's pain has been proved refractory to all appropriate medical therapy. In general, most ablative surgery procedures have somewhat unpredictable outcomes with a risk of further deafferentation resulting in even more pain, and, thus, have been replaced recently by neuromodulatory approaches such as electrical stimulation of the CNS.

- Spinal cord stimulation is most effective for the treatment of pharmacotherapy resistant neuropathic pain that is not infrequently seen in pain clinics. Considering that spinal cord stimulation is a reversible procedure with a very low risk of complications and side effects and the fact that it has been shown to be cost-effective, this treatment seems to be presently underused. The simplicity, safety, and low-cost of percutaneous epidural spinal cord stimulation should favour its further dissemination outside the neurosurgical profession and adaptation by other pain specialists.

## References

1. Merskey H, Bogduk N. Classification of chronic pain: descriptions of chronic pain syndromes and definitions of pain terms. 2nd ed. Seattle, USA: IASP Press, 1994.
2. McCormack K. Signal transduction in neuropathic pain, with special emphasis on the analgesic role of opioids-Part I: The basic science of phenotype expression in normal and regenerating nerve. Pain Rev 1999; 6: 3–33.
3. Devor M, Seltzer Z. Pathophysiology of damaged nerves in relation to chronic pain. In: Wall P, Melzack R. (eds) Textbook of pain. 4th ed. London, UK: Churchill Livingstone, 1999; 129–164.
4. Janig W, Habler HJ. Sympathetic nervous system: contribution to chronic pain. Prog Brain Res 2000; 129: 451–468.
5. Cummins TR, Dib-Hajj SD, Black JA, Waxman SG. Sodium channels and the molecular pathophysiology of pain. Prog Brain Res 2000; 129: 3–19.
6. Black JA, Dib-Hajj SD, McNabola K *et al.* Spinal sensory neurons express multiple sodium channel alpha-subunit mRNAs. Brain Res Mol Brain Res 1996; 43: 117–131.
7. Gurtu S, Smith PA. Electrophysiological characteristics of hamster dorsal root ganglion cells and their response to axotomy. J Neurophysiol 1988; 59: 408–423.
8. Devor M, Keller CH, Deerinck TJ, Levinson SR, Ellisman MH. Na$^+$ channel accumulation on axolemma of afferent endings in nerve end neuromas in Apteronotus. Neurosci Lett 1989; 102: 149–154.
9. England JD, Gamboni F, Ferguson MA, Levinson SR. Sodium channels accumulate at the tips of injured axons. Muscle Nerve 1994; 17: 593–598.
10. England JD, Happel LT, Kline DG *et al.* Sodium channel accumulation in humans with painful neuromas. Neurology 1996; 47: 272–276.
11. Waxman SG, Brill MH. Conduction through demyelinated plaques in multiple sclerosis: computer simulations of facilitation by short internodes. J Neurol Neurosurg Psychiatry 1978; 41: 408–416.
12. Matzner O, Devor M. Na$^+$ conductance and the threshold for repetitive neuronal firing. Brain Res 1992; 597: 92–98.
13. Matzner O, Devor M. Hyperexcitability at sites of nerve injury depends on voltage-sensitive Na$^+$ channels. J Neurophysiol 1994; 72: 349–359.
14. Zhang JM, Donnelly DF, Song XJ, Lamotte RH. Axotomy increases the excitability of dorsal root ganglion cells with unmyelinated axons. J Neurophysiol 1997; 78: 2790–2794.
15. Waxman SG, Kocsis JD, Black JA. Type III sodium channel mRNA is expressed in embryonic but not adult spinal sensory neurons, and is reexpressed following axotomy. J Neurophysiol 1994; 72: 466–470.
16. Dib-Hajj S, Black JA, Felts P, Waxman SG. Down-regulation of transcripts for Na channel alpha-SNS in spinal sensory neurons following axotomy. Proc Natl Acad Sci USA 1996; 93: 14950–14954.
17. Dib-Hajj SD, Tyrrell L, Black JA, Waxman SG. NaN, a novel voltage-gated Na channel, is expressed preferentially in peripheral sensory neurons and down-regulated after axotomy. Proc Natl Acad Sci USA 1998; 95: 8963–8968.
18. Rizzo MA, Kocsis JD, Waxman SG. Selective loss of slow and enhancement of fast Na$^+$ currents in cutaneous afferent dorsal root ganglion neurones following axotomy. Neurobiol Dis 1995; 2: 87–96.

19. Cummins TR, Waxman SG. Downregulation of tetrodotoxin-resistant sodium currents and upregulation of a rapidly repriming tetrodotoxin-sensitive sodium current in small spinal sensory neurons after nerve injury. J Neurosci 1997; 17: 3503–3514.

20. Black JA, Cummins TR, Plumpton C et al. Upregulation of a silent sodium channel after peripheral, but not central, nerve injury in DRG neurons. J Neurophysiol 1999; 82: 2776–2785.

21. Dib-Hajj SD, Fjell J, Cummins TR et al. Plasticity of sodium channel expression in DRG neurons in the chronic constriction injury model of neuropathic pain. Pain 1999; 83: 591–600.

22. Waxman SG, Dib-Hajj S, Cummins TR, Black JA. Sodium channels and pain. Proc Natl Acad Sci USA 1999; 96: 7635–7639.

23. Porreca F, Lai J, Bian D et al. A comparison of the potential role of the tetrodotoxin-insensitive sodium channels, PN3/SNS and NaN/SNS2, in rat models of chronic pain. Proc Natl Acad Sci USA 1999; 96: 7640–7644.

24. Tate S, Benn S, Hick C et al. Two sodium channels contribute to the TTX-R sodium current in primary sensory neurons. Nat Neurosci 1998; 1: 653–655.

25. Chen L, Huang LY. Protein kinase C reduces $Mg^{2+}$ block of NMDA-receptor channels as a mechanism of modulation. Nature 1992; 356: 521–523.

26. Lin Q, Peng YB, Willis WD. Possible role of protein kinase C in the sensitization of primate spinothalamic tract neurons. J Neurosci 1996; 16: 3026–3034.

27. Malmberg AB, Chen C, Tonegawa S, Basbaum AI. Preserved acute pain and reduced neuropathic pain in mice lacking PKCgamma. Science 1997; 278: 279–283.

28. Yu XM, Askalan R, Keil GJ, 2nd, Salter MW. NMDA channel regulation by channel-associated protein tyrosine kinase Src. Science 1997; 275: 674–678.

29. Yu XM, Salter MW. Src, a molecular switch governing gain control of synaptic transmission mediated by N-methyl-D-aspartate receptors. Proc Natl Acad Sci USA 1999; 96: 7697–7704.

30. Woolf CJ, Thompson SW. The induction and maintenance of central sensitization is dependent on N-methyl-D-aspartic acid receptor activation; implications for the treatment of post-injury pain hypersensitivity states. Pain 1991; 44: 293–299.

31. Ma QP, Woolf CJ. Involvement of neurokinin receptors in the induction but not the maintenance of mechanical allodynia in rat flexor motoneurones. J Physiol 1995; 486(Pt 3): 769–777.

32. Traub RJ. The spinal contribution of substance P to the generation and maintenance of inflammatory hyperalgesia in the rat. Pain 1996; 67: 151–161.

33. Smith GD, Wiseman J, Harrison SM, Elliott PJ, Birch PJ. Pre treatment with MK-801, a non-competitive NMDA antagonist, prevents development of mechanical hyperalgesia in a rat model of chronic neuropathy, but not in a model of chronic inflammation. Neurosci Lett 1994; 165: 79–83.

34. Kawamata M, Omote K. Involvement of increased excitatory amino acids and intracellular $Ca^{2+}$ concentration in the spinal dorsal horn in an animal model of neuropathic pain. Pain 1996; 68: 85–96.

35. Yamamoto T, Yaksh TL. Spinal pharmacology of thermal hyperesthesia induced by constriction injury of sciatic nerve. Excitatory amino acid antagonists. Pain 1992; 49: 121–128.

36. Mao J, Price DD, Hayes RL, Lu J, Mayer DJ. Differential roles of NMDA and non-NMDA receptor activation in induction and maintenance of thermal hyperalgesia in rats with painful peripheral mononeuropathy. Brain Res 1992; 598: 271–278.

37. Hudspith MJ, Harrisson S, Smith G *et al.* Effect of post-injury NMDA antagonist treatment on long-term Fos expression and hyperalgesia in a model of chronic neuropathic pain. Brain Res 1999; 822: 220–227.
38. Sotgiu ML, Biella G. Differential effects of MK-801, a N-methyl-D-aspartate non-competitive antagonist, on the dorsal horn neuron hyperactivity and hyperexcitability in neuropathic rats. Neurosci Lett 2000; 283: 153–156.
39. Suzuki R, Matthews EA, Dickenson AH. Comparison of the effects of MK-801, ketamine and memantine on responses of spinal dorsal horn neurones in a rat model of mononeuropathy. Pain 2001; 91: 101–109.
40. Parsons CG. NMDA receptors as targets for drug action in neuropathic pain. Eur J Pharmacol 2001; 429: 71–78.
41. Yamakura T, Shimoji K. Subunit- and site-specific pharmacology of the NMDA receptor channel. Prog Neurobiol 1999; 59: 279–298.
42. Boyce S, Wyatt A, Webb JK *et al.* Selective NMDA NR2B antagonists induce antinociception without motor dysfunction: correlation with restricted localisation of NR2B subunit in dorsal horn. Neuropharmacology 1999; 38: 611–623.
43. Watanabe M, Mishina M, Inoue Y. Distinct spatiotemporal distributions of the N-methyl-D-aspartate receptor channel subunit mRNAs in the mouse cervical cord. J Comp Neurol 1994; 345: 314–319.
44. Urban MO, Gebhart GF. Supraspinal contributions to hyperalgesia. Proc Natl Acad Sci USA 1999; 96: 7687–7692.
45. Pertovaara A, Wei H, Hamalainen MM. Lidocaine in the rostroventromedial medulla and the periaqueductal gray attenuates allodynia in neuropathic rats. Neurosci Lett 1996; 218: 127–130.
46. Kauppila T. Spinalization increases the mechanical stimulation-induced withdrawal reflex threshold after a sciatic cut in the rat. Brain Res 1997; 770: 310–312.
47. Bian D, Ossipov MH, Zhong C, Malan Jr TP, Porreca F. Tactile allodynia, but not thermal hyperalgesia, of the hindlimbs is blocked by spinal transection in rats with nerve injury. Neurosci Lett 1998; 241: 79–82.
48. Pons TP, Garraghty PE, Ommaya AK, Kaas JH, Taub E, Mishkin M. Massive cortical reorganization after sensory deafferentation in adult macaques. Science 1991; 252: 1857–1860.
49. Elbert T, Flor H, Birbaumer N *et al.* Extensive reorganization of the somatosensory cortex in adult humans after nervous system injury. Neuroreport 1994; 5: 2593–2597.
50. Florence SL, Kaas JH. Large-scale reorganization at multiple levels of the somatosensory pathway follows therapeutic amputation of the hand in monkeys. J Neurosci 1995; 15: 8083–8095.
51. Flor H, Elbert T, Knecht S *et al.* Phantom-limb pain as a perceptual correlate of cortical reorganization following arm amputation. Nature 1995; 375: 482–484.
52. Flor H, Elbert T, Muhlnickel W, Pantev C, Wienbruch C, Taub E. Cortical reorganization and phantom phenomena in congenital and traumatic upper-extremity amputees. Exp Brain Res 1998; 119: 205–212.
53. Florence SL, Taub HB, Kaas JH. Large-scale sprouting of cortical connections after peripheral injury in adult macaque monkeys. Science 1998; 282: 1117–1121.
54. Nikolajsen L, Ilkjaer S, Christensen JH, Kroner K, Jensen TS. Randomised trial of epidural bupivacaine and morphine in prevention of stump and phantom pain in lower-limb amputation. Lancet 1997; 350: 1353–1357.
55. Flor H, Denke C, Schaefer M, Grusser S. Effect of sensory discrimination training on cortical reorganisation and phantom limb pain. Lancet 2001; 357: 1763–1764.

56. Shimoji K, Hokari T, Kano T *et al*. Management of intractable pain with percutaneous epidural spinal cord stimulation: differences in pain-relieving effects among diseases and sites of pain. Anesth Analg 1993; 77: 110–116.

57. Parry CB. Pain in avulsion lesions of the brachial plexus. Pain 1980; 9: 41–53.

58. Coderre TJ, Katz J, Vaccarino AL, Melzack R. Contribution of central neuroplasticity to pathological pain: review of clinical and experimental evidence. Pain 1993; 52: 259–285.

59. Ishijima B, Shimoji K, Shimizu H, Takahashi H, Suzuki I. Lesions of spinal and trigeminal dorsal root entry zone for deafferentation pain. Experience of 35 cases. Appl Neurophysiol 1988; 51: 175–187.

60. Kumagai Y, Shimoji K, Honma T *et al*. Problems related to dorsal root entry zone lesions. Acta Neurochir 1992; 115: 71–78.

61. Boas R. Complex Regional Pain Syndromes: Symptoms, Signs, and Differential Diagnosis. In: Janig W, Stanton-Hicks M. (eds) Reflex Sympathetic Dystrophy: A Reappraisal. Seattle, USA: IASP Press, 1996; 79–92.

62. Habler HJ, Janig W, Koltzenburg M. Activation of unmyelinated afferents in chronically lesioned nerves by adrenaline and excitation of sympathetic efferents in the cat. Neurosci Lett 1987; 82: 35–40.

63. McLachlan EM, Janig W, Devor M, Michaelis M. Peripheral nerve injury triggers noradrenergic sprouting within dorsal root ganglia. Nature 1993; 363: 543–546.

64. Chen Y, Michaelis M, Janig W, Devor M. Adrenoreceptor subtype mediating sympathetic-sensory coupling in injured sensory neurons. J Neurophysiol 1996; 76: 3721–3730.

65. Birder LA, Perl ER. Expression of alpha2-adrenergic receptors in rat primary afferent neurones after peripheral nerve injury or inflammation. J Physiol 1999; 515(Pt 2): 533–542.

66. Stanton-Hicks M, Baron R, Boas R *et al*. Complex regional pain syndromes: guidelines for therapy. Clin J Pain 1998; 14: 155–166.

67. Stanton-Hicks M, Raj P, Racz G. Use of regional anesthetics for diagnosis of reflex sympathetic dystrophy and sympathetically maintained pain: a critical evaluation. In: Janig W, Stanton-Hicks M. (eds) Reflex Sympathetic Dystrophy: A Reappraisal. Seattle, USA: IASP Press, 1996; 217–237.

68. Kemler MA, Reulen JP, Barendse GA, van Kleef M, de Vet HC, van den Wildenberg FA. Impact of spinal cord stimulation on sensory characteristics in complex regional pain syndrome type I: a randomized trial. Anesthesiology 2001; 95: 72–80.

69. Tesfaye S, Watt J, Benbow SJ, Pang KA, Miles J, MacFarlane IA. Electrical spinal-cord stimulation for painful diabetic peripheral neuropathy. Lancet 1996; 348: 1698–1701.

70. Kost RG, Straus SE. Postherpetic neuralgia – pathogenesis, treatment, and prevention. N Engl J Med 1996; 335: 32–42.

71. Oaklander AL. The density of remaining nerve endings in human skin with and without postherpetic neuralgia after shingles. Pain 2001; 92: 139–145.

72. Oaklander AL, Romans K, Horasek S, Stocks A, Hauer P, Meyer RA. Unilateral postherpetic neuralgia is associated with bilateral sensory neuron damage. Ann Neurol 1998; 44: 789–795.

73. Sabel BA. Unrecognized potential of surviving neurons: within-systems plasticity, recovery of function, and the hypothesis of minimal residual structure. Neuroscientist 1997; 3: 366–370.

74. Fields HL, Rowbotham M, Baron R. Postherpetic neuralgia: irritable nociceptors and deafferentation. Neurobiol Dis 1998; 5: 209–227.

75. Kanazi GE, Johnson RW, Dworkin RH. Treatment of postherpetic neuralgia: an update. Drugs 2000; 59: 1113–1126.

76. Rowbotham MC, Davies PS, Verkempinck C, Galer BS. Lidocaine patch: double-blind controlled study of a new treatment method for post-herpetic neuralgia. Pain 1996; 65: 39–44.

77. Rowbotham M, Harden N, Stacey B, Bernstein P, Magnus-Miller L. Gabapentin for the treatment of postherpetic neuralgia: a randomized controlled trial. JAMA 1998; 280: 1837–1842.

78. Watson CP, Babul N. Efficacy of oxycodone in neuropathic pain: a randomized trial in postherpetic neuralgia. Neurology 1998; 50: 1837–1841.

*D. Parker   R. Lawton*

# Managing medical mishaps: learning lessons from industry

The promotion of patient safety by reducing medical error is currently at the top of the UK Government's agenda for the National Health Service (NHS).[1,2] Since the publication of *An Organisation with a Memory* in 2000, the practice of healthcare professionals is coming under increasing scrutiny from an anxious public and a scandal-hungry media. Although record keeping is far from comprehensive, attempts to quantify medical error have suggested that the problem is endemic.[3,4] It has been estimated that adverse events occur in 10% of all hospital admissions, at a cost to the UK of £2 billion a year.[2]

All of this means that there is a pressing need for medicine to address patient safety. An attempt will be made in this chapter to outline the factors that influence the likelihood of medical failure, and how other sectors, primarily the safety critical, high-risk industries, have tackled the problem of error. Many lessons have already been learned elsewhere, and medicine should be able to benefit from that hard-earned knowledge, and avoid some potential pitfalls. It has already been recognized that, within medicine, anaesthesiology and analgesiology are most closely analogous to operators in other high-risk situations, e.g. pilots[5] and so it is important that these specialties are at the forefront in addressing human error in medicine.[6]

For the purposes of this chapter, an error may be defined as *the failure of planned actions to achieve their desired ends – without the intervention of some unforeseeable event.*[7] In any consideration of the role of human error in adverse events we always need to keep in mind that to err is human. There is no such thing as error free performance in human terms. Bearing that in mind, it is useful to consider a range of ways in which error defined in this broad way has been categorized by academics with expertise in organizational safety.

## Some Useful Distinctions

### Levels of human performance

One very influential distinction was made in the 1970s by Jens Rasmussen, using the 'think-aloud' verbal protocols of electronics technicians engaged in problem solving. He distinguishes three levels of human performance and describes the types of error likely to occur at each level.[8,9,10]

The *skill-based level* of performance occurs when tasks are familiar and actions are governed by stored sets of instructions, without conscious thought. Performance at this level is generally very good, for example, when we control the way in which we manipulate a vacuum cleaner. Error at this level relates to problems with co-ordination of actions.

The *rule-based level* of performance applies when we try to solve trained-for problems by the application of stored if-then rules. We match the characteristics of the problem to our stored knowledge of solutions, and then consciously check that we have selected the correct solution. If we hear the note of the vacuum cleaner motor is changing, and realize the dust bag is full, we then apply the stored solution of changing the bag. At this level of performance error usually stems from application of the wrong rule, or misremembering of the correct rule. So, for example, we may think the change in note signals a blockage in the pipe, or a twisted cable, and attempt to solve the problem that way.

The third level of performance, known as the *knowledge-based level*, involves consciously thinking the problem through. This level is relevant when the problem faced is novel and conscious effort must be made to construct a plan of action from stored knowledge. In the vacuum cleaning example, this type of performance would be necessary if the person cleaning had never had to change a dust bag before, and had to work out from scratch what the new sound might indicate. Error at this level of performance can arise from incorrect knowledge or from the limitations of our cognitive resources. According to Rasmussen's model, as expertise and familiarity with a problem increases, performance moves from the knowledge-based through the rule-based to the skill-based level. The three levels are not mutually exclusive, but represent a progression, leading to skilled performance.

Rasmussen's model was further developed in 1990, when Reason presented his Generic Error Modelling System (GEMS) framework. This Generic Error Modelling System[7] describes three main error types, and combines Rasmussen's model with the work of Norman[11] on error types. At the skill-based performance level, the kind of errors likely to be made are slips, which are the result of inattention, or lapses, which are the result of overattention. The difference between slips and lapses can be highlighted with reference to the task of starting a car. Chatting to your passenger, and consequently moving off without fastening your seatbelt would be a slip, whereas reaching round to grasp an already fastened seatbelt would be a lapse. In both cases, you are dealing with a routine, straightforward task that demands no conscious thought. Your attention is captured by a distractor, in this case the passenger, and a necessary step in the routine is either omitted or repeated. Mistakes occurring at the rule-based level of performance, on the other hand, are made with the full conscious attention of the individual involved, who is actively trying to solve a problem. The most frequent form of rule-based mistakes involves the misapplication of well-rehearsed problem solving strategies, stored in memory. This can be broken down further into the misapplication of good rules or the application of bad rules. In other words either the correct solution to the problem is applied wrongly, or the wrong solution to the problem is applied correctly. Full attention is also engaged during performance at the knowledge-based level. Mistakes that occur at this level of performance happen when the individual is faced with a problem he or she has never come across before, and so has no pre-stored solutions available, and has to rely on on-line problem-solving to construct a solution. This real-time problem-solving is an effortful process that may be hampered by situational constraints, with the result that error becomes more likely.

## Error and violation

Helpful as these classifications are, they do not tell the whole story. A further distinction, between error and violation, is necessary to capture the complete range of ways in which human performance can and does go astray.[12] According to this distinction the chief characteristic of error is that it is unintentional. Indeed, this characteristic was the focus of the definition offered earlier. Errors arise from information processing problems of various types, which result in a lack of ability to do the job right. In an organizational setting, the likelihood of error can be reduced by training, better information in the workplace etc. When an adverse event occurs as the result of error, it can usually be understood in relation to one or more individuals. On the other hand, violation often has nothing to do with ability, and much more to do with motivation. The chief characteristic of violation is that it represents a deliberate deviation from normal or recommended practice, it is, at least in part, intentional. Therefore the roots of violation are motivational, and can only be understood with reference to the social context within which it occurs. In order to reduce the likelihood of violation, organizations must pay attention to staff morale, and to the prevailing beliefs, attitudes and norms of organizational safety.

In terms of medical practice, errors are more likely to occur when time is short, when the task at hand is unfamiliar, when the task is ill-defined and complex, or when the interface between the individual and the technological system within which he or she operates is poor. Violations are also made more likely by time pressure and high workload, but for different reasons. Here the problem is not that the individual does not know what to do, or is unable to carry out the correct procedures. Rather the individual decides to bend the rules and deviates from the procedure in the full knowledge that they are doing so. The likelihood of violation is also increased when the procedures to be followed are not workable in the prevailing conditions, when the equipment necessary to carry out the procedure is unavailable or when supervision of practice is poor, affording the opportunity to violate.

## Active and latent failures

A third distinction, and one that has proved exceptionally useful in the analysis of organizational accidents, is that between active and latent failures. Active failures involve unsafe acts, be they errors or violations, by those on the front line of operations. So, they might involve the operators of dangerous machinery, the pilot of an aircraft, or the nurses and doctors working at the bedside or in the operating theatre. Active failures tend to have immediate and obvious negative consequences. There is often a tendency to blame the individual at the sharp end, as they are the obvious culprit. However, the sort of blame culture that this engenders brings many problems, including the tendency to look no further than the proximal actions of those involved. A culture of blame leads to low morale among staff who may be working in situations where error is almost inevitable, and an understandable reluctance to report near-misses and incidents that, while not leading to actual accidents, nevertheless would provide invaluable information to those charged with making improvements to safety.

Latent failures, on the other hand, arise from the decisions and actions of those far removed from the front line, in both space and time. These failures, which tend to involve issues such as work planning, resource allocation and staffing levels, have no immediate ill effect, but lie dormant within the organizational system until such time as an unfortunate concatenation of circumstances allows their effect to be felt.[10,13,14]

Latent failures can have two kinds of adverse effect. First, they can translate into error provoking conditions (e.g. time pressure, understaffing, inadequate equipment) which ultimately lead to unsafe acts in the form of errors and violations. Second, they can create long-lasting holes or weaknesses in organizational defences (e.g. untrustworthy alarms, unworkable procedures, design deficiencies). Take the example of the capsize of the cross-channel ferry the Herald of Free Enterprise on its way out of Zeebrugge. Although the latent and active failures in this case were many, a number stand out as being obvious systems failures. One such latent failure that resulted in a total absence of defence against error was the inability to monitor the bow door from the ship's control. Despite numerous previous requests from crew members no alarm had been fitted to indicate whether or not the bow door was closed. On the day of the disaster the bosun, whose responsibility it was to close the door, was asleep in his cabin. Another example of a latent failure that directly lead to errors being made was the tight scheduling of the ferries which did not allow for sufficient turn-around for loading safely and performing all the necessary safety checks. Mr Justice Sheen wrote of the disaster 'At first sight the faults which led to this disaster were the errors of omission on the part of the Master, the Chief Officer and the Assistant Bosun. But a full investigation into the circumstances of the disaster leads inexorably to the conclusion that the underlying faults lay higher up in the company. From top to bottom the body corporate was infected with the disease of sloppiness'.[15]

## Moving the Focus from the Individual: The Systems Approach

The move away from the person-centred approach that seeks to identify individual failures and towards the systems approach necessitated by the search for latent failures has gathered pace in recent years. A crucial early contribution came from the late Barry Turner whose seminal book on *Man Made Disasters*[16] developed the idea of an incubation period for errors within a system, suggesting that errors could lie dormant until circumstances allowed their negative effects to take place. Charles Perrow also made an enormous contribution to this literature, in his book *The Normal Accident*[17] in which he showed how automation, opacity, and the increasingly complex nature of the work in high-risk industries lent themselves to error at all levels of the system. After the event, and with the benefit of hindsight, it is often possible to trace warning signs of an impending adverse event, but foresight is naturally more limited. It is clear from experimental work that people tend to overestimate not only the likelihood that they would have recognized a warning, but also the amount that others actually know before the adverse event.[18] Wagenaar and Groenweg[19] made the point that many accidents seem impossible to those subsequently involved – at least, before they happen. Accidents in complex, highly technical systems, and healthcare would certainly be among them, are often the result of unforeseeable coincidences of unpredictable circumstances. No one individual is privy to all the information that would be necessary to facilitate prediction of the accident. Everyone has only a partial set of information. Therefore, blaming the unfortunate individual who makes what may well be the last in a chain of errors is both unfair and unhelpful.

The basic premise of the systems approach is that human beings are fallible and that errors will always be made.[20] In the context of healthcare, this suggests that errors are just as likely to be the consequences as the causes of poor management of patient safety. This is because, while it is impossible to 'engineer' an error-free human being, it is possible to change the conditions under which humans work. The aim should be to engineer the system to minimise the likelihood of error and violation. When the systems approach is taken, the response to an adverse event is not to find out who made a blunder, but to find out how the defences built into the system to prevent blunders, failed. In order to prevent future adverse events, a proactive approach must be taken, attempting to identify and rectify weaknesses in the system, rather than simply focusing on fixing the individual. Some progress towards the adoption of a systems approach in healthcare is currently being made with the setting up of a national reporting system by the National Patient Safety Agency (NPSA). That agency's brief is to use the lessons that can be drawn from analysis of a wide range of data collected with respect to adverse events, in order to promote patient safety in a blame-free open environment.[1,2]

## Organizational Culture

From the analysis above, it is clear that organizational issues are key to the promotion of patient safety. This is gradually being recognized in the healthcare sector, and it is likely that achieving the right kind of organizational culture will be a focus in the coming years. Organizational culture is a slippery concept, but has been concisely defined as 'a complex framework of national, organizational and professional attitudes and values within which groups and individuals function'.[21] While a good definition of safety culture is even more difficult to come by, most commentators agree that advanced safety cultures have 'a common commitment to safety as a top-level priority, which permeates the entire organization'.[22] This involves (a) the acknowledgement that the organization's activites are intrinsically high-risk, and therefore prone to error, (b) the fostering of an environment in which individuals feel free to report errors, near-misses and incidents without fearing blame, (c) the active involvement of all grades of staff in the development and implementation of solutions to safety problems and (d) the commitment of sufficient time and resources to address safety issues.[21,23,24] Having a strong safety culture need not have an adverse effect on throughput. Indeed, the authors of a recent report to the US Institute of Medicine of the National Academy of Sciences[25] comment that in organizations with a strong safety culture it is 'the most critical underlying feature of their accomplishments'.

This theme is taken up in a recent paper by Reason *et al.*,[26] who suggest that a constant preoccupation with safety is necessary. The vulnerable organization is one characterised by blame, denial and 'the single-minded pursuit of the wrong kind of excellence', the last of which, in healthcare, usually means an unjustified and blinkered focus on a small number of critical indicators such as number of cancelled operations or bed occupancy rates.

## Learning the Lessons

On Tuesday 10th October 1999, at just after 8 am two trains collided two miles from Paddington station in London, UK. Thirty-one people died in the accident, including one newly qualified train driver who passed a signal at red. The Ladbroke Grove Rail Inquiry[27] (HSC, 2001) identified both primary and underlying causes of the event. The primary cause was that one of the drivers drove past the signal at red and then continued under power without recognizing that he was entering an unsignalled route. Adopting a person-centred approach to this incident would result in a focus on the actions of the driver in question. Why did he pass the signal at danger? Was he intoxicated, incompetent, unskilled? Was his training adequate? However, it is only with a much deeper analysis of the latent failures that existed within the system, that the event can be understood and organizational learning achieved.

The following were identified as situational and organizational factors contributing to the accident:

- There was persistent difficulty in the sighting of these particular signals, which had been passed at danger eight times in the previous seven years.
- The training that the novice driver had received which may not have included the particular routing the train took on the day in question.
- The bright sunlight which may have accentuated the yellow 'proceed' signals.
- Problems with communication which meant that new drivers were not made aware of problems with sighting the signal in question.

- The signaler, assuming that the driver would realise his error and stop before he reached the points where the crash occurred, did not act swiftly enough to avoid the collision. This suggests that the same thing had happened before.

The Bristol Royal Infirmary Inquiry[28] in the UK offers another example of an analysis employing the systems approach, and going beyond the failures of the consultant surgeons and managers involved. The report discusses a number of organizational factors, many reflecting the prevailing culture of the NHS at the time, such as poor teamwork, problems of accountability, substandard safety arrangements and a lack of openness about data. The report into the quality of care in paediatric cardiac surgery at Bristol is extensive, but one overriding theme is the inability of the organization to learn, or even recognize the need to learn, from mistakes. In making recommendations about strategies for improvement, the report highlights a need to adopt an 'approach to safety based on designing safer systems and equipment.... The National Patient Safety Agency should bring together interested parties to tackle some of the more *persistent causes of unsafe practices*'.

A final example, of direct relevance to the anaesthetist, is the recent case of Wayne Jowett who died in January 2001 following the intrathecal injection of vincristine. The drug was administered by a doctor in the grade of Senior House Officer (SHO), working under supervision, directly following the correct administration of cytotoxic therapy by the intrathecal route. The UK Department of Health commissioned Professor Brian Toft to undertake the inquiry into this incident using a systems approach. While the immediately proximal error was clear, a wide range of factors that had contributed to the incident were identified, including labelling of syringes, problems with communication between staff and conflicting protocols. Despite all these failures the most dangerous single factor identified in the inquiry was the fact that the syringe containing vincristine could be connected to the spinal needle and that once in place there were no other defensive mechanisms that prevented the drug from being administered.

In the past decade there have been five recorded incidents of intrathecal errors.[29] Furthermore, intrathecal injection errors represent only one form of misconnection error arising from the use of the standard Luer® connector across a wide range of medical devices. Some experts in the field[30] are now calling for a new system of connectors that allows for differentiation between various functions – respiratory, vascular, enteral and neuraxial. In this example, a *persistent cause of unsafe practices* has been identified: the standard Luer® connector. However, redesigning a whole system of connectors is a complex and expensive project and has the potential to lead to other forms of error, e.g. misidentification of connector which, although not fatal in themselves, could lead to delays in care. Thus, if a new system of connectors were to be developed designers, psychologists, risk analysis experts and healthcare professionals would need to be involved in the process. It is the time, effort and expense of eradicating this kind of latent failure that means that disciplining the person to 'blame' is often the easiest and most emotionally satisfying strategy.[31]

## Systems Approaches to Error in Anaesthesia

It is often quoted that the state of anaesthesia is intrinsically unsafe.[32] Moreover, the anaesthetist is in the unusual situation, not unlike that of a pilot, of performing for long periods of time at the automatic, skill-based level identified by Rasmussen,[8] vigilant for long periods of time, yet expected to react quickly and decisively when appropriate. At this stage the anaesthetist may apply existing internalised rules or, if none exists, must solve the problem by relying on experience and knowledge. Thus, the anaesthetist is susceptible to errors at the skill-based level (e.g. missing an important equipment check when distracted), the rule-based level (e.g. assuming that increases in heart rate and blood pressure indicate inadequate anaesthesia rather than disconnection from the ventilator) or the knowledge-based level (e.g. administration of a drug contraindicated in a particular condition). Error is not uncommon in anaesthesia as a number of recent prevalence studies have shown. In one study[33] 89% of 66 respondents had reported at least one error of drug administration, while 12.5% had caused harm to a patient. In another study,[34] one drug administration error was reported for every 133 cases.

While patients expect to experience some pain following surgery they do not expect complications such as physical injury to arise from the anaesthetic. Perhaps as a direct result of these expectations litigation rates against anaesthetists in some countries are high. It is not surprising then that anaesthetics as a specialty has always been forward looking. For example, critical incident reporting was first introduced into medicine in anaesthesia.[35] However, in spite of this, the most influential studies in this area[36,37] have identified situational factors such as inexperience, fatigue, poor communication, failures in planning and checking, but have not investigated the underlying or organizational causes of the individual failures. This is changing rapidly in response to recent UK Government White Papers.[1,2] For example, Battles and Shea[38] used root cause analysis to investigate errors made by graduate medical trainees. They identified deficiencies of educational content, problems of program structure and procedural and management issues. A further study[39] identified root causes and used them to inform the implementation of process changes.

These included policy changes that led to increased use of forcing or constraining functions (for example, removal of concentrated intravenous potassium solutions from floor stocks) and better personnel support (for example, early awareness of and response to localized changes in patient numbers). These changes led to reductions in adverse events from 7.2 to 4.0 per 100,000 patient days. Root cause analysis techniques have also been applied successfully to other indicators of quality such as patient satisfaction[40] and problems with admissions.[41]

A recent study[42] investigated the incidence and nature of organizational failure before urgent and emergency surgery in a district general hospital. This was an unusual study in that the 159 cases were studied prospectively over a 30-day period. Organizational problems were reported to have affected more than half of the cases overall (54%). The most common organizational problems affecting the commencement of anaesthesia were a non-urgent prior case (21 cases) and the inavailability of the results of investigations (16 cases), both of which led to considerable delays to surgery (average 195 and 150 minutes respectively). Other organizational factors included the surgeon being unavailable (14 cases), a clinical emergency (13 cases) and the patient not being prepared for ward (13 cases). While this study did not set out to make the link between organizational factors and mortality and morbidity, a qualitative study of risk factors in anaesthesia did. From deaths reported by anaesthetists in 46 Dutch hospitals, Arbous et al.,[43] identified 119 deaths (from a total of 811) where anaesthesia was implicated. Each death was further analysed to identify the factors contributing to different aspects of anaesthetic management (cardiovascular management, ventilatory management, patient monitoring and other anaesthetic management). Human failure was identified as a contributory factor in between 60% (for patient monitoring) and 77% (for cardiovascular management) of the deaths. Other factors identified in this study were inadequate communication, lack of supervision and inadequate care. Organizational factors were reported to have been a contributory factor in between 11% (for cardiovascular management) and 40% (for patient monitoring) of the deaths. However the authors acknowledge, that the human failures reported may also reflect organizational problems that were not immediately identifiable from the reports. For example, the decision of an anaesthetist not to send a patient to intensive care might stem, not from flawed decision making, but from the knowledge that postoperative facilities are unavailable. It is likely that a large proportion of the human failures identified in this study could be eradicated by system improvements.

Detailed analysis of adverse events which focuses on the task, situational and organizational factors that lead to errors and violations, or allows these active failures to breach the systems defences, is one form of organizational learning. However, for effective safety management this reactive approach is often 'too little and too late'.[44] Moreover, cultural changes are slow and he prevailing belief, of patients and doctors, that fallibility represents incompetence, makes the reporting of one's errors or the errors of others unlikely.[45] Following the edict 'prevention is better than cure' some organizations have adopted a proactive approach to error management. This approach assumes that accidents are only the tip of the iceberg and that treating errors one by one as they are identified in incident reports is inefficient and cost ineffective. Dealing with the source of the outbreak is a much more effective approach. Using a medical metaphor,[44] error management requires the continual monitoring of the 'safety health' of the organization through the measurement of 'vital signs'. The vital signs to be measured and the way this measurement takes place varies between organizations,[13] but usually includes monitoring at the task, workplace and organizational levels. For example, in an error management tool developed for Shell International Exploration and Production[46] 11 General Failure Types were identified through studies of accident records and observations of working practices. These included failures associated with procedures, communications, training, incompatible goals, design and hardware. These 'vital signs' are then assessed via checklists that are constructed from banks of specific indicators (20 items for each failure type) of the presence of the general failure type (e.g. for procedures an indicator might be – is the permit to work schedule available at the work location, while for hardware an indicator might be – in the last month have you had to borrow any equipment from another team or site). These banks of items are developed by task specialists and scored by those people doing the job. The result of this procedure is a profile of the safety health of the organization which identifies those general failure types that are most in need of improvement. These are the organizational factors, the process assumes, that are most likely to give rise to errors in the near future.

## Conclusions

The feeling that 'It won't happen to me' reflects what psychologists term the 'illusion of control'.[47] While it is a comforting philosophy, in actual fact everyone makes errors. Those that occur in medicine are usually not the result of laziness, ignorance or plain lack of professionalism on the part of a few bad doctors and nurses. While there probably are a few bad nurses and doctors, they should normally be identifiable by applying the principles of attribution theory,[48] consistency, distinctiveness and consensus. In practical terms, if a nurse or doctor repeatedly makes errors (high consistency), those errors take different forms and occur in different situations (low distinctiveness) and are errors that other people are unlikely to make (low consensus), then it is more than likely that this pattern of errors reflects some problem with the individual. However, the errors made by these bad nurses and doctors are too few to account for the large numbers recorded in recent studies.[1] As we have seen, errors are a consequence of the systems in which human beings work and the way they are 'wired up' to do the job. Everyone is lazy in the sense that they prefer not to waste information processing resources on routine tasks, but instead rely on heuristics or 'rules of thumb' in problem solving. Everyone is ignorant in that there is so much information available and medicine develops so quickly that it is very difficult to have the most up to date research findings at our fingertips. Health professionals are no better or worse than any other human being in this respect. If we are to learn from mistakes, we must accept our limitations and endeavour to design systems that, by compensating for these limitations, prevent errors arising, as well as detecting and defending against them when they do.

## References

1. Chief Medical Officer. CMO's Update. London: HMSO 2001; 30: 6.
2. Department of Health. An organization with a memory: report of an expert group on learning from adverse events in the NHS. London: HMSO 2000.
3. Vincent C, Neale G, Woloshynowych M. Adverse events in British hospitals: preliminary retrospective record review. BMJ 2001; 3221: 517–519.
4. Reinerstein JL. Let's talk about error. BMJ 2000; 320: 730.
5. Gabba DM. Human error in dynamic medical domains. In: Bogner MS. Human Error in Medicine. Hillsdale, NJ, USA: Erlbaum, 1994; 197–224.
6. Krueger GP. Fatigue, performance and medical error. In: Bogner MS. Human Error in Medicine. Hillsdale, NJ, USA: Erlbaum, 1994; 311–326.
7. Reason JT. Human Error. Cambridge: Cambridge University Press, 1990.
8. Rasmussen J, Jensen A. Mental procedures in real-life tasks: A case study of electronic troubleshooting. Erg 1974; 17: 293–307.
9. Rasmussen J. Human error and the problem of causality in analysis of accidents. Philos Trans R Soc Lond B Biol Sci 1990; 327: 449–460.
10. Rasmussen J. Afterword. In: Bogner MS. Human Error in Medicine. Hillsdale, NJ, USA: Erlbaum, 1994; 385–393.
11. Norman DA. Categorization of action slips. Psych Rev 1981; 88: 1–15.
12. Reason JT, Manstead ASR, Stradling SG, Baxter JS, Campbell K. Errors and violations on the road: A real distinction? Erg 1990; 33: 1315–1332.
13. Reason JT. Managing the risks of organizational accidents. Aldershot, UK Ashgate, 1995.
14. Reason JT. Human error: Models and management. BMJ 2000; 320: 768–770.
15. Sheen, Mr Justice MV Herald of Free Enterprise. Report of Court No. 8074 Formal Investigation. London UK: Dept. of Transport, 1987.
16. Turner BA. Man-made disaster. London UK: Wykeham, 1978.
17. Perrow C. Normal accidents: Living with high-risk technology. New York, USA: Basic Books 1984.
18. Fischoff B. Hindsight does not equal foresight: The effect of outcome knowledge on judgement under uncertainty. J Exp Psych: Hum Perf Perc 1975; 1: 288–299.

19. Wagenaar WA, Groeneweg J. Accidents at sea: Multiple causes and impossible consequences. Int J Man-Mach St 1987; 27: 587–598.

20. Moray M. Error reduction as a systems problem. In: Bogner MS. Human Error in Medicine. Hillsdale, NJ, USA: Erlbaum, 1994; 67–93.

21. Helmreich RL, Merritt AC. Culture at work in aviation and medicine: National, organizational and professional influences. Aldershot, UK: Ashgate; 1998.

22. Pizzi LT, Goldfarb NI, Nash DB. Promoting a safety of culture. 2001; www.ahrq.gov/clinic/ptsafety/chap40.htm

23. Cooper MD. Towards a model of safety culture. Safety Sci 2000; 36: 111–136.

24. Geller ES. Ten leadership qualities for a total safety culture. Prof Safety 2000; 45: 30–32.

25. Kohn L, Corrigan J, Donaldson M. (eds) To Err is Human: Building a Safer Health System. Washington DC, USA: Committee on healthcare in America, Institute of Medicine. National Academy Press; 2000.

26. Reason JT, Carthey J, de Leval MR. Diagnosing 'vulnerable system syndrome': An essential prerequisite to effective risk management. Qual Safety Healthcare; in press.

27. Ladbroke grove.

28. Toft B. External inquiry into the adverse incident that occurred at Queen's Medical Centre, Nottingham, 4th January 2001; www.doh.gov.uk/qmcinquiry/index.htm

29. Woods K. The prevention of intrathecal medication errors: A report to the Chief Medical Officer. 2001; www.doh.gov.uk/imeprevent/index.htm

30. Bickford-Smith PJ. Designing safer medical devices requires financial and political support. BMJ 2001; 322: 548.

31. Wears RL, Janiak B. Moorhead JC et al. Human Error in Medicine: Promise and Pitfalls, Part 1. Ann Emerg Med 2000; 36: 58–60.

32. Davies J, Aitkenhead A. Clinical risk management in anaesthesia. In: Vincent C. Clinical Risk Management: Enhancing Patient Safety. London, UK: BMJ Books, 2001; 111–136.

33. Merry AF, Peck DJ. Anesthetists, errors in drug administration and the law, N Z Med J 1995; 108: 185–187.

34. Webster CS, Merry AF, Larsson L et al. The frequency and nature of drug administration error during anaesthesia, Anaesth Intensive Care 2001; 29: 494–500.

35. Blum LL. Equipment design and human limitations. Anesthesiology 1971; 35: 101–102.

36. Webb RK, Currie M, Morgan CA et al. The Australian Incident Monitoring Study: an analysis of 2000 incident reports, Anaesth Intensive Care 1993; 21: 520–528.

37. Buck N, Devlin HB, Lunn JN. Report on the Confidential Enquiry into Perioperative Deaths. London, UK: Nuffield Provincial Hospitals Trust, The Kings Fund Publishing House, 1987.

38. Battles JB, Shea CE. A system of analyzing medical errors to improve GME curricula and programs. Acad Med 2001; 76: 125–133.

39. Rex JH, Turnbull JE, Allen SJ et al. Systematic root cause analysis of adverse drug events in a tertiary referral hospital, Joint Commission Journal on Quality Improvement 2000; 26: 563–575.

40. Burroughs TE, Cira JC, Chartock P et al. Using root cause analysis to address patient satisfaction and other improvement opportunities. Joint Commission Journal on Quality Improvement 2000; 26: 439–449.

41. Weinberg NS, Stason WB. Managing quality in hospital practice. Int J Quality Health Care 1998; 10: 295–302.

42. Pearse RM, Dana EC, Lanigan CJ, Pook JAR. Organisational failures in urgent and emergency surgery – A potential peri-operative risk factor. Anaesthesia 2001; 56: 684–689.

43. Arbous MS, Grobbee DE, Van Kleef JW *et al*. Mortality associated with anaesthesia: A qualitative analysis to identify risk factors. Anaesthesia 2001; 56: 1141–1153.

44. Reason JT. Understanding adverse events: The human factor. In: Vincent C. Clinical Risk Management: Enhancing Patient Safety. London, UK: BMJ Books, 2001; 9–30.

45. Lawton R, Parker D. Barriers to incident reporting in healthcare systems, Qual in Health Care, in press.

46. Hudson P, Reason J, Wagenaar P *et al*. Tripod-Delta: proactive approach to enhanced safety. J Petroleum Tech 1994; 40: 58–62.

47. McKenna FP. It won't happen to me: Unrealistic optimism or the illusion of control? Br J of Psychol 1993; 84: 39–50.

48. Kelley HH. Attribution theory in social psychology. In: D. Levine. (ed) Nebraska Symposium on Motivation (Vol. 15, pp. 192–241). Lincoln: University of Nebraska Press, 1967.

*E. Hallinan  N.J.H. Davies*

# Legal issues in anaesthesia and intensive care

Anaesthesia today is remarkably safe and generally predictable. Standards of training and equipment are high. Nonetheless adverse incidents still occur, ranging from simple dental damage to catastrophic injury or even death. Patients today are less willing to overlook minor injuries such as a chipped tooth or a broken crown, and will seek compensation far more readily. At the other end of the scale, if a patient has suffered a major adverse consequence of anaesthesia as a result of negligence, it is morally right that he should receive full compensation. In the most serious cases, where the patient dies, the anaesthetist may even face criminal charges. This article will review the principles behind a legal action for clinical negligence, and also consider consent and criminal liability. Finally, we will briefly examine the initial impact of the Human Rights Act.

## Civil Claims

If a patient believes that he has suffered injury, his main remedy is to seek compensation by a civil action. He may have a claim in contract or in tort.

### Contract

A claim for breach of contract is most likely to arise in private practice. There is a contractual agreement to provide medical treatment in return for payment, either directly by the patient or by an insurance company to which the patient has paid premiums. For example, an anaesthetist might undertake to keep a patient free of awareness under general anaesthesia. It is generally accepted that there is no such contract for UK National Health Service (NHS) treatment because this is free and provided by statute. Any contribution made to the NHS by a tax-paying patient does not form the basis of a contract with an individual hospital or doctor.

In practice, a patient's rights to seek compensation for breach of contract will mirror their rights in tort (see below). The contract implies that the doctor will use reasonable care and skill, but does not guarantee success or cure unless the doctor promises this. Any doctor would be foolish to do so. Even the apparently simple operation of vasectomy may fail.[1]

## Tort

Tort is a civil wrong, and it is far more common for an injured patient to bring a claim for the tort of negligence. To succeed, he will need to establish first that the doctor owed him a duty of care, second that there had been a breach of that duty, and third that, as a consequence, the patient sustained an injury which was reasonably foreseeable. This last part, called 'causation', is often disputed. For example would an anaesthetist's failure to use an electrocardiogram (ECG) monitor at induction affect the outcome of, say, sudden severe anaphylaxis occurring at that time?

### Duty of care
It is well established in English law that a doctor owes his patient a duty of care. In a 1925 case,[2] Lord Stewart said, 'if a person holds himself out as possessing special skill and knowledge, and he is consulted, as possessing such skill and knowledge, by or on behalf of the patient, he owes a duty to that patient to use due caution in undertaking the treatment'.

### Breach of duty
A doctor will be negligent if he fails to meet the standard of a responsible colleague. This was first formulated in the 1957 decision of *Bolam v Friern Hospital Management Committee*[3] when Justice McNair stated 'a doctor is not negligent if he has acted in accordance with the practice accepted as proper by a responsible body of medical men skilled in that particular art'. Bolam was a psychiatric patient who suffered a broken hip during electric shock therapy. He alleged that it was negligent to administer this therapy without the use of a muscle relaxant. The Jury (such cases were decided by a Jury in 1957) rejected this allegation after considering the standard set down by Justice McNair.

In anaesthesia, there are often several opinions on how a patient should properly be managed. The Bolam judgment recognized that a particular management might be considered appropriate, even if pursued by only a minority of doctors, provided that it is a *responsible* minority.

A further gloss to this principle, adding the need for *reason*, was applied in the recent case of *Bolitho v City and Hackney Health Authority*.[4] A two-year-old boy was admitted to hospital with croup. Following admission a junior doctor failed to attend when he suffered further episodes of croup. Although the boy seemed to recover quickly, half-an-hour later he stopped breathing, had a cardiac arrest, sustained brain damage and eventually died. It was admitted that the doctor's failure to attend was negligent, but Court considered the question of causation: what was the consequence of this failure, or what would have been the outcome had the doctor attended? The boy's mother argued that if the doctor had attended, she would have passed a tracheal tube and prevented the cardiac arrest. However the Court established that the doctor would have decided *not* to intubate the boy, and so the claim did not succeed.

The mother's argument failed in both the Court of Appeal, and also the House of Lords where the validity of the expert evidence was considered. Lord Brown Wilkinson stated 'if, in a rare case, it can be demonstrated that the professional opinion is not capable of withstanding *logical analysis*, the Judge is entitled to hold that the body of opinion is not *reasonable or responsible*'. The maxim 'I am a responsible doctor and I have always done it this way' is therefore no longer tenable if it cannot stand up to this logical analysis.

The anaesthetist, as a specialist doctor, will be expected to exercise the ordinary skill of his specialty.[5] In law it is acceptable not to reach the highest standards. The required standard is no higher than 'ordinary'.

Trainee anaesthetists, even when relatively junior, often work alone without direct supervision. Nonetheless any trainee, even in a specialist area, is expected to carry out his duties with the skill necessary for safe patient care, and appropriate to the post he fills. Inexperience in that post is no justification for a lower standard. In *Wilsher v Essex Area Health Authority*[6] a neonatal intensive care trainee mistakenly inserted a catheter into the umbilical vein rather than an artery. Lord Justice Mustill said 'the standard is not just that of the averagely competent and well-informed junior houseman (or whatever the position of the doctor) but of such a person who fills a post in a unit offering a highly specialized service'.

Is this too harsh a test in a specialty that can only adequately train and educate through practical experience? Not when examined from a patient's perspective. Any patient expects adequate care under all circumstances. It therefore behoves the profession to teach trainees to recognize when a situation is outside their competence, and ensure they ask for direct supervision if needed.

## Protocols and guidelines

What if an anaesthetist departs from hospital protocols and guidelines, which occurs quite commonly in busy clinical practice? Such documents may not set the appropriate standard of care in a particular case. However in reality the court is likely to rely on them as evidence of accepted practice, and an anaesthetist's reasons for departure will be subject to the court's logical scrutiny.

## Res ipsa loquitur

The burden of proof is normally on the patient to prove the doctor's negligence. However when there is no obvious or ready explanation for an injury, the patient may try to rely on the doctrine of *res ipsa loquitur*. This literally means 'the thing speaks for itself', or in other words, common sense points inexorably to negligence.

*Res ipsa loquitur* is rarely appropriate now because the civil procedure rules allow the patient access to all relevant material. His experts can therefore provide an informed opinion. However, this doctrine may be used in some anaesthesia claims, for example awareness, where it is argued that a patient cannot have been anaesthetized to the appropriate standard. In *Ludlow v Swanson Health Authority*,[7] it was held that if the patient was conscious and experiencing pain during the period of surgery, then negligence can be inferred, even without expert evidence that awareness can only occur if reasonable anaesthetic care is not given (this is not necessarily true under all circumstances, for example in some obstetric cases, or unexpected extreme hypotension). In *Saunders v Leeds Western Health Authority*,[8] a four-year-old suffered cardiac arrest under general anaesthesia. Experts stated that the heart of a fit child does not arrest if proper anaesthetic care is provided. In *Glass v Cambridge Health Authority*[9] the court received similar expert evidence in the case of an adult and applied the doctrine.

*Res ipsa loquitur* was examined at length by the Court of Appeal in *Ratcliffe v Plymouth and Torbay Health Authority, Exeter and North Devon Health Authority*.[10] A patient underwent arthrodesis of his right ankle under both general and spinal anaesthesia, and suffered an unexplained serious neurological defect on the right side below his waist. Magnetic resonance imaging (MRI) showed a lesion in the spinal cord at T11–T12, and another less distinct lesion at T9. The anaesthetist maintained that since the spinal was given at L3–L4, it could not have caused damage consistent with the clinical findings nor the lesions seen on MRI. The judge found that the anaesthetist's care had been appropriate, and that although the spinal injection had caused the nerve damage the mechanism could not be identified. It was possible that the operation had triggered an unexplained reaction in the central nervous system (CNS). The patient's claim failed.

At appeal the patient argued that the judge had incorrectly dismissed the application of *res ipsa loquitur* and should have found that the patient's condition inferred negligence. The patient further argued that once the doctrine was raised it was the defendants' responsibility to rebut the inference, and they could not do so by suggesting an explanation that could only be considered a possibility. The Court of Appeal considered whether *res ipsa loquitur* had any place in clinical negligence claims. Although it had merit in some circumstances, for example an operation on the wrong limb or a retained swab, even if the doctrine was raised, the patient's case was likely to be supported by expert evidence. The appeal failed. It should therefore be sufficient for a doctor to show that he took all reasonable care, although it is naturally helpful if he can also offer a plausible (even if improbable) explanation for any injury.

Lord Justice Hobhouse said '*res ipsa loquitur* is no more than a convenient Latin phrase used to describe the proof of facts which is sufficient to support an inference that a Defendant was negligent and therefore to establish a *prima facie* case against him'. He went on to say '...*res ipsa loquitur* should be dropped from the litigator's vocabulary and replaced by the phrase a *prima facie* case. *Res ipsa loquitur* is not a principle of law, it does not relate to or raise any presumption. It is merely a guide to help to identify when a *prima facie* case is being made out. Where expert and factual evidence has been called on both sides at trial its usefulness will normally have long since been exhausted'.

### Causation
Once the patient has established that a breach of duty has occurred, he must then prove that the breach caused the injury. The Courts generally apply the 'but for' test: but for the negligence would the injury have occurred in any event? This may be obscure as many patients have co-existing illnesses, and so the full harm caused by the negligence may be difficult to assess. This area can give rise to much argument between the parties involved. If an injury is judged more likely than not to have resulted anyway from co-existing disease, the patient cannot recover any damages. This was the case in *Hotson v East Berkshire Area Health Authority*[11] where there was a delay in the diagnosis of a slipped epiphysis, but no damages were awarded for the loss of a 25% chance of recovery.

*Contributory negligence*

Are there circumstances in which the actions of the patient can be said to have contributed to his injuries? In principle, if a patient fails to give a full history at assessment or comply with postoperative instructions, the defence of contributory negligence should be available. However, we have been unable to find any reports where a finding of contributory negligence was made against a patient. This may reflect a reluctance by the Court to limit an award if there is evidence that the patient did not appreciate the consequences of failing to answer questions or follow the doctor's advice. However, in a recent unreported County Court decision, *Pidgeon v Doncaster Health Authority*, the Health Authority was found to be negligent in the reporting of a cervical smear test, but two-thirds of the liability was attributed to the patient's negligence in failing to attend for follow-up smears, despite clear written instructions to do so.

## Consent

It is unlawful to administer medical treatment to an adult who is conscious and of sound mind without his consent. Refusal by a competent adult to accept treatment (even mechanical ventilation), no matter how illogical or unreasonable, must be respected. Unlike some other jurisdictions, in this country we have no doctrine of 'informed consent'. Nonetheless the doctor has a duty to inform the patient, in a way he understands and without pressure, the reason for the treatment, its nature, the likely outcomes, and the likely consequence of refusing treatment. Sufficient information should be given to enable him to make an educated choice, and time allowed for any questions. The precise amount of information is a matter for professional opinion, taking account of what a reasonable patient might expect. The General Medical Council suggests that good practice demands a level of information above that determined by existing caselaw.

Some patients are unable to give consent. Parents give consent for their very young children. However even quite young children may have a good understanding and insight into their condition, and it is good practice to involve both child and parents. The situation is more complicated for an older child, who may well have a full understanding of his condition, perhaps even more than his parent, and a keener appreciation of the consequences of treatment. Section 8 of the UK Family Law Reform Act 1969 provides that a minor who has attained the age of 16 years is able to give consent for any surgical, medical or dental treatment, putting him in the same position as an adult.

The issue of consent with children who had not yet reached 16 years was considered in *Gillick v West Norfolk and Wisbech Area Health Authority*[12] which held that a child under 16 years could consent to treatment, in this case contraception, if they understood what was involved. By contrast in *Re S (a minor: consent to medical treatment)*[13] the Court considered the ability of a 15½-year-old patient (S) to give consent, and found that S was not 'Gillick competent'.

For the adult psychiatrically ill patient, the same principles apply. Competence to give consent requires the patient to be able to understand the information given by the doctor and to use it to make a reasoned judgment. Even the most severe psychiatric illness may not preclude insight into a physical condition and therefore competence to give consent. This was underlined in *Re C (adult: refusal of treatment)*[14] where a schizophrenic was held competent to refuse the amputation of his foot. In *Re F (mental patient: sterilization)*[15], the UK House of Lords held that the test to be applied for any operation or treatment in adults incapable of giving consent is the same as the test laid down in Bolam – a doctor will not be negligent if he or she acts in accordance with a responsible body of medical opinion.

What are the consequences of failing to obtain valid consent for medical treatment? In principle, the patient could claim for battery (touching intentionally without consent), but the Courts have severely limited such an action in medical cases, unless consent was fraudulently obtained. *Chatterton v Gerson*[16] involved a patient who consulted a chronic pain specialist for treatment of a painful hernia scar. Following a phenol nerve block, she had an area of numbness down one leg which affected her mobility. She bought an action for battery on the grounds that she had not given full consent to the procedure because she had not been warned of the risk of numbness. Justice Bristow said 'once the patient is informed in broad terms of the nature of the procedure which is intended, and gives her consent, that consent is real, and the cause of the action on which to base a claim for failure to go into risks and implications is negligence, not trespass'. The House of Lords endorsed this approach in *Sidaway v Bethlem Royal Hospital Governors*.[17] Lord Scarman said 'it would be deplorable to base the law in medical cases of this kind on the torts of assault and battery'.

What is the position of the patient who is temporarily incompetent, for example already under general anaesthetic and requiring further surgery to which he has not consented? If that need arises as an emergency, surgical procedures can be lawfully carried out. In *Re F*[15] the House of Lords considered that, as a matter of public policy, clinicians should be able to give necessary treatment in emergencies without risking an action in tort. This treatment should be limited to what is necessary and cannot be reasonably delayed.

## Overview of Recent Claims

In an internal unpublished review by the UK Medical Protection Society of 150 anaesthetic claims the commonest serious incidents were:

- Absent or inadequate supply of fresh gases.
- Difficulty with laryngoscopy.
- Misplacement, displacement or blockage of an endotracheal tube.
- Disconnection or misconnection of the breathing circuit.
- Failure of intravenous access.
- Awareness under general anaesthesia.

There was a broad spectrum of injuries. Dental damage was the basis for claim in as many as 58 cases. Under most circumstances dental damage is avoidable with the careful use of the laryngoscope. Almost all such cases will be settled promptly, usually for no more than the costs of appropriate remedial dental treatment.

There were just six cases of awareness under general anaesthesia, which are unlikely to be defensible if there is any question of faulty equipment, divergence from accepted practice, or poor standard of record keeping. Any patient is entitled to expect to be safely and adequately anaesthetized during surgery. Sometimes the patient genuinely confuses events during emergence from anaesthesia with those during the operation itself. The compensation awarded may be much higher if the claim is not limited to pain and discomfort during the procedure, but the patient develops some sort of psychiatric injury as a result of the traumatic experience. This more serious injury can be greatly mitigated by an early sympathetic reaction from the anaesthetist and other hospital staff to any complaint of awareness.

Other claims include nerve injuries allegedly sustained during anaesthesia. Some will be indefensible, but ulnar nerve lesions can occur despite the most careful positioning and monitoring of the patient. However, once again, such a claim will be disappointingly difficult to defend if there is any question of departure from usual practice or inadequate record keeping.

In 11 claims, the patient sadly suffered a fatal or catastrophic brain injury during the course of general anaesthesia. Sometimes the cause is obvious, but there may be occasions where there is no obvious explanation. The court is then faced with a range of expert evidence from both sides, and the judge will have to decide on the most likely explanation. This arose recently in *Williams v South Glamorgan Health Authority*,[18] where a patient became cyanosed during general anaesthesia, and suffered a cardiac arrest resulting in very severe hypoxic ischaemic encephalopathy. In the absence of any other likely explanation, the claimant alleged that the anaesthetist, a Senior House Officer (SHO), allowed an excessive flow of anaesthetic gas into the breathing circuit causing barotrauma and bilateral pneumothoraces. The claim failed. The Judge preferred the evidence of the Senior House Officer, and found it more likely that the claimant's injuries were caused by an anaphylactic reaction to suxamethonium.

## No Fault Compensation Schemes

In the Williams case, the Claimant suffered devastating personal injury as a result of anaesthesia, yet will receive no compensation and will probably have to rely on the State for long-term care. Since many claims in clinical negligence fail, is there any room for a no fault compensation scheme in the UK?

It is easy to see the attraction of such a scheme. If a patient has trusted himself to the care of doctors and suffers injury, why should he have to prove that this was caused by negligence in order to receive compensation? Legal processes are lengthy and costly, and especially for claims arising from UK NHS treatment, there are obvious arguments that these costs would be better directed towards improving patient care.

However, there is resistance to such schemes. Claimant lawyers point out that it is unlikely that the State would be able to fund compensation for all patients to the level of awards currently allowed by the courts. Patients who are successful under the present scheme would therefore be at an advantage.

Possible models include schemes allowing tariffs of awards for specific classes of injuries. This type of scheme will not provide compensation for financial losses, such as loss of earnings, and is more likely to cover minor injuries. Alternative models could cover the serious injuries related to events around the time of birth. For example, the American states of Virginia and Florida have created no fault schemes for these injuries, funded by a levy on obstetricians and hospitals. This effectively removes the patient's right to sue, and raises concerns as to whether the negligent doctor is held properly accountable for his actions. It is still necessary for the patient to prove causation, i.e. that the medical care of the birth caused the injury, and relatively few patients receive compensation through these schemes.

In New Zealand, a no fault scheme covers all injuries resulting from medical mishap or error, with the exception of mental injury. However, since the scheme was originally conceived, it has undergone review as the compensation it provided was inadequate and the medical profession was perceived as escaping censure. There is now mandatory reporting by doctors of medical errors resulting in personal injury, which has resulted in a complex and multi-layered complaints system. The merits of no fault scheme for the UK will no doubt continue to be debated.

## Criminal Culpability

There may be occasions where a patient dies as a result of a doctor's error that is so outside the scope of responsible practice that the doctor faces a criminal investigation. The question is then what distinguishes an error which might be considered negligent from an error for which society demands a criminal conviction and punishment? A charge of murder is unlikely because of the need to prove the *mens rea*, or intent, to kill the patient. However several doctors have been charged with manslaughter, and anaesthetists are particularly vulnerable since an apparently minor error may result in the swift and newsworthy death of a previously fit patient.

An anaesthetist has the dubious distinction of being at the heart of a case in which The House of Lords defined the criteria for involuntary manslaughter by doctors in *Regina v Adomako* (UK).[19] Previously, the tests for such cases were similar to that used in prosecutions involving careless driving – was the defendant reckless to the risk of causing death or injury by dangerous driving? To be proved reckless, the defendant must have created an obvious and serious risk, without having given thought to the possibility of there being any such risk, or having recognized the risk, nonetheless gone on to take it. The House of Lords felt that this test was not appropriate for medical cases because doctors treat patients whose lives may already be at high risk, and in such an expert field the criteria of what the ordinary prudent individual would appreciate would not be applied in the same way.

The House of Lords held that the appropriate test in medical manslaughter based on breach of duty is whether the doctor had been grossly negligent. The ingredients of involuntary manslaughter in such cases are therefore, firstly, the existence of a duty, secondly, breach of that duty causing death, and thirdly, gross negligence justifying a criminal conviction of manslaughter. The third limb of the test defines the criminal nature of the prosecution, and is a question solely for the jury, considered against the background of all the facts of the case. In this case, Dr Adomako was a locum anaesthetist who failed to notice that his paralyzed patient had become disconnected from the ventilator during eye surgery. The House of Lords upheld the conviction.

They found that the jury was entitled to conclude that his failure to monitor the patient's breathing (the disconnect alarm failed to sound) was more than 'mere inadvertence' to an obvious serious potential risk. Dr Adomako's failure therefore constituted gross negligence of the degree necessary for manslaughter.

## The Human Rights Act 1998

The Human Rights Act came into force in the UK in October 2000, and provides that the rights set out in the European Convention of Human Rights will affect domestic law. The rights most likely to impact on medical law are the right to life (Article 2), the right not to be subjected to torture or to inhuman or degrading treatment or punishment (Article 3), and the right to respect for private and family life (Article 8).

Under the Act, it is unlawful for a public authority to act in a manner incompatible with a convention right. Although there has been some debate as to what constitutes a public authority, there seems little doubt that it will include a Health Authority or Trust. It will also include 'any person certain of whose functions are public in nature'. The definition of a public body still needs clarification in these early days, but there seems to be doubt as to whether it would apply to treatment given in the private sector, or by General Practitioners.

Article 2 (the right to life) raises interesting questions about the validity of 'do not resuscitate' orders, or the obligation of a state to provide lifesaving treatment. If a lack of resources led to inadequate provision of intensive care beds, would the resulting death of a patient form the basis of a claim under the Act? The answer appears to be 'possibly'. In *Osman v UK*,[20] the European Court accepted that the effect of Article 2 was that there would be a violation of the article if authorities did not take 'measures' within the scope of their powers which, judged reasonably, might have been expected to avoid a real and immediate risk to the life of an identified individual or individuals. However, the Court also held that obligations imposed by this article should not be interpreted so as to 'impose an impossible or disproportionate burden on the authorities'.

The European Court has never considered whether Article 2 could require the state to provide lifesaving treatment. However, prior to the enactment of the Human Rights Act, our domestic courts considered the issue of funding lifesaving treatment in *Regina v Cambridgeshire Health Authority ex parte B*.[21] The Master of the Rolls, Sir Thomas Bingham stated 'difficult and agonizing judgments have to be made as to how a limited budget is best allocated to the maximum advantage of the maximum number of patients. That is not a judgment which the Court can make. In my judgment, it is not something that a Health Authority such as this Authority can be fairly criticized for not advancing before the Court'. It would appear that, although the Court will be reluctant to interfere with a Health Authority's allocation of resources in relation to medical treatment, the Health Authority may be required to justify its choices.

Article 3 deals with the prohibition of torture. In *D v UK*,[22] the European Court was asked to considered the case of a person who was being deported to St Kitts where he would no longer receive the life prolonging treatment for AIDS that he had been receiving in the UK. The Court considered that his deportation would amount to inhuman treatment and would violate Article 3. More recently in *Regina v (Pretty) v Director of Public Prosecutions and others*, involving a patient with motor neurone disease, the Court considered the impact of Article 3. Lord Steyn recognized that the final stages of this disease might be inhuman and degrading, but was certain there was no action or inaction on the part of the authorities that was subjecting her to inhuman and degrading treatment. The House of Lords also suggested that the failure to provide pain relief might amount to an infringement of the Act. This raises the possibility that a right to treatment that relieves pain, but not that necessarily saves life, could be established.

This is a fast developing area of law and there is little doubt it will impact on issues relating to the provision of medical services. It may be used to highlight the increasing demands placed on our finite NHS.

## References

1. Thake v Maurice [1986] 1 All ER 497.
2. R v Bateman [1925] 94 LJKB 791 (CA).
3. [1957] 2 All ER 118; [1957] 1 WLR 582.
4. [1997] 4 All ER 771 (HL).
5. Maynard v West Midlands Health Authority [1985] 1 All ER 635.
6. [1987] QB 730; [1986] 3 All ER 801 (CA).
7. [1989] 1 Med LR 104.
8. [1993] 4 Med LR 355.
9. [1995] 6 Med LR 91.
10. [1998] Lloyds Report Med 162 (CA).
11. [1987] AC 750; [1987] 2 All ER 909 (HL).
12. [1985] 3 All ER 404, [1986] AC 112.
13. [1994] 2 FLR 1065.
14. [1994] 1 All ER 819.
15. [1990] 2 AC 1.
16. [1981] QB 432; [1981] 1 All ER 257 (QBD).
17. [1984] 1 All ER 1018 (CA); [1985] 1 All ER 643 (HL).

18. [2000] MLC 0277.
19. [1995] 1 AC 171 (HL).
20. [1998] 29 EHRR 245.
21. [1995] 1 WLR 898.
22. [1997] 24 EHRR 423.

*G. Stanley   J.N. Cashman*

# Education and training in anaesthesia

Education and training are terms that are used loosely and interchangeable in medicine, but which encompass different concepts. Indeed a comparison of education and training reveals them to have almost diametrically opposed attributes (table 1) and yet both are equally important in the development of doctors.[1,2] Education has been defined as the process which results in a persistent, predetermined alteration in behaviour usually reflected by the acquisition of new knowledge, skills or attitudes by the learner.[3] Increasingly traditional techniques for instruction with their emphasis on factual learning are being replaced by the teaching of professional competencies such as communication and problem solving skills. It has been suggested that the following common themes should be addressed when considering education in anaesthesia.[3]

- Whom do we teach?

- What do we teach?

- What are the most effective teaching methods?

- How do we measure the effectiveness of our teaching?

- Can we improve the effectiveness of our teachers?

This chapter will examine aspects of the educational process relevant to the practice of anaesthesia. The various components of the training process, beginning with medical student education and progressing through the training grade to the established practitioner, will be considered. Much of the discussion will be based on the US and European (particularly UK)

**Table 1** Comparison of education and training

| Education | Training |
| --- | --- |
| Intrinsically valuable | Practically useful but without intrinsic worth |
| Broad | Circumscribed |
| Open ended | Closed ended; focuses on specific skills |
| University objectives | Professional objectives |
| Promotes further growth | Inhibits further growth |
| Difficult to teach, learn | Easy to teach, learn |
| and examine | and examine |

Adapted from McManus I, 1995.[2]

experience but the overall content of the chapter is relevant to anaesthesia and education regardless of geographical location. There is a geographical variation in the roles of academic departments of anaesthesia. In North America, Australia, South Africa and much of Europe, university departments of anaesthesia are responsible for postgraduate training in anaesthesiology. In contrast in the UK and the Republic of Ireland university departments of anaesthesia are primarily responsible for the education of undergraduates and of postgraduates studying for higher degrees. Many academic departments of anaesthesia in the UK provide a great deal of support to the schools of anaesthesia in the training of anaesthetic trainees. However, some distinction between institutions dedicated to education from those dedicated to training is thought to be desirable.[4]

## Undergraduate Education and Training in Anaesthesia

### The undergraduate medical curriculum

The length and content of the undergraduate medical curriculum varies widely between countries and even within any one country.[5] The structure of medical education in North America differs from that of the UK and Australasia, being very similar in the US and Canada. The length of training required for a medical degree in member states of the European Union is stipulated in Article 23 of European Community directive 93/16/EEC but this directive provides little detail regarding the content of the training.[5]

The Institute for International Medical Education is a newly established institution entrusted with the development of 'global minimum essential (core) requirements' for medical education. The institute has developed a three-phase plan for the introduction of a global medical curriculum and has collected together a glossary of Medical Education Terms (www.iime.org).[6]

*Duration of the undergraduate medical curriculum*

The main difference between medical education in North America compared with the UK and Australasia is that, on the whole, a prior baccalaureate degree is required before admission into medical school. As a result there is a corresponding reduction in the total duration of study, which has implications for anaesthesia as a topic in the undergraduate curriculum. In the US over 95% of medical graduates have completed at least 4 years of a previous degree consequently the duration of the medical course is only 3 years.[7] However, there are a few North American schools that provide a combined college and medical school programme. In these schools the overall duration of study is a little over 5 years,[7] which is very similar to the duration of study in Europe and Australia. In Europe European Community directive 93/16/EEC specifies that the length of training for a medical degree leading to full registration (i.e. including pre-registration posts) should be 5500 h or 6 years.[5] In a move towards the North American model a number of medical schools in Australia and in the UK have introduced Graduate Entry Medical Programmes – GEMPs. Typically such courses last 4 years, which is similar to the duration of medical courses in North America.[8,9] Selection to graduate entry medical programmes is based on performance in a common entry test such as the Graduate Australian Medical School Admission Test, which tests understanding of scientific language and reasoning in social sciences, the humanities, biology, chemistry and physics.[10]

*Anaesthesia and the undergraduate medical curriculum*

It is recommended that for each member state of the European Union there should be a single 'Competent Authority' charged with regulating the primary medical qualification (European Community directive 93/16/EEC).[5] The Education Committee of the General Medical Council (GMC) has been discharging that role for more than a century within the UK, although it is the universities that are primarily responsible for the delivery of medical student training. In the UK anaesthesia was included as a subject that should be a component of every course of professional study and examinations by the GMC in 1912. However, 35 years later anaesthesia as a subject was omitted from the GMCs recommendations and another 33 years elapsed before it was reinstated into the curriculum by the GMC. This change of recommendation by the GMC was brought about because of the expansion of the specialty of anaesthesia into the fields of resuscitation, pain relief, intensive and perioperative care. At the time the Education Committee of the GMC proposed that students during their clinical clerkships should be taught by a specific period of instruction and clinical attachment in a Department of Anaesthesia.[11] In a refinement of its recommendations on the undergraduate medical curriculum the GMC introduced the concept of a system-based core curriculum founded on a series of core goals and objectives which covered:[12]

- Knowledge

- Skills

- Attitudes and behaviours.

This has now become the established format for training. Basic and advanced life support, intensive care medicine, perioperative management of the surgical patient and the relief of pain (acute and chronic), are all included in this new systems-based approach. Nevertheless, the role of anaesthesia within the undergraduate curriculum has not been clearly defined with the result that anaesthesia has not figured very prominently in the medical school curriculum.[13] In the US, most medical schools include pharmacology lectures, in relation to anaesthesia in the pre-clinical years and then have brief rotations through the anaesthesia department, often as part of a surgical block and sometimes only on an elective basis. Few medical schools incorporate a visit to the operating room to reinforce physiological and pharmacological principles at the pre-clinical as opposed to clinical level. The use of multimedia in the form of a pre-recorded CD-ROM presentation or even interactive DVD has become increasingly common. European universities provide more formal lecture time than UK medical schools but fewer provide a regular period of attachment to an anaesthesia department than UK medical schools. In contrast UK establishments provide more in-theatre teaching than their European counterparts.[14]

One topic that the medical school curriculum currently fails to address adequately relates to the impaired physician and the issue of chemical dependency. This topic is of considerable importance to anaesthetists. One in 15 doctors in the UK may suffer from some form of dependence on alcohol or drugs during their lifetime.[15] In Australia and New Zealand 1.3% of all registrars in anaesthesia suffer from a drug related problem requiring intervention during their training.[16] Whether the prevalence of drug addiction is higher in anaesthetists compared to other medical specialists remains controversial. One study has suggested that anaesthetists are not the highest risk group amongst doctors[17] whereas another study suggests that anaesthesiologists are three times more likely to become substance abusers than other physician groups.[18] Mortality in addict anaesthetists is more than 15% over 5 years[19] and more than a quarter of all cases of fentanyl abuse present for the first time as a fatal overdose.[18] Rehabilitation programmes succeed in 60–80% of the cases but residents in anaesthesia need to be redirected to another medical specialty.[19]

## New teaching techniques for undergraduates

Innovation in the medical curriculum has been accompanied by development in teaching techniques. In particular a paradigm shift from the methodologies of structure- and process-based to problem- and evidence-based learning and measurements of outcome.[20] One such explicit analytical approach is Clinical Problem Analysis (CPA), which aims to assist students not only in problem solving but also in organizing learning.[21] This technique addresses the topic of how medical students learn to cope with complex clinical cases and how they construct differential diagnoses for such cases. Novice students may learn to solve clinical problems by emulating experts' behaviour. However, experts use efficient strategies for discriminating among alternative hypotheses in an organized step-wise manner, whilst non-experts typically generate large numbers of possible diagnostic hypotheses belonging to widely different disease categories.[21,22] By repeated use of clinical problem analysis as well as accumulation of clinical experience, students gradually develop finely tuned knowledge structures that they learn to apply when appropriate. Clinical problem analysis is claimed to have a number of advantages over traditional clinical presentations:[23]

- Explicitly addresses co-morbidity and drug–drug interactions

- Geared to treatment

- Takes into account both causes and consequences of the patient's current condition

- Can (even) be used in unsolved cases.

## Promoting anaesthesiology to medical students as a career choice

Relatively few studies have addressed the importance of undergraduate education for future recruitment into the specialty. In the UK, graduates at entry to medical school are more likely than non-graduates to choose general practice as a career whereas those who took an intercalated degree are more likely than others to choose a hospital medical specialty.[24] The duration of the undergraduate anaesthetic exposure and the level at which it occurs seems to have very little influence on graduates' subsequent choice of anaesthetics as a career. In particular a well-structured anaesthetic rotation does not appear to make anaesthesiology more appealing for the potential future anaesthesiologist. The career choices of graduates from two London Medical schools was not significantly affected by whether or not they had undergone a comprehensive undergraduate anaesthetic training programme.[25] Furthermore experiences in anaesthesia during internship and residency were important for only a minority of graduates (1-in-5 female graduates and 1-in-7 male graduates).[26] Whilst anaesthesia recruitment is not related to the duration of undergraduate anaesthesia exposure it is influenced by other factors such as perceived life-style, the application of physiology and pharmacology to patient care, practical and procedural aspects of practice, specific role models who were influential and encouraging, and chance.[26–28]

## Postgraduate Education and Training in Anaesthesia

The UK has one of the smallest anaesthetic workforces in Europe with 9.6 trained anaesthetist per 100,000 head of population, the figure rises to 14.5 per 100,000 when trainees are included.[29] In contrast within the US, there is a six-fold variation in anaesthetic manpower; with 4.3 anaesthesiologists per 100,000 head of population in parts of Texas rising to 25.5 per 100,000 in parts of Illinois.[30] In the US, where there has been a huge expansion of the so-called hospital specialist or 'hospitalist', the number of anaesthesiologists may well increase. Such hospital specialists have a background in general medicine and have become the surrogate care provider once a patient is admitted to the hospital. It is likely that anaesthesiologist may function in an hospitalist-type role in the future, especially in predominantly surgical units.

### Trainee anaesthesiologists

#### Choosing anaesthetics as a career
There does not seem to be any association between technical orientation and a tendency to gravitate to technologically orientated specialties such as anaesthetics.[31] Nevertheless a number of attempts have been made to develop career selection instruments to assist doctors in their career choice. One such instrument Sci45 has been shown to be valid in matching individuals' personal and professional preferences to possible career specialty choices.[32]

*Pre-anaesthesia experience*: In the US, it was traditionally accepted that most trainees would do a preliminary year of either general surgery or internal medicine, with the bias towards surgery before they start the anaesthetic programme. With the emergence of so-called transitional programmes that offer rotations through a number of specialties, including paediatrics, these have started to become more popular with future anaesthesiologists. The emergence of the perioperative physician in anaesthetic practice has also tended to move some of the bias away from surgery back to medicine. In the UK, the mandatory 6-month's pre-registration clerkship in both medicine and surgery may make the decision-making process a little easier. Recently the UK GMC has accepted a proposal from the UK Royal College of Anaesthetists for a 4-month module in anaesthesia, pain management and intensive care for pre-registration house officers. As a result there are now several pre-registration rotations that offer some anaesthesia and/or intensive care experience. The Australian and New Zealand College of Anaesthetists stipulates a period of 24 months in general hospital appointments, which must not comprise more than 6 months in anaesthetics or intensive care medicine before anaesthetic specialty training can commence.[33] In contrast, in Canada there has been a move towards direct entry into residency training from medical school for all graduates.[34]

*Selections of trainees for anaesthetic rotations*
There is a clear need to attract trainees of the highest quality into anaesthetics. Already some medical schools are attempting to psychologically 'profile' students into specialties virtually from day one! While it is certain that not everyone will agree with this new approach it has to be recognized as one possible strategy for the future. This could lead to a focusing of medical education on a sub-specialty right from the outset and a 'general' medical school education could become a thing of the past. With the ever-increasing costs of healthcare and the development of 'super-specialties', there may be a strong political and economic motivation to support this approach.

The challenge is to recognize at time of application those individuals who are likely to attain a measure of success in anaesthetics but, unlike in industry, formalized personality assessment is not a commonly used tool. The observation that there is significant heterogeneity in the personality of anaesthetists[35] has recently been confirmed.[36] Nevertheless it has been suggested that attributes such as empathy, strong internalization of pro-normative values, and the ability to work well within either structured or open settings are conducive to superior performance in the specialty.[37,38] Psychological profiling such as the 16PF personality questionnaire and the California Psychological Inventory (CPI) have been used to identify those personality traits associated with success.[38,39] The most important traits would seem to be social skills assertiveness, sensitivity and emotional maturity. In contrast, assessment of motor skills as part of an anaesthesiology selection process has attracted little attention. Tests such as the Crawford small-part dexterity test and the steadiness hole test can predict motor skills in surgical trainees.[40]

Pre-interview screening can assist in the ranking of applicants ahead of interview. Such screening may combine academic measures such as scores and grades, performance measures and prior achievement/experience. Computer-assisted data management has been used to provide automatic sorting of selection parameters and calculation of ranking as well as maintenance of a concise information profile for each candidate.[41] The process is subject to other variables such as candidate preferences, particularly in respect of the perceived prestige of a particular training programme.[28] Furthermore the potential for bias to be introduced at interview has led to the suggestion that the interview should be conducted 'blind'.[42]

*Training in anaesthesia and the postgraduate medical curriculum*
Until 1987, the duration of residency training in anaesthesia in the US was 3 years. This included the internship year in medicine or surgery. At the time, this duration of training was one of the shortest in the world for the specialty. After 1988, a fourth year was added, making the specific anaesthesia training period 3 years, still a relatively short time, certainly by UK standards. Since then, fellowship programmes have grown considerably in areas such as critical care, pain management, paediatrics, obstetrics and cardiac anaesthesia. There are certification examinations in the first three of these subspecialties and many trainees complete 4 years of anaesthesia training. In Europe there is much greater diversity than in the US in the organizational background of postgraduate medical education. European Community directive 93/16/EEC lays down the minimum standards for specialist postgraduate training but this directive is the consolidation of several previous directives and parts of it are more than 20 years old.

Currently the overall duration of training (Basic, Intermediate and Advanced) in anaesthesiology in western European countries (5 years) is in line with the US. The duration of training in central and eastern European countries is shorter (4 years) and longer in the UK (7 years).[29,43]

With such a widely diversified specialty it is particularly challenging to decide how to use the relatively short training period to its best advantage. In addition to clinical education, the Accreditation Council for Graduate Medical Education (ACGME) mandates that a programme should emphasize interpersonal skills, effective communication, and professionalism.[44] Graduating residents should be able to work independently, responsibly, with integrity and must demonstrate a commitment to excellence and the ethical principles of clinical care. They must learn to develop a relationship with patients, engage in active listening and provide an opportunity for input and questions. They should always remain sensitive and responsive to cultural differences, including awareness of how these differences can affect the perioperative course on a number of levels e.g. extent of family involvement and cultural differences in pain perception.[45]

It is important that new trainees have a broad framework on which to build (table 2). Yet despite attempts to produce a clearly defined curriculum for residency programmes, formalized nationally accepted objectives have not

**Table 2** European Academy of Anaesthesiology anaesthetic training programme

General surgery
Obstetrics
Gynaecology
Orthopaedics
ENT and other forms of surgery within the mouth
Neonatal/paediatrics
Neurosurgery
Cardiac surgery
Ambulatory surgery
Intensive care/internal medicine
Resuscitation and emergency medicine
Preoperative assessment and postoperative care including management of
  acute pain
Management of chronic pain
Training to teach others
Administration/budgeting
Research

ENT – ear, nose and throat.

been devised with the result that each residency programme adapts to provide its own programme of study and this leads to incongruence.[3] In Canada, each residency programme is required to have clear educational goals with respect to knowledge, skills, and other attributes for residents at each level of training and for each major rotation.[46] Residents must be afforded a reliable system for communication and interaction with supervisory physicians. In the US, the Residency Review Committee (RRC) has mandated that a trainee carry out a certain minimum number of procedures (table 3).[44] For the majority of programmes, these numbers are not difficult to attain and their role is probably more to provide a secondary framework for programmes to work with rather than as a basis for punitive action. Residents are also required to keep a detailed log of their cases. This logging system has recently become internet-based and it allows for very sophisticated data analysis, not just of individual residents but of programmes as a whole. However, the value of the anaesthetic log-book has been questioned.[47]

Modern technology is now a clear element in medical education. The use of interactive CD-ROMs and internet-based learning modalities are playing an ever-increasing role,[48,49] and departments must decide how to incorporate these advances into their curriculum.[50] These computer-based learning tools still need to be fully evaluated.[51] One novel aspect of training that is being incorporated into the US programmes relates to the emerging role of the anaesthesia provider in areas of business management, career planning, hospital politics and operating room dynamics.

**Table 3** Clinical components for residency education in anaesthesiology[44]

*Cardiothoracic and vascular*
Anaesthesia for 20 patients undergoing surgical procedures involving
cardiopulmonary bypass
20 intrathoracic (thoracotomy, thoracoscopy) noncardiac cases
20 other major vascular cases (including endovascular cases)

*Neurosurgery*
20 procedures involving an open cranium, some of which must include
intracerebral vascular procedures

*Obstetrics*
40 anaesthetics for vaginal delivery
A minimum of 20 anaesthetics for cesarean section
Evidence of direct involvement in cases involving high-risk obstetrics

*Orthopaedic and trauma*
10 major trauma cases

*Paediatrics*
Anaesthesia for 100 children under the age of 12 including anaesthesia for 15 infants
<1 year of age and neonates <45 weeks postconceptual age

*Pain: acute and non-acute*
25 nerve blocks for management of patients with acute, chronic, or cancer pain
disorders
Documented involvement in the management of acute postoperative pain, including
familiarity with patient-controlled intravenous techniques, neuraxial blockade, and
other pain-control modalities

*Practical procedures*
Significant experience with certain specialized techniques for airway management
(such as fibreoptic intubation, double lumen endotracheal tube placement, and
laryngeal mask airway management), central vein catheter placement, pulmonary
artery catheter placement, peripheral artery cannulation, transoesophageal
echocardiography, evoked potentials, and electroencephalography

*Pre and postoperative care*
Documented involvement in the systematic process of the preoperative management
of the patient
A postanaesthesia-care experience of 2 contiguous weeks, which must involve
direct care of patients in the postanaesthesia-care unit and responsibilities for
management of pain, haemodynamic changes, and emergencies related to the
postanaesthesia-care unit. Designated faculty must be readily and consistently
available for consultation and teaching

*Regional techniques*
50 epidural anaesthetics for patients undergoing surgical procedures, including
caesarean sections
50 subarachnoid blocks performed for patients undergoing surgical procedures
40 peripheral nerve blocks for patients undergoing surgical procedures

*Intensive care*
A critical care rotation, including active participation in patient care by anaesthesia
residents in an educational environment in which participation and care extend
beyond ventilatory management, and active involvement by anaesthesiology faculty
experienced in the practice and teaching of critical care
This training must take place in units in which the majority of patients have
multisystem disease

*Sub-specialty training in anaesthesia*: If time is a limiting factor in general anaesthetic training, then it is a critically scarce commodity when it comes to sub-specialty training. The need for particular sub-specialty training has led, quite appropriately, to the development of fellowship programmes, which commonly occur in the fifth and final year of training.[33]

### Evaluation of training programmes

It is extremely important that all training programmes are held to some level of standardized performance and regulated by members of our own profession. In the US, all programmes have to be visited and accredited at regular intervals by the Accreditation Council for Graduate Medical Education. Within the Accreditation Council for Graduate Medical Education, each specialty has its own oversight Residency Review Committee, which will visit programmes on a regular basis every 3–5 years or more frequently, depending on the reports from previous visits. These visits are carried out by a designated 'field-operative' who has been specially trained to critically appraise a residency programme and compare it with acceptable benchmarks. The Residency Review Committee may put a programme 'on probation' if there are a number of deficiencies or citations in that programme and it even has the power to close a programme if there are serious deficiencies or recurrent citations in key areas.[44] A European Hospital Visitation Programme was created in 1989 by the European Academy of Anaesthesiology and since 1996 has been administered jointly with the European Board of Anaesthesiology. However, unlike in North America, Australia and the UK this programme is entirely voluntary. The visitation team of three includes one member from the host country. The main criteria for assessment are similar to those of the Residency Review Committee and a registration certificate is normally valid for up to 5 years. So far 38 institutions have been visited in various European countries.[52]

### Assessing the competence of trainees in anaesthesia

The competent clinician possesses the intellectual capacity to make valid medical judgements and the technical expertise to implement such judgements.[53] The objective of assessment should be the development of reliable measures of performance which have predictive value for clinical competence and also have a formative educational role.[54] Miller has proposed a pyramid of competence that conceptualizes the essential facets of clinical competence (fig. 1).[55] According to this model competence encompasses basic facts ('knows'), applied knowledge ('knows how'), behavioural rather than cognitive performance ('shows how') and actual performance ('does'). Thus competence embraces knowledge, cognitive and clinical skills and cannot be assessed by any one test of performance. Performance-based testing aimed at assessing 'does' and 'shows how' using standardized patients, simulated

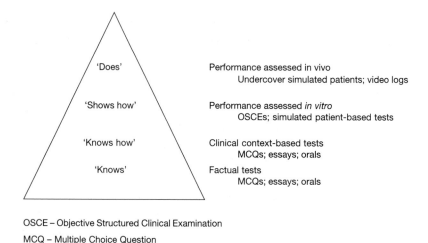

'Does'                    Performance assessed in vivo
                             Undercover simulated patients; video logs

'Shows how'              Performance assessed *in vitro*
                             OSCEs; simulated patient-based tests

'Knows how'              Clinical context-based tests
                             MCQs; essays; orals

'Knows'                 Factual tests
                             MCQs; essays; orals

OSCE – Objective Structured Clinical Examination

MCQ – Multiple Choice Question

**Figure 1** Pyramid of competence.[55]

patients and Objective Structured Clinical Examinations (OSCEs) is prefer-able to old style testing assessing 'knows' using Multiple Choice Questions (MCQs) in evaluating clinical performance.[56] The combination of at least three different forms of assessment and their collation ('triangulation') provides a much more reliable index of performance. Furthermore bench-marks for defining competence and thresholds for attaining competence must be clearly delineated.[54] Unfortunately criterion-referenced standard-setting procedures are time consuming and simpler less transparent methods may find wider acceptance.[57] In the context of assessing competence the evalua-tion of trainees' progress falls into two categories:

- In-training examinations

- In-training assessment

*In-training examinations*: Despite much concern examinations can be con-sidered to have a variety of useful functions.[2] These include:

- Licensing function

- Graduating function

- Ranking function

- Motivating function

- Integrative function

- Informing function

The graduating function is a surrogate for the licensing function, which in turn ensures a minimal level of competence (summative assessment), whereas the informing function (formative assessment) provides feedback.

One of the most widely used tools for measuring factual knowledge is the MCQ format. Advantages of the MCQ format include: high reliability and feasibility, tests much knowledge in a short time, quick and accurate marking and low cost. Whereas disadvantages include: low face validity especially if used as the sole assessment, test factual recall not judgement, difficult to set with potential for confusion/ambiguity and encourages guessing. Different formats and marking schemes have been devised for MCQs but pass standards should be determined using criterion-based rather than norm-based referencing. It has been suggested that negative marking, a technique almost entirely confined to medical and dental examinations in the UK, should be rejected because it discriminates between students on the basis of their risk-taking behaviour[58] although not everyone agrees with this premise.

Oral (*viva voce*) examinations are a component of many certification processes, but despite their popularity they lack reliability and validity and do not correlate well with other measures of performance. The development of techniques for modification of the oral examination may address some of the concerns regarding reliability and validity. Much greater structure can be achieved in the clinical case oral examination using formats such as Chart-Simulated Recall[59] and Structured Question Grid[60] but neither format seems to be a substantially better than the traditional clinical case oral examination format. A structured oral examination format using standardized questions, global rating scales and anchored performance criteria has been found to perform more favourably than traditional formats in both surgical[61] and anaesthetic[62] oral examinations.

The American Board of Anesthesiology and American Society of Anesthesiologists jointly have developed an annual in-training MCQ examination that has a formative role. The examination is similar to the former's MCQ which is the first step towards Board Certification (i.e. summative role).[63] The European Academy of Anaesthetists also conducts an in-training examination to provide feedback to trainees and programme directors. The examination is based on the Academy's Part I MCQ examination.[52] In the UK and in Ireland there is no formative in-training examination but the respective fellowship exams are in effect mid-training exams. In contrast the Diploma examination of the European Academy and the fellowship examination of the Australian and New Zealand College of Anaesthetists are end-training examinations. Indeed the Australasian examination is a required pre-requisite for progress to the final year of the residency programme.[33]

While the American Board of Anesthesiology's Diploma examination for graduating residents in the US and the Royal College of Anesthetists Fellowship examination in the UK are clear examples of milestones in the evaluation process, such benchmarks cannot tell the whole story. Written and oral assessments of knowledge and clinical practice in the examination setting are important but will always be criticized as not truly evaluating performance in a 'real-world' setting. Increasingly more sophisticated methods such as the use of real patient or simulated patient interactions and objective structured clinical examinations are being employed to assess clinical performance.[54] Nevertheless, the Accreditation Council for Graduate Medical Education is beginning to recognize the value of more meaningful real-world assessment processes. In their 10-year Outcomes Project, initiated in 2000, the ACGME aims to radically change the way trainees are evaluated in every specialty using a much more goal-oriented approach to learning and evaluation.[44] Finally it is interesting to report that the Nordic Federation for Medical Education has expressed the view that specialist training in Europe should follow a comprehensive formative evaluation process rather than an American style Board examination system.[64]

*In-training assessment*: It is a key component of residency training programmes in North America, Europe and Australia. At the present time in the US, all residents in anaesthesia are formally evaluated at least every 6 months. The methods by which programmes do this are extremely varied but usually it involves faculty within the department submitting written reports on residents progress during the preceding 6 months.[65,66] Many programmes now conduct these evaluations 'on-line' using the Internet or a departmental intranet. Some programmes have developed a points system to grade the trainees on what they consider key characteristics, usually refinements of the original elements of clinical competence defined by the American Board of Anesthesiology.[63] These include:

- Essential attributes such as ethical and moral behaviour, honesty and integrity

- Acquired professional skills, such as communication, adaptability and an advocacy for quality care

- Knowledge acquisition

- Judgement

- Clinical skills.

Some departments have even introduced weighting systems to refine the process further. Thus in a survey of over 100 programmes, it was found that judgement was rated somewhat higher than knowledge, although both were considered important attributes. The scores related to judgement were therefore weighted slightly higher than knowledge in the final evaluation analysis.[65] Finally residents are required by the Accreditation Council for Graduate Medical Education to make an anonymous, confidential, evaluation of faculty and the programme as a whole, at least once a year. In some departments residents numerically grade the faculty in key areas and then aggregate scores are used to either reward or chastise those that deviate from an accepted norm!

*Anaesthesia simulators*

Simulation and role-play form one of the most important techniques in the area of experiential learning and currently the use of sophisticated anaesthesia simulators is undergoing extensive evaluation. Gredler has proposed two major classes of simulation: tactical-decision simulations and social-process simulations.[67] In tactical-decision simulations the emphasis is on the collection and interpretation of data and the development of a strategy to achieve a specific goal. In social-process simulations the emphasis is on the study of human interactions and communication. Medical simulators are mainly of the tactical-decision type and can be further sub-divided into comprehensive 'realistic' simulators, small-scale computer-based trainers and manikins.[3] Manikins have an established place in teaching and assessing manual skills such as Basic Life Support whilst interactive computer simulation allow clinical problems to be attempted in an interactive environment.[3] In comprehensive simulator design a number of key issues need to be addressed in order to assess complex cognitive and interpersonal skills.[68] Thus the evaluation techniques must:

- Define what constitutes the skill and specify the criteria against which performance can be assessed

- Develop evaluation procedures that permit accurate and reliable observations of these activities

- Standardize the content and format of the evaluation procedures

- Establish standards for identifying individuals who do not achieve acceptable levels of proficiency

An assessment of the validity (the degree to which the test truly measures what it is intended to measure), the reliability (measure of consistency and precision) and the feasibility (basically cost) of the evaluation procedures are also important. Simulated patients (actors programmed to portray the roles of patients) have also been shown to satisfy the requirements for validity, fairness and reliability.[69] Not everybody is convinced that it is possible to separate out and assess separately different skills from the content of the problem.[70]

Setting up a simulator is an expensive proposition but they are being used with increasing frequency and, in some US programmes, they have become a mandatory component of the training of residents and have also been validated as an assessment tool in medical student evaluation.[71] Simulators have numerous advantages. Residents can work through repeatedly a variety of potentially life-threatening clinical scenarios without compromising patient safety. There are even a few departments that use the simulator as part of the resident selection process at the time of medical student interview!

## Board certified anaesthesiologists

The perception of specialty board certification as a standard of excellence would appear to be valid as an association between board certification status and positive clinical outcome has been demonstrated.[72] However, continuous professional development, the process of life-long systematic learning, is necessary for the maintenance of competence of all practitioners.[51] An appreciation is needed of what, how and why clinicians learn and change; how better programmes of education can be designed; and ways in which organizations can provide such education.[73] Two different systems to ensure that anaesthesiologists maintain their clinical competence have been devised in North America although both require participation in continuing medical education activities in order to accrue points.[74] In contrast to the Canadian system (Maintenance of Competence Program; MOCOMP)[75] the American approach to recertification (Continued Demonstration of Qualifications; CDQ)[76] includes a written examination. Schemes similar to the Canadian scheme are being introduced in Australia (Maintenance of Standards; MOS)[77] and in the UK.

### Recertification

The member boards of the American Board of Medical Specialties including the American Board of Anesthesiology have set up a recertification procedure to encourage doctors to continue learning and keep up to date.[63] Prompted by initiatives at the federal, state and local levels, the American Board of Anesthesiology announced in 1989 its intention to introduce a system for voluntary recertification of its diplomats and in 1995 introduced the concept of time-limited certification. All diplomates who were certified on or after January 1st, 2000, would be required to re-certify 10 years after their original certification date. Those diplomates who received certification prior to this date would be encouraged to volunteer for recertification, but it would not be mandatory. The recertification process involves the candidate being a practicing anaesthesiologist with a permanent, unrestricted medical license, documentation from their facility chief of staff (or equivalent), which attests that their clinical performance is commensurate with acceptable standards of practice and the accrual of sufficient credit hours of Continuing Medical Education. Candidates are then eligible to take a written MCQ examination that assesses basic and sub-specialty knowledge, but it is not necessary to answer all questions to achieve a passing grade. In contrast the Maintenance of Competence Program, which is designed to be more flexible and non-coercive is based on self directed education, peer evaluation and scholarly contribution but does not include any summative assessment.

In the UK anaesthesiologists have up to now been required to attend recognized courses of Continuing Medical Education (now Continuing Education and Professional Development (CEPD)) for a minimum number of hours (50 per year) but recently a more stringent, revalidation process with a 5 year cycle has been proposed.[78,79] This requires not only attendance at Continuing Education and Professional Development approved courses (annual target of 50 CEPD points) but also peer and patient evaluation together with the keeping of a log-book.

## Conclusion

Over the last few years there has been a significant change in the role and image of the anaesthesiologist. We are being increasingly respected as perioperative physicians and as leaders in operating room and hospital management. It only seems appropriate that this role should extend increasingly into the realm of education. For the medical student there is much to be gained from spending time with anaesthesiologists, either by reinforcing basic principles of physiology and pharmacology in the real-time operating room setting or by introducing important practical techniques such as line placement and airway support. For trainees new to our profession we need to make a commitment to afford them the highest quality educational experience and to mentor and evaluate them in a logical and meaningful manner. We have a responsibility to fuel the renaissance in our specialty from the ground up by producing impeccable role models today for the anaesthesiologists of tomorrow.

### References

1. Calman KC, Downie RJ. Education and training in medicine. Med Educ 1988; 22: 488–491.
2. McManus IC. Examining the educated and the trained. Lancet 1995; 345: 1151–1153.
3. Eagle C. Anaesthesia and education. Can J Anaesthesiol 1992; 39: 58–65.
4. Moran Campbell EJ. On education and training (letter). Lancet 2000; 356: 1116.
5. Prys-Roberts C. Role of anaesthesiologists in undergraduate medical education. Curr Opin Anaesthesiol 2000; 13: 653–657.
6. Institute of International Medical Education (undated). Available from http://www.iime.org

7. Crowley AE, Etzel SI, Petersen ES. Undergraduate medical education. JAMA 1982; 248: 3245–3252.
8. McCrorie P. Tales from Tooting: reflections on the first year of the MBBS Graduate Entry Programme at St George's Hospital Medical School. Med Educ 2001; 35: 1144–1149.
9. Australian Medical Workforce Advisory Committee (AMWAC). Innovations in medical education to meet workforce challenges. Aust Health Rev 2000; 23: 43–59.
10. Aldous CJ, Leeder SR, Price J, Sefton AE, Teubner JK. A selection test for Australian graduate-entry medical schools. Med J Australia 1997; 166: 247–250.
11. General Medical Council Education Committee. Recommendations on basic medical education. London: General Medical Council, 1980.
12. General Medical Council Education Committee. Tomorrow's doctors: recommendations on undergraduate medical education. London: General Medical Council, 1993.
13. Cheung V, Critchley LA, Hazlett C, Wong EL, Oh TE. A survey of undergraduate teaching in anaesthesia. Anaesthesia 1999; 54: 4–12.
14. Cooper G, Prys-Roberts C. Anaesthesia and resuscitation in the undergraduate curriculum. Baillière Clin Anaes 1988; 2: 243–252.
15. Working group on the misuse of alcohol and drugs by doctors. London: British Medical Association, 1998.
16. Weeks AM, Buckland MR, Morgan EB, Myles PS. Chemical dependence in anaesthetic registrars in Australia and New Zealand. Anaesth Intens Care 1993; 21: 151–155.
17. Hughes PH, Storr CL, Brandenburg NA, Baldwin DC, Anthony JC, Sheehan DV. Physician substance abuse by medical speciality. J Addict Dis 1999; 18: 23–37.
18. American Society of Anaesthesiologists Committee on Occupational Health. Model Curriculum on Drug Abuse and Addiction for Residents in Anesthesiology. www.asahq.org//curricrevFINAL040501.htm
19. Czernichow S, Bonnet F. Risk of drug dependence for anesthesiologists. Ann Fr Anesth 2000; 19: 668–674.
20. Carraccio C, Wolfsthal SD, Englander R, Ferentz K, Martin C. Shifting paradigms: from Flexner to competencies. Acad Med 2002; 77: 361–367.
21. Custers EJFM, Stuyt PMJ, De Vries Robbé PF. Clinical problem analysis (CPA): a systematic approach to teaching complex medical problem solving. Acad Med 2000; 75: 291–297.
22. Van der Vluiten CPM, Newble DI. How can we test clinical reasoning? Lancet 1995; 345: 1032–1034.
23. Custers EJFM, Stuyt PMJ, De Vries Robbé PF. Clinical problem solving and the clinical presentation curriculum (letter). Acad Med 2000; 75: 1043–1045.
24. Lambert TW, Goldacre MJ, Davidson JM, Parkhouse J. Graduate status and age at entry to medical schools as predictors of doctors' choice of long-term career. Med Educ 2001; 35: 450–454.
25. Cashman JN. Anaesthetic training for medical undergraduates. Proc Eur Cong Anaesth Warsaw, 1990, p286–290.
26. Roberts LJ, Khursandi DC. Career choice influences in Australian anaesthetists. Anaesth Intens Care 2002; 30: 355–359.
27. Yang H, Wilson-Yang K, Raymer K. Recruitment in anaesthesia: results of two national surveys. Can J Anaesthesiol 1994; 41: 621–627.
28. Wass CT, Rose SH, Faust RJ, Offord KP, Harris AM. Recruitment of house staff into anesthesiology: factors responsible for house staff selecting anesthesiology as a career and individual training program. J Clin Anesth 1999; 11: 150–163.

29. Saunders D. Anaesthetic manpower, special article 1. The anaesthetic workforce in the United Kingdom. Eur Acad Anaesthesiol Newsletter 2002; 16: 11–13.

30. Wennberg JE, Cooper MM. (eds) The Dartmouth Atlas of Health Care. Chicago, American Hospital Publishing, 1998.

31. Zeldow PB, Devens M, Daugherty SR. Do person-orientated medical students choose person-orientated specialties? Do technology-orientated medical students avoid person-orientated specialties? Acad Med 1990; 65: S45-S46.

32. Gale R, Grant J. Sci45: the development of a specialty choice inventory. Med Educ 2002; 36: 659–666.

33. Australian and New Zealand College of Anaesthetists. The process of specialist education and training. Structure and duration of training of ANZCA. www.anzca.edu.au/publications/reports

34. Tweed WA, Donen N. The experiential curriculum; analternative model for anaesthesia education. Can J Anaesth 1994; 41: 1227–1233.

35. Reeve PE. Personality characteristics of a sample of anaesthetists. Anaesthesia 1980; 35: 559–568.

36. Kluger MT, Laidlaw T, Khursandi DS. Personality profiles of Australian anaesthetists. Anaesth Intens Care. 1999; 27: 282–286.

37. Gough HG, Bradley P, McDonald JS. Performance of residents in anesthesiology as related to measures of personality and interests. Psychol Rep 1991; 68: 979–994.

38. McDonald JS, Lingam RP, Gupta B, Jacoby J, Gough HG, Bradley P. Psychological testing as an aid to selection of residents in anesthesiology. Anesth Analg 1994; 78: 542–547.

39. Lebovits AH. The identification of factors predictive of anesthesiology resident outcome. Anesth Analg 1990: 70: S231.

40. Hoffer MM, Hsu SCC. Hand function in the selection of orthopedic residents. Acad Med 1990; 65: 661.

41. Baker JD 3rd, Bailey MK, Brahen NH, Conroy JM, Dorman BH, Haynes GR. Selection of anesthesiology residents. Acad Med 1993; 68: 161–163.

42. Robin AP, Bombeck CT, Pollak R, Nyhus LM. Introduction of bias into residency-candidate interviews. Surgery 1991; 110: 253–258.

43. Kübler A. Anaesthesia in countries of central and eastern Europe – towards the EU (Guest Editorial). Eur Acad Anaesthesiol Newsletter 1999; 11: 4–5.

44. Accreditation Council for Graduate Medical Education. Residency Review Committee. Program requirements for residency education in anaesthesia. www.acgme.org/RRC

45. Ortega RA, Youdelman BA, Havel RC: Ethnic Variability in the treatment of pain. Am J Anesth 1999; 26: 429–432.

46. The Royal College of Physicians and Surgeons of Canada. General Standards of Accreditation. Ottawa, 1989.

47. Nixon MC. The anaesthetic logbook: a survey. Anaesthesia 2000; 55: 1076–1080.

48. Ruskin KJ. The internet. A practical guide for anesthesiologists. Anesthesiol 1998; 86: 1003–1014.

49. Rampil JJ. Medical information on the internet. Anesthesiology 1998; 86: 1233–1245.

50. Ortega RA, Arkoff H, Havel RC. The use of multimedia to teach new cardiac anaesthesia procedures. J Cardiothor Anesth 1998; 12: 695–700.

51. Scherpereel PA. Continuous professional development for anaesthetists. Curr Opin Anaesthesiol 1999; 12: 689–693.

52. Joint Committee of EAA and UEMS-section Anaesthesiology. Hospital visiting programme. www.eaa.euro-anaesthesiology.org/

53. Siker ES. Assessment of clinical competence. Curr Opin Anaesthesiol 1999; 12: 677–684.
54. Wass V, Van der Vluiten C, Shatzer J, Jones R. Assessment of clinical competence. Lancet 2001; 357: 945–949.
55. Miller GE. The assessment of clinical skills/competence/performance. Acad Med 1990; 65: 563–567.
56. Dauphinee WD. Assessing clinical performance: where do we stand and what might we expect (editorial). JAMA 1995; 274: 741–743.
57. Searle J. Defining competency. The role of standard setting. Med Educ 2000; 34: 363–366.
58. Fowel S, Jolly B. Combining marks, scores and grades: reviewing common practices reveals some bad habits. Med Educ 2000; 34: 785–786.
59. Solomon DJ, Reinhart MA, Bridgham RG, Munger BS, Starnaman S. An assessment of an oral examination format for evaluating clinical competency in emergency medicine. Acad Med 1990; 65: S43–S44.
60. Olson LG, Coughlan J, Rolfe I, Hensley MJ. The effect of a Structured Question Grid on the validity and perceived fairness of a medical long case assessment. Med Educ 2000; 34: 46–52.
61. Anastakis DJ, Cohen R, Reznick RK. The structured oral examination as a method of assessing surgical residents. Am J Surg 1991; 162: 67–70.
62. Kearney RA, Puchalski SA, Yang HY, Shakun EN. The inter-rater and intra-rater reliability of a new Canadian oral examination format in anesthesia is fair to good. Can J Anaesth 2002; 49: 232–236.
63. American Board of Anesthesiology. Defining clinical competence as the first step toward board certification in anesthesiology and maintenance of certification. www.abanes.org/booklet
64. Karle H, Nystrup J. Comprehensive evaluation of specialist training: an alternative to board examinations in Europe. Med Educ 1995; 29: 308–316.
65. Rosenblatt MA. Schartel SA. Evaluation, feedback, and remediation in anesthesiology residency training: a survey of 124 United States programs. J Clin Anesth 1999; 11: 519–527.
66. Schubert A. Tetzlaff JE, Tan M, Ryckman JV, Mascha E. Consistency, inter-rater reliability, and validity of 441 consecutive mock oral examinations in anesthesiology: implications for use as a tool for assessment of residents. Anesthesiology. 1999; 91: 288–298.
67. Gredler M. Designing and evaluating games and simulation: A process approach. London: Kogan Page, 1992.
68. Andrew BJ. Interviewing and counselling skills. Techniques for their evaluation. J Am Diet Assoc 1975; 66: 576–580.
69. Evensen SA, Karterud SW, Mathisen P, Sekkelsten A. Assessment of medical students' ability to communicate unpleasant news. Tidsskr Nor Laege 1997; 117: 2804–2806.
70. Norman G. The long case versus objective structured clinical examinations (editorial). Brit Med J 2002; 324: 748–749.
71. Morgan PJ, Cleave-Hogg DM, Guest CB, Herold J. Validity and reliability of undergraduate performance assessments in an anaesthesia simulator. Can J Anaesth 2001; 48: 225–233.
72. Sharp LK, Bashook PG, Lipsky MS, Horowitz SD, Miller SH. Specialty board certification: the missing link. Acad Med 2002; 77: 534–542.
73. Fox RD. New horizons for research in continuing medical education. Acad Med 1990; 65: 550–555.

74. Bashook PG, Parboosingh J. Recertification and the maintenance of competence. Brit Med J 1998; 316: 545–548.

75. Campbell CM. The maintenance of competence programme of the Royal College of Physicians and Surgeons of Canada (MOCOMP). Postgrad Med J 1996; 72 (Suppl. 1): S41–S42.

76. Eggers GWN. Continued demonstration of qualifications. Am Soc Anesth Newsletter 1990; 54: 4–6.

77. Phillips GD. Defining moments in medicine. Anaesthesia. Med J Australia 2001; 174: 17–18.

78. Wilkinson G. The future of continuing education and professional development. Roy Coll Anaesth Newsletter 1999; 45: 63–69.

79. Wilkinson G. Continuing education and professional development April 2000. The revised system. Roy Coll Anaesth Bulletin 2000; 1: 19–22.

*E. Rowland   H. Binns*

# Resuscitation

## Introduction

Resuscitation from cardiopulmonary arrest is one of the most cost-effective interventions in medicine. Unfortunately, survival after cardiac arrest remains poor despite several decades of research in advanced cardiac life support. Research itself is a highly sensitive issue in a group of patients in this situation. The ethical dilemmas of lack of informed consent, and possible withdrawal of accepted treatments in randomized trials designed to investigate new interventions are paramount. Mammalian models, primarily canine and porcine, provide one avenue for prior exploration, but definitive trial evidence in human beings requires meticulous planning, to prevent mere inclusion in a trial compromising the clinical outcome. In cardiopulmonary resuscitation, time is the crucial denominator of success, and delay created by randomization or choice of therapy is clearly unacceptable.

Despite these constraints there have been a number of significant advances in resuscitation in the last decade. There has been a change in emphasis on where, who by and with what resuscitation takes place. In recognition that the majority of arrests take place outside hospital, and that ventricular fibrillation remains the commonest rhythm at the time of arrest, resuscitation by first responders and bystanders has become the target in both the USA and Europe. Defibrillators have evolved to accommodate this ethos. Automatic External Defibrillators (AED) are capable of analyzing the surface electrocardiogram reliably and will discharge semi-automatically for an appropriate recognized rhythm so that they can be used by minimally trained individuals. Biphasic, and perhaps triphasic defibrillation waveforms are superceding the traditional monophasic waveforms, with equivalent or greater efficacy at lower energies. Pharmacological therapy built into most advanced life support protocols are being tested against alternatives for vasopressor and antidys-rhythmic action. There is also a growing recognition that a return of spontan-eous circulation (ROSC) is not the end of resuscitation, and that many interventions during and immediately after initial advanced life support have the potential to improve long-term survival and neurological outcome.

## Defibrillation

Of all interventions designed to improve survival from cardiac arrest, defib-rillation from pulseless ventricular dysrhythmia is the most efficacious. Issues of when, how, with what waveform and energy the heart is defibrillated are the focus of many new developments in cardiopulmonary resuscitation.

## Biphasic Defibrillators

Since 1962 when Lown et al.[1] showed that the human heart could be safely defibrillated with a transthoracic countershock, the majority of defibrillators have employed monophasic waveforms. Although experiments with biphasic waveforms were conducted in these early days, for the last 40 years the monophasic shock has been universal in clinical practice. Monophasic defib-rillators remain standard in the vast majority of UK hospitals and ambulances. A monophasic waveform consists of current in the positive direction only. This current either decays exponentially to give the monophasic truncated wave-form; or takes the form of a damped sine wave (fig. 1a). These different forms of monophasic waveform have similar efficacy. In biphasic waveforms the current polarity is reversed midway through the discharge to give both positive and negative current. Again this takes two forms, the truncated exponential decay (BTE) (fig. 1b) and one where the decay is attenuated to give a recti-linear biphasic waveform (BRL) (fig. 1c).

### Animal studies

Biphasic defibrillation has been studied since the early 1980s[2,3] and used increasingly since then because of the need to provide effective shocks with low energy. Implantable cardiovertor defibrillators require low energy, high efficacy waveforms to reduce generator size and increase longevity. Biphasic waveforms were shown first in animal models to have superior defibrillating properties.[4,5] Tang et al. used a pig model of ventricular fibrillation of 4 and 7 min duration to compare the efficacy and safety of biphasic (three 150-J

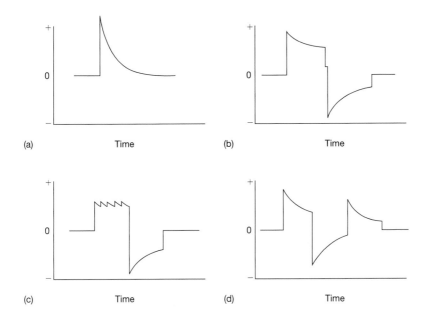

**Figure 1** Defibrillator waveforms a) damped sine wave monophasic, b) truncated exponential biphasic, c) rectilinear biphasic, and d) triphasic.

shocks) and monophasic (200-, 300-, 360-shocks) waveforms.[6] Biphasic shocks were associated with a higher rate of successful defibrillation, and significantly less impairment of myocardial function. Other workers have examined the relative effectiveness in terminating prolonged ventricular fibrillation of 10 min duration in dogs,[7] and of 5 min duration in pigs.[8] Both defibrillation threshold and resuscitation times were significantly lower in the biphasic groups.

## Electrophysiology studies in human beings

As implantation of automatic internal cardiac defibrillators has increased, so studies performed in the electrophysiology laboratory during their testing have increased our knowledge of biphasic defibrillation in man.[9,10] Randomized trials demonstrate equivalent or greater efficacy of biphasic over monophasic waveforms at the same or lower energy requirements both for internal and external defibrillation.[11–13]

In 1998, the American Heart Association reviewed the evidence for a statement on the use of biphasic defibrillation applied to advanced life support.[14] At this time there were only three reports of the use of biphasic defibrillation in out-of-hospital cardiac arrest and only one comparative study which was not randomized.[15] While they gave a class IIa recommendation ('acceptable

and useful, fair-to-good evidence provides support') for biphasic defibrillators, they emphasized that this did not imply a higher recommendation than
that for traditional monophasic devices. Despite this, biphasic automatic
external defibrillators have replaced earlier models for emergency team use
in the USA.

Further experimental work randomizing therapy between biphasic and
monophasic waveforms in implantable cardioverter defibrillator patients
supports this change.[16] Observational studies in populations where biphasic
automatic external defibrillators are now standard for out-of-hospital arrest
report higher efficacy in termination of ventricular fibrillation than from
monophasic defibrillators and comparable patient outcomes.[17,18]

### Randomized clinical trials

Finally, a randomized trial in the clinical setting of out-of-hospital ventricular
fibrillation cardiac arrest has compared fixed 150-J biphasic shocks to accelerating 200–360 monophasic shocks.[19] Automatic external defibrillators
were randomly preset to one or other waveform on a daily basis in four
emergency medical services systems. Of 338 patients with cardiac arrest, 115
had a cardiac aetiology, presented with ventricular fibrillation and received
at least one shock from an automated external defibrillator. Biphasic waveforms were more effective at terminating ventricular fibrillation (100% vs
84%, $P = 0.003$) and achieving return of spontaneous circulation (76% vs
54%, $P = 0.01$). There was a non-significant trend towards increased
survival to hospital admission, and no difference in survival to discharge.
Despite this, those defibrillated using the biphasic technology were more
likely to have good cerebral function.

The rapidly accumulating data in favour of biphasic waveforms over
monophasic waveform justify replacement of both in- and out-of-hospital
defibrillators. Research into the potential merits of triphasic waveforms
(fig. 1 d) is under way.[20]

## Myocardial Dysfunction and Defibrillation

Defibrillation is not a benign therapy. The recognition of myocardial
dysfunction after resuscitation from ventricular fibrillation has prompted
research into whether this is caused by the ischaemia or treatment given to
reverse the dysrhythmia. Early death following initial return of spontaneous
circulation can be largely attributed to heart failure and/or recurrent ventricular fibrillation. This post-resuscitation myocardial dysfunction was initially
observed in controlled studies in both pigs and rats.[21,22]

Whether the number of shocks applied, the energy level used, or the cumulative energy given is most strongly related to myocardial damage is also important clinically. Xie *et al.* performed a series of experiments on rats to investigate this.[23] Animals received precordial compression and manual ventilation of the lungs after 4 min of ventricular fibrillation and after a further 6 min were defibrillated with a single shock at either 2J, 10J, or 20J. Myocardial function, expressed as dP/dt at 40 mmHg arterial pressure, was decreased, and left ventricular diastolic pressure was increased in close relation to the energy level. Survival was also prolonged by lower defibrillation energies with means of 5, 15 and >24 h for 20, 10, 2J shocks respectively. In the same Sprague-Dawley model, Gazmuri *et al.* showed that repetitive shocks, if low energy, do not accentuate systolic dysfunction but impair diastolic function by left ventricular dilatation.[24,25]

Animal studies comparing myocardial function after monophasic waveform shocks with lower energy biphasic shocks are consistent with observations in human beings during implantation of implantable cardioverter defibrillators.[26] Reddy found significantly more ST elevation after a 200-J monophasic defibrillation than a 115- or 130-J biphasic waveform.[27]

Defibrillation at the lowest energy sufficient to terminate ventricular fibrillation should be the objective in order to reduce post-resuscitation mortality. Early work on triphasic currents suggests that 80% tilt waveforms may have lower defibrillation thresholds than biphasic ones,[20,28] but further work is needed before these waveforms are used routinely in human beings.

## Analysis of Ventricular Fibrillation Waveform

The chances of successful defibrillation from ventricular fibrillation decrease by 10% each minute from the onset.[29] As the vast majority of arrests occur outside hospital, the time needed to bring a device to the patient is likely to be at least 5 min, but more commonly 10 min or more. Ventricular fibrillation matures from coarse to fine over time, and this can help predict the likelihood of success at defibrillation. Increasing evidence suggests that in ventricular fibrillation of longer duration, perhaps as short as 4 min, the likelihood of defibrillation to a pulse-generating rhythm is increased if perfusion with chest compressions precedes the initial shock. Hence an analysis of ventricular fibrillation from the surface electrocardiogram which correlates with duration and likely outcome of defibrillation would enable emergency teams to differentiate which patients should be shocked immediately and which receive cardiopulmonary resuscitation for a few minutes first. One such form of analysis is the 'scaling exponent' which is an estimate of the fractal self-similarity dimension of the ventricular fibrillation waveform,

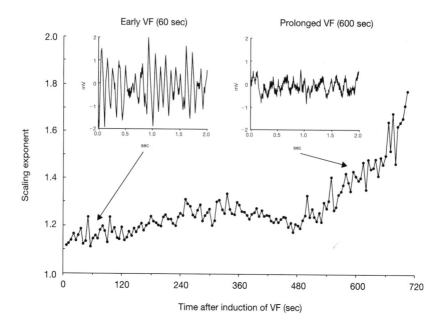

**Figure 2** Scaling exponent with early and late ventricular fibrillation (Modified from Angelos MG et al.,[30] with permission).

based on the recognition that ventricular fibrillation is chaos[30,31] (fig. 2). The scaling exponent rises gradually from onset of ventricular fibrillation (1.18 ± 0.03) through the first 5 min (1.29 ± 0.06) to a plateau at 12–14 min (1.75 ± 1.89), and is independent of variables which affect amplitude including body habitus, electrode type and placement, etc. It has been shown to predict defibrillation success for out-of-hospital ventricular fibrillation arrest in man.[32] Future automatic external defibrillators may have the ability to read and interpret the scaling exponent and direct resuscitation attempts accordingly.

## Perfusion Prior to Defibrillation

Although defibrillation is often capable of terminating ventricular fibrillation of even prolonged duration, it frequently does so by conversion to pulseless electrical activity or asystole. It is for this reason that return of spontaneous circulation and survival to arrival and discharge from hospital are the only important endpoints for any new resuscitation intervention. In one series of 1497 patients who received at least one of the first three stacked shocks as part of their resuscitation attempt ventricular fibrillation was terminated in 76%, but in 76% of these converted to a pulseless rhythm.[33] The likelihood of defibrillating to a pulse-generating rhythm declines with duration of ventricular fibrillation, and this is thought to result from prolonged myocardial ischaemia due to unperfused coronary arteries. A study in dogs compared immediate defibrillation with defibrillation after epinephrine and 90 s of cardiopulmonary resuscitation for 7.5 min of ventricular fibrillation.[34] Immediate defibrillation gave return of spontaneous circulation in 21% of animals against 64% in the pretreated group, with demonstrable increase in coronary perfusion. In swine with 8 min of ventricular fibrillation, immediate defibrillation was compared against 2 min of cardiopulmonary resuscitation and a cocktail of drugs before the first shock. This pre-perfused group resulted in a higher degree of return of spontaneous circulation (77% vs 22%) and 1 h survival (44% vs 0%).[35] Further work in pigs using both biphasic and damped sinusoidal monophasic waveforms showed greater termination of ventricular fibrillation with 6 min of prior cardiopulmonary resuscitation. 46% of pre-treated animals converted to a pulse-generating rhythm, while none of those shocked immediately did.[36]

Recently work further demonstrates the importance of prior cardiopulmonary resuscitation treatment by actually re-inducing ventricular fibrillation after defibrillation to pulseless rhythms and then defibrillating again after cardiopulmonary resuscitation.[37] Fifteen dogs were randomized into three groups after 12 min of untreated ventricular fibrillation. Group 1 was defibrillated immediately, Group 2 received 4 min of advanced cardiac life support and then defibrillated, Group 3 was defibrillated at 12 min, electrically re-fibrillated and then given 4 min of advanced cardiac life support before repeat defibrillation. All animals in Groups 1 and 3 were converted to pulseless electrical activity or asystole at first defibrillation. After 4 min of advanced cardiac life support all Group 2 and 3 animals were converted to sinus rhythm. Although Group 1 had 4 min less ventricular fibrillation, Groups 2 and 3 paradoxically had shorter resuscitation times (251 and 245 vs 459 s) and improved 1 h survival (10 of 10 vs 1 of 5).

Cobb et al. introduced a 90 s cardiopulmonary resuscitation algorithm into the standard automatic external defibrillator protocol for a population-based study of human ventricular fibrillation arrest. They compared the survival and neurological status of patients receiving this treatment to historical controls in the same emergency services catchment area.[38] Survival was improved from 24–30% ($P = 0.04$), with the majority of the benefit seen in patients for whom the initial response time was greater than 4 min (17–27%, $P = 0.01$). The proportion who survived with favourable neurological outcome also increased (17–23%, $P = 0.01$).

The cut-off for duration of ventricular fibrillation after which perfusion therapy prior to defibrillation is beneficial is not clearly defined, but believed to be around 5 min.[39] This would then apply to the majority of out-of-hospital cardiac arrests that do not receive bystander cardiopulmonary resuscitation.

## Automated External Defibrillators

The majority of cardiac arrests occur in the community and defibrillation of ventricular fibrillation remains the most efficacious intervention for improving survival.[40] It is exquisitely time-sensitive, hence the need to improve speed of access to life-saving defibrillating equipment. The automated external defibrillator has been developed to provide public access to a device that accomplishes much of the decision-making in whether a shock is appropriate, and can therefore be operated by minimally or even untrained personnel. Following spoken commands and diagrams, electrocardiogram electrodes are fitted to the chest wall of the victim and the automated external defibrillator interprets the electrocardiogram and instructs the operator to discharge a shock if applicable. These devices are now standard for many paramedical services, and available in selected public places. Specific settings in which their viability and safety have been tested are on airplanes[41,42] and in casinos.[43]

Automated external defibrillators need to have as high a sensitivity and specificity for shockable rhythms as possible.[44,45] Failure to achieve high specificity will result in pulseless electrical activity and asystole being treated inappropriately with the resultant myocardial damage as well as delay in more effective treatment. A low sensitivity would prevent patients from getting their best chance of survival. A recent retrospective analysis examined these variables by analysis of automated external defibrillator readings from cardiac arrest over a 3 year period.[46] Data was examined by both paramedics and physicians and each case individually and independently reviewed. A total of 3,448 automated external defibrillator rhythms were studied, with the primary objective the correct identification and defibrillation of ventricular fibrillation or ventricular tachycardia. Sensitivity and specificity for appropriate management of a shockable rhythm were 81 and 99.9% respectively. Positive and negative predictive values were 99.6 and 95.5%. Of the 132 errors found, 42% were automated external defibrillator dependent, the others due to operator factors.

To justify their placement in public places, and access to the lay first responder, automated external defibrillators have to be straightforward and safe to use. Gundry *et al.* undertook a study comparing the response of naïve sixth-grade children to trained paramedic teams to a mock cardiac arrest scenario.[47] The endpoint was time to successful delivery of a shock from an automated external defibrillator for simulated ventricular fibrillation. Performances were also videotaped to ensure safety of use including complying with automated external defibrillator prompts to remain clear of the mannequin. Mean time to defibrillation was $90 \pm 14$ s for the children and $67 \pm$ seconds for the paramedics. Although this difference is highly significant statistically ($P \leq 0.0001$), the real-time increase of 23 s is so small that the possibility of a successful resuscitation attempt by the children remains comparable to that of the trained personnel.

Automated external defibrillators have been shown in numerous observational studies to improve return of spontaneous circulation and survival.[48,49] In the setting of existing emergency services[50,51] and using non-medical first responders including police[52,53] there is further evidence of their efficacy, with some randomized data. Their increasing availability in the public domain for operation by lay first responders requires changes in the law limiting liability for bystander resuscitators.[54] In the United Kingdom the Defibrillatory Advisory Committee has been set up early in 2002 to implement deployment of automated external defibrillators.[55]

One outstanding issue with automated external defibrillators is what the delay time should be from a delivered shock to re-analysis that may direct a further shock. Most devices are programmed for immediate rhythm analysis, yet commonly there is a short period of electrical silence or poorly organized activity before the re-initiation of ventricular fibrillation or before sinus rhythm supervenes. Blouin *et al.* examined data from automated external defibrillators over an 18 month period in all patients who received at least one shock from an automated external defibrillator and in whom ventricular fibrillation/ventricular tachycardia recurred.[56] Twenty percent of all recurrences were within the first 6 s, 73% by 60 s and 90% by 200 s. Automated external defibrillators need to have the capacity for repeated re-analysis, and be programmed to advise their operators on contemporaneous measures such as chest compressions.

## Drugs in Resuscitation

The advanced cardiac life support drugs include epinephrine, atropine, bicarbonate, calcium and arguably lidocaine, amiodarone, procainamide and bretylium. The benefit of each of these is uncertain, in fact a prospective study of the use of these drugs during in-hospital arrest demonstrated significantly decreased survival from primary cardiac arrest for all of them ($P < 0.001$) except lidocaine ($P = 0.01$) and amiodarone which was not used.[57] Obviously, the greatest chance of a desirable outcome from cardiac arrest exists when the rhythm is ventricular fibrillation or tachycardia and defibrillation is immediately performed. These patients may achieve return of spontaneous circulation before any drugs are administered and this will greatly bias the findings of this study. As cardiac arrest becomes prolonged, the possibility of a favourable result declines and the potential for varied rhythms, aetiological diagnoses and acidosis will lead to more pharmacological input. This trial therefore, serves merely to highlight the need for randomized trials for individual drugs in the Advanced Life Support (ALS) armamentarium.

## Vasopressors

### Epinephrine

The role of epinephrine in resuscitation arises from two actions: peripheral vasoconstriction and myocardial inotropy. The former action focuses the limited cardiac output available from chest compressions into the organs of high oxygen dependency, the brain and heart. The second β-agonist mediated action makes sense for a few causes of cardiac arrest, but in most cases results in an even higher demand for work from an already ischaemic myocardium. Even in cardiac arrest of non-cardiac cause, myocardial tissue highly sensitive to reductions in coronary flow will be ischaemic post arrest. Any advantage in myocardial oxygen delivery may be offset by an increase in myocardial oxygen demand. These concerns lead to two questions: should we use high-dose epinephrine as an adjunct in resuscitation attempts unresponsive to the first few cycles of treatment? And is epinephrine the vasopressor of choice or would another vasopressor be preferable?

### High-dose epinephrine

Until the most recent resuscitation guidelines, patients not responding to the first three cycles of CPR +/− defibrillation might receive high-dose epinephrine. Early experimental work on animals and uncontrolled human studies encouraged this practice, and in a swine model it was shown that the balance between myocardial oxygen supply and demand was improved.[58] High-dose epinephrine has been shown to improve arterial diastolic pressure,[59] coronary perfusion pressure[60] success rates of resuscitation[61,62] and neurological outcome. These results motivated two randomized trials presented in the same issue of the New England Journal of Medicine in 1992. Brown et al.[63] enrolled all patients with primary cardiac arrest excepting those felt to be secondary to overdose. They were randomized to receive either epinephrine $0.02\,\mathrm{mg\,kg^{-1}}$ or epinephrine $0.2\,\mathrm{mg\,kg^{-1}}$ as their first vasopressor medication, equivalent to 1.4 mg vs 14 mg for a 70 kg man. Comprehensive outcome measures of return of spontaneous circulation, survival to hospital admission and discharge, and neurological outcome showed only a small, insignificant trend to improvement in the high-dose group. Stiell et al.[64] used higher doses still of epinephrine. Victims of cardiac arrest both in- and out-of-hospital were randomized to receive up to five doses of epinephrine either 7 mg or 1 mg at 5 min intervals according to existing protocols. Again, no significant difference was found between the high-dose group (n = 317) and the standard-dose group (n = 333) in patients surviving for 1 h (18% vs 23%), or surviving to hospital discharge (3% vs 5%). Among survivors, there was no significant difference in the proportion recovering the best category of cerebral performance (90% vs 94%). Subgroup analysis, including out-of-hospital and in-hospital cohorts, failed to identify any groups who appeared to benefit from high-dose epinephrine, and suggested that some may have worse outcomes. These two studies have largely discredited the use of high-dose epinephrine in cardiac arrest, although as an inotrope and vasopressor in peri-arrest and hypotensive crises it still has a role. A retrospective cohort study shows that the total cumulative dose of epinephrine clearly predicts unfavourable neurological outcome after cardiac arrest with ventricular fibrillation.[65]

## Alternative Vasopressors

Epinephrine has been the vasopressor of choice for over 40 years of cardiopulmonary resuscitation. Its $\beta$- and $\alpha_1$-adrenergic effects increase myocardial oxygen consumption, magnify global myocardial ischaemia and increase the severity of post-resuscitation myocardial dysfunction. Recent work searching for an alternative has concentrated on vasopressin (human anti-diuretic hormone), and $\alpha_2$-adrenergic agonist agents.

### $\alpha_2$-agonists

Early work in the 1960s used asphyxia-induced ventricular fibrillation in the dog model of cardiac arrest. Redding and Pearson studied the effects of epinephrine versus a selective $\alpha$-agonist methoxamine and found greater success with the latter.[66,67] More recently Roberts et al. examined each drug's effect on myocardial and cerebral blood flow during cardiopulmonary resuscitation in dogs.[68] Both were higher after methoxamine and were associated with significantly greater post-resuscitation cardiac output and survival.

In animals Sun et al.[69] compared the effect of $\alpha$-methylnorepinephrine (aMNE), a selective $\alpha_2$-agonist, with epinephrine and placebo in Sprague-Dawley rats. The animals were subjected to 8 min of untreated ventricular fibrillation before ventilation and chest compressions commenced. The study drugs were administered 2 min later, and at 4 min all animals were successfully defibrillated. There was no difference in resuscitation rates or coronary perfusion pressure between animals receiving aMNE and epinephrine. However, left ventricular diastolic pressure, cardiac index and $dP/dt_{40}$ were all improved by the new drug and post-resuscitation survival was significantly

**Table 1** Resuscitability and survival from VF arrest of 4 and 8 min duration after four drug regimes given during cardiac arrest

| VF | Resuscitability | Survival, h | J |
|---|---|---|---|
| 4 min | | | |
| Epinephrine | 5/5 | 8.2 ± 4 | 20 ± 8 |
| Phenylephrine | 5/5 | 41 ± 10[a,b] | 3 ± 1[a,b] |
| Epi+esmolol | 5/5 | 31 ± 11[a,b] | 6 ± 2[a,b] |
| Saline placebo | 4/5 | 12 ± 11 | 12 ± 9 |
| 8 min | | | |
| Epinephrine | 5/5 | 6.6 ± 4.9 | 26 ± 9 |
| Phenylephrine | 5/5 | 38 ± 14[a,b] | 5 ± 3[a,b] |
| Epi+esmolol | 5/5 | 30 ± 10[a,b] | 9 ± 5[a] |
| Saline placebo | 3/5 | 2.5 ± 1 | 16 ± 10 |

VF, ventricular fibrillation; epi, epinephrine.
[a]$P < 0.01$ vs epi; [b]$P < 0.01$ vs saline.

Modified from Tang W et al.,[70] with permission.

greater (all aMNE animals survived >72 h, epinephrine mean of 19 h, placebo mean of 16 h). Pre-treatment with an adrenoreceptor blocking drug-, yohimbine, abolished the effect. They conclude that aMNE is as effective for initial cardiac resuscitation and associated with markedly improved myocardial function and survival.

A further elegant study on Sprague-Dawley rats analyzed the mechanisms of post-resuscitation myocardial dysfunction seen with epinephrine.[70] Tang et al. used four different drug regimes in 40 animals after either 4 or 8 min untreated ventricular fibrillation. Ventilation and precordial compression was initiated at the time of drug administration and defibrillation was attempted 4 min later. Myocardial function, expressed as dP/dt$_{40}$, coronary perfusion pressure, number of shocks needed to terminate ventricular fibrillation and survival were the outcomes. The four drug regime were epinephrine, epinephrine with $\beta_1$-adrenoreceptor blocker, a selective $\alpha$-agonist phenylephrine, and saline placebo. The results are shown in table 1 and figure 3. Myocardial dysfunction and total energy required to defibrillate was significantly higher in the epinephrine alone group, and effect this was partially abolished by the addition of esmolol. Duration of survival was decreased in line with this. The longest survival and lowest degree of myocardial dysfunction was seen with phenylephrine. There have been no recent comparisons of $\alpha$-agonists and epinephrine in man.

## Vasopressin

Vasopressin is known to improve cerebral blood flow during cardiopulmonary resuscitation[71] but whether this is beneficial to neurological recovery

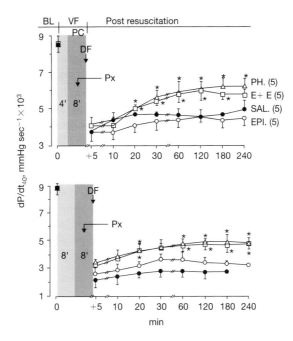

**Figure 3** Effects on recovery of myocardial function after resuscitation (expressed as dP/dt$_{40}$) of four drug regimes given during cardiac arrest. VF = ventricular fibrillation; PC = pre-cordial compression; Px = time of drug administration; DF = defibrillation; PH = phenylephrine; E = epinephrine and esmolol; SAL = saline; EPI = epinephrine alone (Modified from Tang W *et al.*,[70] with permission).

is uncertain. It has also been shown to increase coronary perfusion during human cardiopulmonary resuscitation[72] and to achieve survival in patients with cardiac arrest refractory to epinephrine.[73]

Wenzel *et al.* performed a study in the porcine model.[74] After 4 min of cardiac arrest and 3 min of cardiopulmonary resuscitation they randomly assigned animals to accelerating doses of vasopressin (0.4, 0.4, 0.8 units/kg), epinephrine (45, 45, 200 mg kg$^{-1}$ μg/kg) or placebo at 5 min intervals. As a marker of cerebral perfusion aortic diastolic pressure was recorded. This was significantly higher in the active drug versus placebo groups, and in vasopressin over epinephrine. After 22 min of arrest (with CPR from 4 min) defibrillation was attempted. All the pigs receiving epinephrine or placebo died, all on vasopressin survived ($P < 0.05$). Neurological examination at 24 h showed only an unsteady gait in these survivors. Magnetic resonance imaging of the brain showed no cerebral pathology at 96 h.

The first trial comparing vasopressin to epinephrine in man recruited 40 patients who had not responded to three countershocks in the pre-hospital setting.[75] The group that received vasopressin had 50% more admitted to hospital, and a 66% increase in those alive at 24 h.

Recently a larger randomized controlled trial in man has refuted the advantage of vasopressin over epinephrine. Stiell *et al.* tested 40 units vasopressin against 1 mg epinephrine as the initial vasopressor for in-hospital cardiac arrest, using epinephrine for all subsequent vasopressor doses.[76] No advantage was shown in survival to 1 h, to hospital discharge or neurological outcome. The authors concluded that vasopressin is not a viable alternative to epinephrine, perhaps a little surprising when there was no adverse change in outcome, and only a single dose was given such that 88% of the patients received some epinephrine. Further work substituting vasopressin for epinephrine throughout the resuscitation attempt is needed, but this is now greatly hampered in the USA by the withdrawal of the waiver of informed consent for trials of this nature.

As yet therefore, there are no large-scale comparative trials of epinephrine against alternative vasopressors in man. The animal and small human studies above provide a compelling argument for work of this nature to be undertaken. Given that over 60% of patients achieving return of spontaneous circulation in out-of-hospital cardiac arrest do not survive to hospital discharge, new pharmacology that reduces the cardiac and neurological sequelae of cardiac arrest has great potential to improve mortality.

## Antidysrhythmias

Except for the use of atropine for asystole, which itself has not been shown to improve outcome, antidysrhythmic drugs are given in cardiac arrest for ventricular fibrillation or pulseless ventricular tachycardia. Lidocaine has long been employed in this regard for resistant and recurrent ventricular dysrhythmia. This has arisen due to its proven Class 1A activity in pulse-generating ventricular tachycardia, but it has never been shown to improve outcome in cardiac arrest. Numerous other antidysrhythmics have come in and out of favour in resuscitation. Bretylium, $Mg^{2+}$, procainamide have all been used, but there is increasing evidence that they do not alter outcome, in part because of their prodysrhythmic action.

### Lidocaine

Lidocaine, while effective at terminating ventricular tachycardia, has significant negative inotropic effects on the myocardium which can be prolonged. In animal models of myocardial ischaemia lidocaine may be prodysrhythmic.[77] There is no randomized trial of lidocaine versus placebo in out-of-hospital cardiac arrest. Herlitz *et al.* performed a retrospective, non-randomized analysis of all patients with ventricular fibrillation cardiac arrest in Goteburg during a 12 year period.[78] Of 1,212 cases, lidocaine was given in 405 (33%). Factors affecting its use included whether individual staff present were authorized for its administration. Those who received lidocaine for sustained ventricular fibrillation had significantly higher return of spontaneous circulation and survival to hospital (38% vs 18%, $P < 0.001$), but survival to discharge was no different. Even in the subgroup who achieved a pulse-generating rhythm, survival to arrival at hospital (94% vs 84%, $P < 0.05$) but not discharge was improved.

## Amiodarone

Amiodarone has proven efficacy in preventing recurrent ventricular and atrial tachycardia.[79] It is one of very few dysrhythmics not associated in randomized controlled trials with an increased mortality.[80–82] In reducing mortality in survivors of sudden cardiac death and those with sustained syncopal ventricular tachycardia, it falls short of the efficacy of the implantable defibrillators,[83,84] but is safer than placebo.[85] Chronic amiodarone administration increases the energy requirements for both biphasic[86] and monophasic[87] defibrillation of ventricular dysrhythmias, shown well in patients with implantable defibrillators. This might suggest it would reduce the potential for successful resuscitation from cardiac arrest, but the electrophysiological and antidysrhythmic properties of the drug differ greatly between chronic oral administration and acute intravenous use. Intravenous amiodarone is widely used for frequent or incessant, destabilizing ventricular dysrhythmias in the hospital setting,[88–90] particularly when unresponsive to lidocaine or procainamide.[88,89]

Initial animal studies suggested that amiodarone might give additional benefit in cardiac arrest.[91] Encouraged by this, Kudenchuk et al.[92] set up the large multi-centre ARREST trial comparing amiodarone to placebo in out-of-hospital cardiac arrest due to ventricular fibrillation. Patients received either 300 mg of amiodarone or its diluent, polysorbate 80, as placebo. The hypotensive effects of amiodarone are in part due to this solvent. Qualifying criteria in 504 patients were continuing ventricular fibrillation or pulseless ventricular tachycardia resistant to the first stack of three defibrillating shocks, or recurrent after this. Average time to drug administration was greater than 20 min after multiple shocks, endotrachea intubation and epinephrine had failed to restore a viable rhythm. This seminal paper showed that recipients of amiodarone were more likely to survive to hospital admission (44% vs 34%, $P = 0.03$). It was underpowered to detect an advantage in survival to hospital discharge, but there was not even a trend to improvement (13.4% vs 13.2% for placebo). One argument against using amiodarone routinely for refractory ventricular fibrillation/ventricular tachycardia is that in this study costs are raised by higher admission rates to hospital without providing long-term benefit to patients.[93] The prolonged delay before amiodarone was given clearly raises the possibility of a Type II error, where a real and sustained survival advantage of the drug, if given early, has not been detected. ARREST is the first large randomized trial to show a benefit of any antidysrhythmic drug against placebo in out-of-hospital cardiac arrest.

## Amiodarone versus lidocaine

The amiodarone compared with lidocaine for shock-resistant ventricular fibrillation (ALIVE) trial from Toronto was published in March 2002.[94] This randomized 347 patients with ventricular fibrillation out-of-hospital cardiac arrest who either remained in the rhythm after three shocks, one dose of epinephrine and a further shock, or had recurrent ventricular fibrillation. Trial drugs were administered in a 'double dummy' fashion so that each patient received either amiodarone and lidocaine placebo or amiodarone placebo and lidocaine. Doses were $5 \, \mathrm{mg \, kg^{-1}}$ amiodarone and $1.5 \, \mathrm{mg \, kg^{-1}}$ lidocaine. The primary study endpoint was survival to admission to intensive care, with deaths recorded in the emergency department not considered admitted. Survival was 22.8% in the amiodarone group, 12.0% in the lidocaine group, $P = 0.009$. This absolute survival advantage of 10.8% equates to a number needed to treat of 10. This remarkable result was consistent across subgroups, and is despite an average time from dispatch of the emergency services to arrival on the scene of 7 min, and to drug administration of 25 min. This study provides convincing evidence for the use of amiodarone as first line antidysrhythmic medication in shock-refractory VF (fig. 4).

## Magnesium

Magnesium dilates coronary arteries, suppresses automaticity and inhibits calcium influx into myocytes, all actions that suggest magnesium supplementation could be cardioprotective.[95] This is supported by an association of low serum magnesium concentration with cardiac dysrhythmias, sudden death and reduced survival after myocardial infarction.[96] Two major studies of magnesium supplementation after myocardial infarction have had opposing conclusions. The LIMIT-2[97] study, with a remarkable sample size of 2,300 from a single centre in the UK, found a 24% improvement in mortality with magnesium sulphate given within 24 h of a myocardial infarction as bolus followed by infusion. The much larger ISIS-4[98] study found a non-significant trend to higher mortality. One proposed explanation for the failure of ISIS-4 to prove a benefit is that the magnesium was given too late, after thrombolysis, such that it was not present to protect from reperfusion injury. Subgroup analysis of the ISIS patients does not yield any significant benefit, either for those with early treatment, or for those without

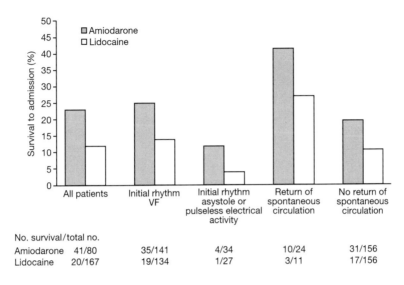

| No. survival/total no. | | | | |
|---|---|---|---|---|
| Amiodarone | 41/80 | 35/141 | 4/34 | 10/24 | 31/156 |
| Lidocaine | 20/167 | 19/134 | 1/27 | 3/11 | 17/156 |

**Figure 4** Effect of treatment with amiodarone or lidocaine on the rate of survival to hospital admission of patients with refractory or recurrent VF cardiac arrest (ALIVE study). VF denotes ventricular fibrillation. Return of spontaneous circulation refers to transient return before the administration of the study drug (Modified from Dorian P et al.,[94] with permission).

thrombolysis. LIMIT-2 did not show a reduction in dysrhythmias. Despite this, magnesium remains recommended for recurrent and refractory ventricular tachycardia, particularly in the context of hypomagnesaemia.

As an adjunct to resuscitation from cardiac arrest $Mg^{2+}$ has been tested now in both in- and out-of-hospital settings. The MAGIC trial randomized 156 patients with any rhythm cardiac arrest to receive 8 mmol $Mg^{2+}$ bolus plus 32 mmol over 24 h or placebo.[99] Standard advanced life support protocols were followed in tandem with the study drug. There was no significant difference between $Mg^{2+}$ and placebo groups in return of spontaneous circulation (54% vs 60%, $P = 0.44$) or survival to hospital discharge (21% vs 21%, $P = 0.98$). In the pre-hospital setting, Allegra et al.[100] studied 109 patients with ventricular fibrillation refractory to the first three shocks. Epinephrine and either 2 g of $MgSO_4$ or placebo were given from pre-filled syringes and acute life support protocol continued. Again, no benefit could be shown for return of spontaneous circulation (25.5% vs 18.5%, $P = 0.38$), survival to hospital admission or to discharge (3.6% vs 3.7%, $P = 1.0$). A further randomized double-blind placebo controlled study has been performed in Leeds, UK.[101] One hundred and five patients with out-of-hospital cardiac arrest and refractory ventricular fibrillation received 2–4 g of $MgSO_4$ or placebo. They found a non-significant trend to greater return of spontaneous circulation at the scene or in the Accident and Emergency Department (17% vs 13%), and to survival to hospital discharge (4% vs 2%), with an odds ratio for return of spontaneous circulation of 1.69 for patients treated with magnesium.

## Buffers

Sodium bicarbonate has been part of the arsenal of advance life support for around 35 years, but in the last decade doubts about its efficacy and indeed safety have greatly reduced its use. The 1992 American Heart Association guidelines for cardiac arrest gave it Class I status for pre-existing hyperkalaemia, Class IIa status (likely to be beneficial) for pre-existing metabolic acidosis or tricyclic overdose, Class IIb (no well-established evidence) after prolonged cardiac arrest.[102] The latest edition of AHA/ESC Guidelines do not clearly allocate sodium bicarbonate to any class, but discuss its use in various cardiac arrest scenarios.[103] This reflects the uncertainty and controversy surrounding the use of buffers.[104,105]

Severe blood acidaemia (pH < 7.1–7.2) suppresses myocardial contractility, predisposes to ventricular dysrhythmias, causes venoconstriction, and impairs oxygen delivery.[106] It is not illogical therefore, to administer exogenous buffer as an adjunct to resuscitation from cardiac arrest, in which a combination of metabolic and lactate acidosis is usual. This assumes that acidosis resulting from ischaemic injury is itself detrimental to successful resuscitation. However, there is evidence that acidification of the cellular milieu protects the myocardium from further ischaemia.[107] Furthermore, far from reversing myocardial intracellular acidosis, bicarbonate has been shown in pigs to increase the intracellular acidosis,[108,109] reduce cardiac output and lead to neurologically detrimental hypernatraemia and hyperosmolality. It also shifts the oxyhaemoglobin curve to the left, which could reduce oxygen delivery to the tissues.

## Experimental work

Animal work in recent years has aimed to resolve this dilemma. In part, the impetus for this is a realization that the massive post-resuscitation mortality from myocardial dysfunction is related to the degree of acidosis. Sun *et al.* compared three different buffers to placebo in a rat model of untreated ventricular fibrillation cardiac arrest lasting 4 and 8 min.[110] Cardiopulmonary resuscitation was commenced and either $NaHCO_3$ as a $CO_2$-generating buffer, Carbicarb® or tromethamine as $CO_2$-consuming buffers or saline placebo injected into the right atrium. After a further 2 min of cardiopulmonary resuscitation the rats were all successfully defibrillated. There was no difference in energy requirement for defibrillation. In the 4 min ventricular fibrillation group left ventricular function was significantly decreased in all animals, but less so in the Carbicarb® and tromethamine arms. This was mirrored by an increase in survival time. With 8 min of untreated ventricular fibrillation these effects were magnified and survival improved by all buffer agents against placebo. The authors conclude that while buffers may not improve return of spontaneous circulation, they may ameliorate post-resuscitation myocardial dysfunction and hence improve survival. Nevertheless, later work by the same group in the same model yielded conflicting results. In this series the degree of myocardial impairment was increased, and survival foreshortened.[111]

Bar-Joseph et al. studied the same three buffers in a dog model of prolonged ventricular fibrillation.[112] After 10 min of untreated cardiac arrest, cardiopulmonary resuscitation was commenced and epinephrine given at 5 min intervals. Buffer or placebo preceded defibrillation. Resuscitation was continued until return of spontaneous circulation for 40 min. Buffer-treated animals had higher return of spontaneous circulation (7/9 $NaHCO_3$, 6/10 Carbicarb®, 2/10 saline), and this was achieved twice as fast with sodium bicarbonate than with saline. Other workers using the dog model have confirmed these results, finding the best level of return of spontaneous circulation and survival in subjects given sodium bicarbonate in combination with epinephrine and cardiopulmonary resuscitation before defibrillation is attempted.[113]

Overall, the tide of experimental evidence is again moving towards the view that buffers improve both return of spontaneous circulation and survival in cardiac arrest. The scenarios that most support their use are in combination with vasopressors, after prolonged ventricular fibrillation arrest from 4 to 12 min, and with a short period of cardiopulmonary resuscitation before defibrillation is attempted. This picture is close to the reality of most out-of-hospital cardiac arrests.

## Human studies

Data in human beings is highly limited. A retrospective study looked at 273 patients successfully resuscitated out of a series of 619 arrests.[114] Arterial blood-gases were recorded at admission to the emergency department. Of these 273 patients, 215 received an average of 79 mmol$^{-1}$ sodium bicarbonate, while 58 had no exogenous buffer. Those receiving buffer had had resuscitation 3 times longer, and were less likely to have had ventricular fibrillation as their initial rhythm. Despite these two greatly differing prognostic factors there was no difference in survival between the groups.

The most recent prospective randomized trial performed in 1995 used the buffer mixture Tribonat[115] compared to saline placebo in out-of-hospital asystolic or ventricular fibrillation arrests not responding to the first shock. Survival to discharge was 10% in the buffer group versus 14% for saline.[116] Further randomized trials in out-of-hospital cardiac arrest setting are needed to define if and when buffers should be used.

## Out-of-Hospital Cardiac Arrest and Bystander Resuscitation

The majority of cardiac arrests take place outside the hospital, and survival in this setting can be an order of magnitude less than in hospital. Out-of-hospital arrests are less likely to be witnessed and the availability of medically trained personnel, defibrillators and drugs which may alter outcome are all subject to delays. Numerous studies have shown that survival is increased in victims of cardiac arrest who receive cardiopulmonary resuscitation from bystanders.[117–119] In the Swedish Cardiac Arrest Registry of 10,966 individuals survival rate was 2.7 times higher for those for which bystander cardiopulmonary resuscitation was attempted.[120] The King County, Washington cohort of 7,265 cardiac arrests from 1983 to 2000 report a multivariate-adjusted odds ratios of 1.45 and 1.69 for dispatcher-assisted and non-assisted cardiopulmonary resuscitation compared to no bystander cardiopulmonary resuscitation.[121]

Questions which arise from this are how to encourage bystanders to offer cardiopulmonary resuscitation, how to educate bystanders in basic life support techniques, and how to make available the necessary technology, in particular public access defibrillators. Factors likely to increase the offering of bystander cardiopulmonary resuscitation are public awareness and attitude, and the aesthetic advantage of not having to give mouth-to-mouth rescue breathing, as discussed below. Anyone is potentially a witness to cardiac arrest, hence if cardiopulmonary resuscitation training is to be prior to witnessing an event it must be universal. The only feasible way to achieve this is in schools, as suggested by Zipes.[122] As both the knowledge and the practical proficiency needed for quality cardiopulmonary resuscitation are attenuated with time, refresher courses would have to be available for individuals willing to retain these skills.

Alternatively, bystanders can be offered instructions of basic life support at the time of witnessing an arrest by the emergency services dispatchers. Dispatcher-assisted cardiopulmonary resuscitation has not been universally shown to improve outcome, due mainly to the inherent time delay in explaining techniques. When compared to outcome for victims who receive bystander cardiopulmonary resuscitation without instructions, dispatcher-assisted cardiopulmonary resuscitation gives a trend to decreased survival.[121] This however, is not a randomized study, and it is clear that bystanders feeling able to offer cardiopulmonary resuscitation without instruction may have already had some experience or training, and will begin cardiopulmonary resuscitation earlier. What is certain is that dispatcher advice greatly increases the proportion of victims who do receive bystander cardiopulmonary resuscitation, and that this therefore increases survival.

Factors that modify the effect of bystander cardiopulmonary resuscitation on survival have also been studied, and although these findings are largely predictable, they do help define where the focus on education should be.[123] Factors associated with the effects of bystander cardiopulmonary resuscitation include: the response time if the interval between collapse and the start of bystander cardiopulmonary resuscitation is short, if both chest compressions and ventilation are performed rather than either alone, if the bystander is a non-lay person, the response time of emergency medical services, the age of patients and if the arrest is outside of home. The latter is perhaps surprising given that cardiac arrest in the home has the worst outcome, in part because it is often unwitnessed.

## Alternatives to Traditional Manual CPR

The impetus to develop new protocols and new techniques for cardiopulmonary resuscitation is to improve perfusion of the heart and brain while the circulation is arrested. Approaches include interposed abdominal compression (IAC-CPR), active compression-decompression (ACD-CPR), phased thoracic-abdominal compression-decompression (PTACD-CPR), and invasive forms of cardiopulmonary resuscitation. All of these require additional personnel and/or equipment, and in most cases intensive training is necessary for effective and safe usage. Convincing evidence for their efficacy lies largely in the in-hospital setting.

## Interposed Abdominal Compression CP1R

Abdominal compressions interspersed with chest compressions can double the effective circulating volume for cardiopulmonary resuscitation alone.[124] Abdominal compression should be sited in the midline equidistant from xiphi-sternum and umbilicus, and aim to produce a pressure of 100 mmHg, similar to that needed to palpate the abdominal aorta. The technique is simplest in practice with abdominal and chest compressors either side of the patient (fig. 5). Of 17 controlled animal studies using this technique, 16 have confirmed positive haemodynamic effects compared to standard cardiopulmonary resuscitation.[125] Initial concerns over the safety of the technique, in particular a possible increased risk of vomiting or visceral trauma, have not been borne out by practice in over 400 patients.[126] In human beings there

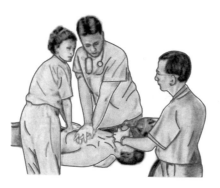

**Figure 5** Interposed abdominal compression cardiopulmonary resuscitation.

have been four randomized trials of IAC-CPR, three in hospital. The first of these showed significant improvement in return of spontaneous circulation, and survival to 24 h and to hospital discharge.[127] The second also shows improved return of spontaneous circulation and 24 h survival. Pooled data from these two studies gives a 24 h survival of 33% versus 13% for standard cardiopulmonary resuscitation. Neurological outcome was also better in the in-hospital trial patients. The pre-hospital study showed no difference in outcome.[129] The technique is not recommended as a last-ditch therapy when standard cardiopulmonary resuscitation fails. The American Heart Association recommend the use of IAC-CPR in the in-hospital environment where personnel sufficiently trained in the technique exist.[130]

## Active Compression-Decompression

The principle behind this technique is that active decompression reduces intra-thoracic pressure and hence increases venous return, 'priming the pump' for the next compression. A hand-held suction device is applied to the chest wall, and this requires some skill in its use, as well as a greater expenditure of energy on the rescuer's part. Early data showed improved haemodynamic variables of arterial pressure and vital organ perfusion, but the results from clinical trials are inconsistent. On the positive side, a French study showed one year survival rates improved from <2% to 5% by the use of ACD-CPR.[131] Other large studies[132–134] have found no significant benefit, with equal resuscitation success scores and survival of 12% and 13% for CPR and ACD-CPR groups respectively. Factors associated with improved outcome include rigorous and repetitive training. There is some concern over safety, and certainly women with large breasts and those with chest wall deformities are not suitable for this device. Overall 4 clinical studies have been favourable and 4 neutral, and it is felt that ACD-CPR has a role with suitably trained rescuers.

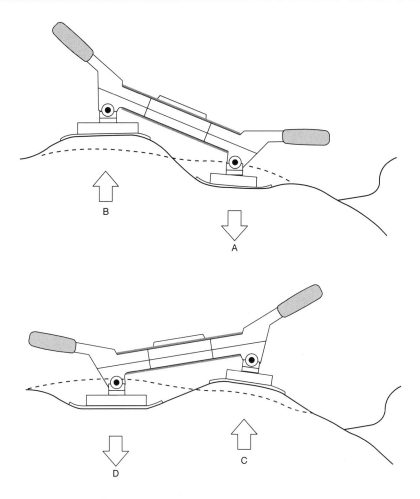

**Figure 6** The Lifestick® for phased chest and abdominal compression-decompression CPR. Chest compression (A) is coincident with abdominal decompression (B). This is followed by chest decompression (C) and abdominal compression (D) (Modified from Tang W *et al.*,[135] with permission).

## Phased Chest and Abdominal Compression-Decompression

This technique improves circulation and vital organ perfusion by combining the latter two principles. The Lifestick® (Datascope, Fairfield, New Jersey) has been devised to provide alternate thoracic and abdominal compression and decompression using a see-saw action between the two suction pads.[135] (fig. 6). Experimental studies demonstrate impressive haemodynamic effects of three-fold increase in coronary perfusion pressure, and improved cerebral blood flow and minute ventilation. This is mirrored by improved resuscitation and 72 h survival rate.[136,137] Large-scale clinical trials are underway. A German pilot study was unable to show improved survival using Lifestick CPR compared to standard CPR in human beings, but the sample size was small and there were incidental significant differences in presenting dysrhythmia and cause of cardiac arrest between the groups.[138]

## Invasive CPR Techniques

Open chest direct cardiac massage is highly dependent on experienced trained personnel present both at the time of arrest, and subsequently for aftercare. The haemodynamics of direct cardiac massage are superior to closed chest cardiopulmonary resuscitation[139] but there is no convincing evidence that this translates into improved survival, not surprising given the inevitable morbidity of urgent thoracotomy.[140–142] The few small trials in human beings emphasize that any advantage from direct cardiac massage requires that it is applied early after cardiac arrest commences, not as an endstage rescue attempt.[142] In one series of 49 patients, no survival benefit was seen from open-chest cardiopulmonary resuscitation, but this was not commenced until over 20 min of cardiac arrest had elapsed. In specific situations: cardiac arrest due to pericardial tamponade, pulmonary embolism and penetrating chest trauma, direct cardiac massage has life-saving potential and can be used by appropriately trained personnel.[144,145]

New devices for minimally invasive direct cardiac massage are under development, aiming to reduce the morbidity from a large, rapidly performed thoracotomy.[146] Through a 2 cm incision a wand-like instrument is inserted into the thorax to directly compress the heart. This technique has been shown to be relatively easily learnt by physicians of varying disciplines.[147] In animal models it produces better organ perfusion and is a promising new development in cardiopulmonary resuscitation.[148]

Emergency cardiopulmonary bypass has been used both experimentally and in small human studies.[144,145] It can be applied through the femoral vessels without need for thoracotomy. In certain situations including hypothermic arrest and that due to drug overdose, it has shown promise. There are no significant outcome studies to date.

## Ventilation Issues

### Is mouth-to-mouth breathing necessary in out-of-hospital cardiac arrest?

In the out-of-hospital setting where the majority of cardiac arrests occur, initial basic life support is likely to be provided by family, friends and other bystanders. Traditionally Basic Life Support intersperses mouth-to-mouth artificial respiration with chest compressions. The technical difficulty of performing rescue breathing in this way, combined with concerns about its aesthetic acceptability, prevent a significant proportion of victims of cardiac arrest receiving bystander cardiopulmonary resuscitation. Studies show that frequently only a third, and as low as 16% of patients suffering witnessed arrest receive cardiopulmonary resuscitation from bystanders.[149–151] Anonymous questioning of healthcare providers consistently reveals a strong reluctance to give mouth-to-mouth breathing.[152–154] From this, the question arises of whether artificial ventilation is necessary in the early stages of an arrest. Furthermore, there is increasing evidence that pauses in chest compressions necessary to allow rescue breathing result in rapid falls in coronary perfusion pressure, which then takes significant time to re-establish. Central arterial oxygenation actually remains relatively high for a substantial period after cardiac arrest.[155]

Numerous animal models have shown that although rescue breathing improves arterial oxygen saturation and pH over chest compressions alone, in ventricular fibrillation cardiac arrest there is no resultant improvement in survival.[156] In pigs, direct comparison of chest compressions interrupted for breathing (CCRB) with chest compressions alone (CC) demonstrated higher coronary perfusion pressures, marked increase in the number of chest compressions received per minute and improved left ventricular blood flow in the chest compressions group.[157] Other work in swine shows that these differences translate into a greatly improved outcome, with 12 of 15 versus 2 of 15 ($P < 0.0001$) pigs surviving neurologically intact to 24 h.[158]

Not surprisingly, in asphyxial cardiac arrest the converse is true. Experimental data strongly supports the combined use of chest compression with simulated mouth-to-mouth breathing over each intervention alone.[159,160] In real life, the cause of an arrest is rarely obvious, even to trained personnel, but nevertheless, the majority of out-of-hospital events are not primarily asphyxial, and those which are have a high chance of full recovery of around 80%.

Bystander cardiopulmonary resuscitation is often under the instruction of a telephone dispatcher. Explaining the technique of rescue breathing is complex and lengthy compared to that for chest compressions alone, prolonging downtime with no basic life support before the emergency services arrive at the scene. Studies in training lay persons on mannequin mock arrests show great advantages in the chest compression only protocol, both in circulation achieved and the time taken for cardiopulmonary resuscitation to commence.[161]

A large randomized trial has now been performed in the setting of out-of-hospital cardiac arrest in Seattle, with bystanders offered instruction by telephone dispatchers either for chest compressions alone, or with rescue breathing.[162] Survival to hospital discharge was 14.6% chest compressions compared to 10.4% rescue breathing $P = 0.18$. Instruction could be completed in 81% of the chest compression only group and 62% in the traditional cardiopulmonary resuscitation group ($P = 0.005$), and took 1.4 min longer.

Computer simulations of blood flow and gas exchange have been used to predict the quality of cardiopulmonary resuscitation with chest compressions alone, and with 5:1 and 15:2 compression:ventilation ratios.[163] As chest compressions increase blood flow and ventilation increases arterial oxygen values, an appropriate measure of cardiopulmonary resuscitation efficiency should combine these as oxygen delivery. In the early stages of cardiopulmonary resuscitation the best oxygen delivery is provided by chest compression alone, but by 4 min, hypoxia tips the balance to favouring combined cardiopulmonary resuscitation, with a 15:2 ratio better than 5:1.

Overall the prevailing opinion is that in the context of bystander cardiopulmonary resuscitation in out-of-hospital cardiac arrest chest compressions alone are at least, if not more, effective than combined with mouth-to-mouth breathing. This is in a scenario where medical help is on the way, and there is no obvious respiratory cause of circulatory arrest. In the above trial, patients who were subsequently felt to have had a respiratory primary arrest had a survival to hospital discharge of 75.7% versus 80.7% for the CC and CCRB groups respectively, $P = 0.39$. It would be ideal if it were possible to determine quickly by telephone the likelihood of a primary respiratory cause, perhaps on the basis of age. A move to this simpler protocol of cardiopulmonary resuscitation for lay bystander use increases the willingness to offer victims this life-saving intervention from 50% to over 90%.[162]

## Inspiratory Impedance Threshold Valve

The inspiratory impedance threshold valve (ITV) is a small plastic device that attaches to an endotracheal tube in situ (fig. 7). It was developed for use with active compression-decompression cardiopulmonary resuscitation. It allows the rescuer to freely ventilate the patient's lungs but impedes airflow during the decompression phase of cardiopulmonary resuscitation, hence reducing intrathoracic pressure and increasing venous return.[164] The device has been shown to improve bloodflow throughout the heart and brain when used with standard CPR[165] and especially with ACD-CPR[166] (fig. 8). In experimental studies in pigs, 24 h survival rates (17 of 20 vs 11 of 20 in control) and neurological recovery were significantly improved.[167]

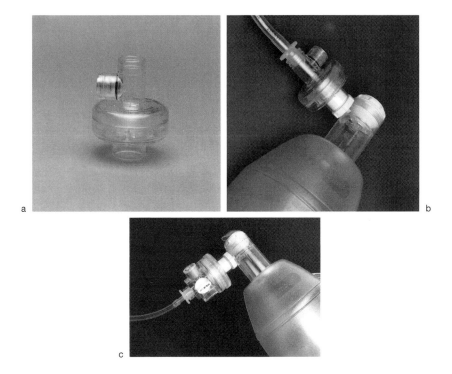

**Figure 7** Inspiratory impedance threshold valve (From Lurie K *et al.*,[164] with permission).

Work in human beings is at an early stage, but there is one randomized study in patients receiving ACD-CPR for out-of-hospital cardiac arrest.[168] Here 400 patients had either an active or a sham inspiratory impedance threshold valve attached immediately following endotracheal intubation. There were significant improvements in return of spontaneous circulation and 24 h survival and a positive trend in survival to hospital discharge. This device is likely to become common practice in cardiac arrest management, and may even be of use in the absence of endotracheal intubation.

## After Return of Spontaneous Circulation

### Aims of resuscitation

Advanced life support measures discussed above essentially concentrate on achieving a return of a pulse-generating rhythm. Success in attaining return of spontaneous circulation in out-of-hospital cardiac arrest varies in different settings from less than 3% to 33% in the USA.[149,169] However, only around 20% of these patients survive to hospital discharge, and only around 50% of these without significant neurological impairment.[170] Deaths after return of

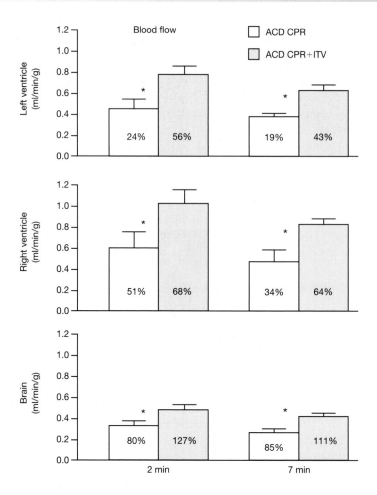

**Figure 8** Blood flow during cardiopulmonary resuscitation in a porcine model of ventricular fibrillation. Bar graphs show mean organ blood flow. CPR = cardiopulmonary resuscitation; ITV = inspiratory impedance threshold valve; ACD = abdominal compression-decompression (Modified from Lurie K *et al*. Circulation 1995; 91(6): 1629–32, with permission).

spontaneous circulation are almost invariably due to cardiovascular or neurological failure, and most occur in the first 48 h of intensive care.[171] As the organs most sensitive to nutrient and oxygen deprivation, the heart and brain function deteriorate both with circulatory arrest of increasing duration and as a result of reperfusion injury.[172] Therapies aimed at protecting these tissues in the time immediately after return of spontaneous circulation have the potential to improve survival five-fold. These therapies may be better applied during initial resuscitation, such that their protective and regenerative properties are present at the onset of reperfusion. Resuscitation can hence be thought of in two phases, return of spontaneous circulation and support for heart and brain to prevent early mortality and morbidity.[30]

> **Table 2** Potential treatments for preservation of cardiac and brain function after return of spontaneous circulation in cardiac arrest
>
> ---
>
> Use of lower energy defibrillation energies to reduce myocardial dysfunction
> Alternative vasopressors that do not increase myocardial oxygen consumption
> Hypothermia of high oxygen dependency tissues, especially brain
> Inspiratory impedance valves
> Mechanical circulatory support: Intra-aortic balloon pumps
> Cardiopulmonary bypass
> Minimally invasive direct cardiac massage
> Inotropic support (dobutamine)
> Metabolic support (Glucose-insulin-K$^+$, amino acids)
> $K_{ATP}$ channel openers
> Na$^+$/H$^+$ exchange blockers (cariporide)
> Calpain inhibitors
> Antioxidants
> Regulation of gene expression

## Potential Therapy for Preservation of Cardiac and Brain Function

Many of these treatments are experimental, in some cases theoretical without even convincing animal evidence for efficacy. Potential avenues for future development are listed in table 2. The more experimental approaches in the second half of this list are reviewed in detail in the excellent summary on resuscitation from prolonged ventricular fibrillation by Angelos, Menegazzi and Callaway.[30] Of special mention is the use of mild hypothermia, discussed below.

## Hypothermia

Several studies have shown that mild hypothermia markedly reduces cerebral damage arising from cardiac arrest in dogs.[173–176] The mechanism for this is not clear but a reduction in cerebral oxygen consumption, suppression of free radical formation, preservation of ATP content,[178] and reduction in acidosis[179] have all been postulated. Early clinical work in human beings has shown encouraging improvements in neurological recovery.[180,181] Nagao used a combination of emergency cardiopulmonary bypass, coronary reperfusion therapy and mild hypothermia in patients unresponsive to initial conventional cardiopulmonary resuscitation.[182] Mild hypothermia was induced in those with systolic blood pressures of over 90 mmHg and Glasgow Coma Scores of 3–5, and continued at 34°C for at least two days. Fifty-two percent of patients receiving hypothermia survived with good recovery. Feasibility and safety studies using external cooling blankets to induce mild hypothermia in human beings revealed no adverse outcome.[183]

The first two randomized trials to use hypothermia as an adjunct to resuscitation were reported in February 2002.[184,185] Both trials found a significant

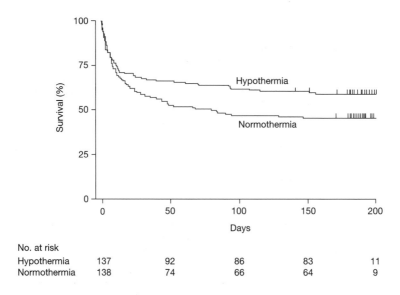

No. at risk

| | | | | | |
|---|---|---|---|---|---|
| Hypothermia | 137 | 92 | 86 | 83 | 11 |
| Normothermia | 138 | 74 | 66 | 64 | 9 |

**Figure 9** Survival of victims of cardiac arrest successfully resuscitated and alive at admission to hospital treated with and without mild hypothermia (HACA study) (Modified from ref. 184, with permission).

improvement in survival to hospital discharge with good neurological function. In the Austrian study[184] 273 patients with ventricular fibrillation cardiac arrest were included if they responded to initial resuscitation attempts achieving return of spontaneous circulation and survival to hospital admission. They were randomized to receive mild hypothermia of 32–34°C over 24 h or standard treatment with normothermia. Outcome was assessed in a blinded manner and primary endpoint was a favourable neurological outcome at 6 months. This was defined as good recovery or moderate disability and was seen in 55% of the hypothermia group, 39% of controls. Mortality at 6 months was also improved (41% vs 55%) with no increase in complications (fig. 9).

The Australian study[185] enrolled 77 patients who remained unconscious after return of spontaneous circulation from ventricular fibrillation arrest and similarly randomized them to hypothermia of 33°C or normothermia, in this study for 12 h. Outcome was sufficient recovery to allow discharge from hospital to home or a rehabilitation facility. This endpoint was reached by 43% of the hypothermic group and 26% of the normothermic patients. After adjusting for base-line differences and length of resuscitation, the odds ratio for a good outcome with hypothermia as opposed to normothermia was 5.25 ($P = 0.001$).

These two studies represent the first demonstration of clinical efficacy of any therapy in preventing brain damage after cardiac arrest.

## References

1. Lown S, Amarasingham R, Neuman J. New method for terminating cardiac arrhythmias – use of synchronised capacitor discharge. JAMA 1962; 182: 548–555.

2. Schuder JC, Gold JH, Stoeckle H, McDonald WC, Cheung KN. Transthoracic ventricular defibrillation in the 100 kg calf with symmetrical one cycle bi-directional rectangular wave stimuli. IEEE Trans Biomed Eng 1983; 30: 415–422.

3. Jene JL, Jones RE, Balasky G. Improved cardiac cell excitation with symmetrical biphasic defibrillator waveforms. Am J Physiol 1987; 253: H1418–H1424.

4. Chapman PD, Vetter JW, Souza JT, Wetherbee JW, Troup PJ. Comparison with monophasic with single and dual capacitor biphasic waveforms for nonthoracotomy canine internal fibrillation. J Amer Coll Cardiol 1989; 14: 242–245.

5. Gliner BE, Lyster TE, Dillion SM, Bardy GH. Transthoracic defibrillation of swine with monophasic and biphasic waveforms. Circulation 1995; 92: 1634–1643.

6. Tang W, Weil MH, Sun S, Yamaguchi H, Povoas HP, Pernat AM, Bisera J. The effects of biphasic and conventional monophasic defibrillation on post-resuscitation myocardial function. J Amer Coll Cardiol 1999; 34: 815–822.

7. Leng CT, Paradis NA, Calkins H, Berger RID, Laid AC, Rent KC, Kalpern HR. Resuscitation after prolonged ventricular fibrillation with use of mono- and biphasic waveform pulses for external defibrillation. Circulation 2000; 101: 2968–2974.

8. Niemann JT, Burian D, Garner D, Lewis RJ. Monophasic versus biphasic transthoracic countershock after prolonged ventricular fibrillation in a swine model. J Amer Coll Cardiol 2000; 36: 932–938.

9. Wyse DG, Kavanagh KM, Gillis AM et al. Comparison of biphasic and monophasic shocks for defibrillation using a non-thoracotomy system. Am J Cardiol 1993; 71: 197–202.

10. Winkle HL, Mead RH, Ruder MA et al. Improved low energy defibrillation efficacy in man with the use of a biphasic truncated exponential waveform. Am Heart J 1989; 117: 122–127.

11. Bardy GH, Gliner BE, Kudenchuk PJ, Poole JE, Dulack GZ, Lones GK, Anglerson J, Troutman C, Johnson G. Truncated biphasic pulses for transthoracic defibrillation. Circulation 1995; 91: 1768–1774.

12. Mittal S, Ayati S, Stein KM et al. Comparison of a novel rectilinear biphasic waveform with a damped sine-wave monophasic waveform for transthoracic ventricular defibrillation. J Amer Coll Cardiol 1999; 34: 1595–1601.

13. Greene HL, Dimarco JP, Kudenchuk PJ et al. Comparison of monophasic and biphasic defibrillating pulse waveforms for transthoracic cardioversion. Am J Cardiol 1995; 75: 1135–1138.

14. Cummins RO, Haziniski MF, Kerber RE et al. Low-energy waveform defibrillation: Evidence-based review applied to emergency cardiovascular care guidelines. Circulation 1998; 97: 1654–1667.

15. Gliner BE, Jorgenson D13, Poole JE et al. Treatment of out-of-hospital cardiac arrest with a low-energy, impedance-compensating biphasic waveform automatic external defibrillator. The LIFE Investigators Biomedical Instrumentation & Technology 1998; 32(6): 631–644.

16. Higgins SL, Herre JM, Epstein AE et al. A comparison of biphasic and monophasic shocks for external defibrillation. Prehosp Emerg Care 2000; 4: 305–313.

17. White RID, Hawkins DG, Atkinson EJ. Patient outcome following defibrillation with a low energy biphasic truncated exponential waveform in out-of-hospital cardiac arrest. Resuscitation 2001; 49: 9–24.

18. Poole JE, White RD, Kanz KG *et al.* Low-energy, impedance-compensating biphasic waveforms terminate ventricular fibrillation at high rates compared with a high-energy monophasic waveform in victims of out-of-hospital cardiac arrest. The LIFE investigators. J Cardiovasc Electrophys 1997; 8(12): 1373–1385.

19. Schneider T, Martens PR, Paschen H *et al.* Multicentre, randomized, controlled trial of 150-J biphasic shocks compared with 200- to 360-J monophasic shocks in the resuscitation of out-of-hospital cardiac arrest victims. Optimized Response to Cardiac Arrest (ORCA) Investigators. Circulation 2000; 102: 1780–1787.

20. Huang J, Kenknight BH, Roilins DL, Smith WM, Ldeker RE. Ventricular defibrillation with triphasic waveforms. Circulation 2000; 101: 1324–1328.

21. Tang W, Weil MH, Sun S *et al.* Progressive myocardial dysfunction after cardiac resuscitation. Crit Care Med 1993; 21: 1046–1050.

22. Gazmuri RJ, Weil MH, Bisera J, Tang W, Fukui M, McKee P. Myocardial dysfunction after successful resuscitation from cardiac arrest. Crit Care Med 1996; 24: 992–1000.

23. Xie J, Weil MH, Sun S, Tang W, Sato Y, Jin X, Bisera J. High energy defibrillation increases the severity of post-resuscitation myocardial dysfunction. Circulation 1997; 96(2): 683–686.

24. Gazmuri RJ, Deshmukh S, Shah PR. Myocardial effects of repeated electrical defibrillation in the isolated fibrillating rat heart. Crit Care Med 2000; 28: 2690–2696.

25. Gazmuri RJ. Effects of repetitive electrical shocks on post-resuscitation myocardial function. Crit Care Med 2000; 28(Suppl): N228–N232.

26. Tang W, Weil MH, Sun S. Low-energy biphasic waveform defibrillation reduces the severity of post-resuscitation myocardial dysfunction. Crit Care Med 2000; 28(Suppl 1): N222–N224.

27. Reddy RK, Gleva MJ, Gliner BE *et al.* Biphasic transthoracic defibrillation causes fewer ECG ST-segment changes after shock. Ann Emerg Med 1997; 30: 127–134.

28. Jung W, Manz M, Moosdorf R. Comparative defibrillation efficacy of biphasic and triphasic waveforms. New Trends Arrhythmia 1993; 9: 765–766.

29. Larsen MP, Eisenberg MS, Cummins RO, Hallstrom AP. Predicting survival from out-of-hospital cardiac arrest: a graphic model. Ann Emerg Med 1993; 22: 1652–1658.

30. Angelos MG, Menegazzi JJ, Callaway CW. Bench to bedside: Resuscitation from prolonged ventricular fibrillation. Acad Emerg Med 2001; 8: 909–924.

31. Kaplan DT, Cohen RJ. Is fibrillation chaos? Circ Res 1990; 67: 886–892.

32. Clifton W, Callaway CW, Sherman LP, Mosesso VN, Dietrich TJ, Holt E, Clarkson MC. Scaling exponent predicts defibrillation success for out-of-hospital ventricular fibrillation cardiac arrest. Circulation 2001; 103: 1656–1661.

33. Hergarten KM, Steuven HA, Waite EM *et al.* Pre-hospital experience with defibrillation of coarse ventricular fibrillation: a ten-year review. Ann Emerg Med 1990; 19: 57–62.

34. Niemann JIT, Cairns C13, Sharma J, Lewis RJ. Treatment of prolonged ventricular fibrillation; immediate countershock versus high-dose epinephrine and CPR preceding countershock. Circulation 1992; 85: 281–287.

35. Menegazzi JT, Davis EA, Yealy DM *et al.* An experimental algorithm versus standard Advanced Cardiac Life Support in a swine model of out-of-hospital cardiac arrest. Ann Emerg Med 1993; 22: 235–239.

36. Garcia LA, Allan JIT, Kerber RE. Interactions between CPR and defibrillation waveforms: effect on resumption of a perfusing rhythm after defibrillation. Resuscitation 2000; 47: 301–305.

37. Leng CT, Berger RID, Calkins H, Lardo AC, Paradis NA, Halperin HR. Electrical induction of ventricular fibrillation for resuscitation from postcountershock pulseless and asystolic cardiac arrests. Circulation 2001; 104: 723–728.

38. Cobb LA, Fahrenbruch CE, Walsh TR *et al*. Influence of cardiopulmonary resuscitation prior to defibrillation in patients with out-of-hospital ventricular fibrillation. JAMA 1999; 281: 1182–1188.

39. Cruz B, Niemann JT. Experimental studies on precordial compression or defibrillation as initial intervention for ventricular fibrillation. Crit Care Med 2000; 28 (suppl): N225–N227.

40. Cummins RO, Ornato JP, Thies WH, Pepe PE. Improving survival from cardiac arrest: the chain of survival concept. Circulation 1991; 83: 1832–1847.

41. O'Rourke MF, Donaldson EE, Geddes JS. An airline cardiac arrest program. Circulation 1997; 96: 2849–2853.

42. Page RL, Joglar JA, Kowal RC *et al*. Use of automated external defibrillators by a U.U. airline. N Engl J Med 2000; 343: 1210–1216.

43. Valenzuela TD, Roe DJ, Nichol G, Clark LL, Spaite DW, Hardman RG. Outcomes of rapid defibrillation by security officers after cardiac arrest in casinos. N Engl J Med 2000; 343: 1206–1209.

44. Jekova 1, Cansell A, Dotsinsky 1. Noise sensitivity of three surface ECG fibrillation detection algorithms. Physiological Measurement 2001; 22: 287–297.

45. Varon J, Sternbach GL, Marik PE, Fromm RE. Automatic external defibrillators: lessons from the past, present and future. Resuscitation 1999; 41: 219–223.

46. MacDonald RD, Swanson JM, Mottley JL, Weinstein C. Performance and error analysis of automated external defibrillator use in the out-of-hospital setting. Ann Emerg Med 2001; 38: 262–267.

47. Guadry J, Comess K, Ed Rook F, Jorgensen D, Bardy G. Comparison of naive sixth-grade children with trained professionals in the use of an automated external defibrillator. Circulation 1999; 100: 1703–1707.

48. Nichol G, Stiell IG, Laupacis A *et al*. A cumulative meta-analysis of the effectiveness of defibrillator-capable emergency medical services for victims of out-of-hospital cardiac arrest. Ann Emerg Med 1999; 34: 517–525.

49. Marenco JP, Wang PJ, Link MS, Homoud MK, Estes NAM. Improving survival from sudden cardiac arrest: the role of the automated external defibrillator. JAMA 2001; 285: 1193–1200.

50. Auble TE, Menegazzi JL, Paris PM. Effect of out-of-hospital defibrillation by basic life support providers on cardiac arrest mortality: a meta-analysis. Ann Emerg Med 1995; 25: 642–648.

51. Watts DD. Defibrillation by basic emergency medical technicians: effect on survival. Ann Emerg Med 1995; 26: 635–639.

52. Mosesso VN, Dam EA, Auble TE, Paris PM, Yealy DM. Use of automated external defibrillators by police officers for treatment of out-of-hospital cardiac arrest. Ann Emerg Med 1998; 32: 200–207.

53. White RD, Asplin BR, Bugliosi TF, Hankins DG. High discharge survival rate after out-of-hospital ventricular fibrillation with rapid defibrillation by police and paramedics. Ann Emerg Med 1996; 28: 480–485.

54. SoRelle R. States set to pass laws limiting liability for lay users of automated external defibrillators. Circulation 1999; 99: 2606–2607.

55. Davis CS, Colquhoun M, Graham S, Evans T, Chamberlain D. Defibrillation Advisory Committee. Defibrillators in public places: the introduction of a national scheme for public access defibrillation in England. Resuscitation 2002; 52: 13–21.

56. Biouin D, Topping Q, Moore S, Stiell I, Afilalo M. Out-of-hospital defibrillation with automated external defibrillators: post-shock analysis should be delayed. Ann Emerg Med 2001; 38: 256–261.

57. Van Walraven Q, Stiell IG, Wells GA, Hebert PC, Vandemheen KI. Do advanced cardiac life support drugs increase resuscitation rates from in-hospital cardiac arrest? The OTAC Study Group. Ann Emerg Med 1998; 32(5): 544–553.

58. Brown CG, Taylor RB, Werman HA, Luu T, Ashton J, Hamlin RC. Myocardial oxygen delivery/consumption during cardiopulmonary resuscitation: a comparison of epinephrine and phenylephrine. Ann Emerg Med 1988; 17: 302–308.

59. Gonzalez ER, Ornato JP, Ganett AR, Levine RL, Young DS, Racht EM. Dose dependent vasopressor response to epinephrine during cardiopulmonary resuscitation in human beings. Ann Emerg Med 1989; 18: 920–926.

60. Paradis NA, Martin GB, Rosenberg J et al. The effect of standard and high-dose epinephrine on coronary perfusion during prolonged cardiopulmonary resuscitation. J Amer Med Assoc 1999; 265: 1139–1144.

61. Barton CW, Callaham M. High-dose epinephrine significantly improves resuscitation rates in human victims of cardiac arrest. Ann Emerg Med 1990; 19: 490-1 Abstract.

62. Kuscove EM, Paradis NA. Successful resuscitation from cardiac arrest using high-dose epinephrine therapy: report of two cases. J Amer Med Assoc 1988; 259: 3031–3034.

63. Brown CG, Martin DR, Pepe PE et al. A comparison of standard-dose and high-dose epinephrine in cardiac arrest outside the hospital. N Engl J Med 1992; 327: 1051–1055.

64. Stiell IG, Hebert PC, Weitzman BN et al. High-dose epinephrine in adult cardiac arrest. N Engl J Med 1992; 327: 1045–1050.

65. Behringer W, Kittler H, Sterz F et al. Cumulative epinephrine dose during CPR and neurologic outcome. Ann Intern Med 1998; 129: 450–456.

66. Redding JS, Pearson JW. Resuscitation for ventricular fibrillation. JAMA 1968; 203: 255–260.

67. Redding JS, Pearson JW. Evaluation of drugs for cardiac resuscitation. Anaesthesia 1963; 24: 203–207.

68. Roberts D, Landolfo K, Dobson K, Light BR. The effects of methoxamine and epinephrine on survival and regional distribution of cardiac output in dogs with prolonged ventricular fibrillation. Chest 1990; 98: 999–1005.

69. Sun S, Weil MH, Tang W, Kamoham T, Klouche K. Alphal-methylnorepinephrine, a selective alpha2-adrenergic agonist for cardiac resuscitation. J Amer Coll Cardiol 2001; 37(3): 951–956.

70. Tang W, Weil MH, Sun S, Noc M, Yang L, Gazmuri RJ. Epinephrine increases the severity of post-resuscitation myocardial dysfunction. Circulation 1995; 92: 3089–3093.

71. Lindner KH, Brinkmann A, Pfenninger EG, Lurie KG, Goertz A, Lindner IM. Effect of vasopressin on haemodynamic viability, organ blood flow and acid-base status in a pig model of cardiopulmonary resuscitation. Anaesth Analg 1993; 77: 427–435.

72. Morris DC, Dereczyk BE, Gryborski M et al. Vasopressin can increase coronary perfusion pressure during human cardiopulmonary resuscitation. Acad Emerg Med 1997; 4: 878–883.

73. Lindner KH, Prengel AW, Brinkmann A, Strohmenger HU, Lindner IM, Lurie KG. Vasopressin administration in refractory cardiac arrest. Ann Intern Med 1996; 124: 1061–1064.

74. Wenzel V, Lindner KH, Krismer AC *et al.* Survival with full neurological recovery and no cerebral pathology after prolonged cardiopulmonary resuscitation with vasopressin in pigs. J Amer Coll Cardiol 2000; 35(2): 527–533.

75. Lindner KH, Dirks B, Strohmenger HU, Prengel AW, Lindner IM, Lurie KG. Randomized comparison of epinephrine and vasopressin in patients with out-of-hospital ventricular fibrillation. Lancet 1997; 349: 535–537.

76. Stiell IG, Hebert PC, Wells GA *et al.* Vasopressin versus epinephrine in in-hospital cardiac arrest: a randomized controlled trial. Lancet 2001; 258(9276): 105–109.

77. Aupetit JF, Timour Q, Loufoua-Moundanga J *et al.* Pro-fibrillatory effects of lidocaine in the acutely ischaemic porcine heart. J Cardiovasc Pharmacol 1995; 25: 810–816.

78. Herlitz J, Ekstr6m IL, Wennerblom B *et al.* Lidocaine in out-of-hospital ventricular fibrillation: does it improve survival? Resuscitation 1997; 33: 199–205.

79. Lee KIL, Tai YT. Long-term low-dose amiodarone therapy in the management of ventricular and supraventricular tachyarrhythmias: efficacy and safety. Clin Cardiol 1997; 20(4): 373–377.

80. Julian DG, Camm AJ, Frangin G, Janse MJ, Munoz A, Schwatz PJ, Simm P. Randomized trial of effect of amiodarone on mortality in patients with left-ventricular dysfunction after recent myocardial infarction: EMIAT: European Myocardial Infarct Amiodarone Trial Investigators. Lancet 1997; 349(9053): 667–674.

81. Cairns JA, Connolly SJ, Roberts R, Gent M, for the Canadian Amiodarone Myocardial Infarction Arrhythmia Trial (CAMIAT) Investigators. Randomized trial of outcome after myocardial infarction in patients with frequent or repetitive ventricular premature depolarizations. Lancet 1997; 349: 675–682.

82. Kuck K-H, Cappato R, Siebels J, Ruppel R. Randomized comparison of antiarrhythmic drug therapy with implantable defibrillators in patients resuscitated from cardiac arrest: The Cardiac Arrest Study Hamburg (CASH) Circulation 2000; 102: 748–754.

83. The AVID Investigators. A comparison of anti-arrhythmic-drug therapy with implantable defibrillators in patients resuscitated from near-fatal ventricular arrhythmias. N Engl J Med 1997; 337: 1576–1583.

84. Moss AJ, Hall WJ, Cannom DS *et al.* Improved survival with an implanted defibrillator in patients with coronary disease at high risk for a ventricular arrhythmia. N Engl J Med 1996; 335: 1933–1940.

85. Sim I, McDonald KM, Lavori DW, Norbutas CM, Hlatky MA. Quantitative overview of randomized trials of amiodarone to prevent sudden cardiac death. Circulation 1997; 96(9): 2823–2827.

86. Nielsen JD, Hamden MH, Kowal RC, Barbera SJ, Page RL, Joglar JA. Effect of acute amiodarone loading on energy requirements for biphasic ventricular defibrillation. Am J Cardiol 2001; 88: 446–448.

87. Zhou L, Chen BP, Kluger J, Fan C, Chow MS. Effects of amiodarone and its active metabolite desethylamiodarone on the ventricular defibrillation threshold. J Amer Coll Cardiol 1998; 31: 1672–1678.

88. Kowey PR, Levine JH, Herne JM *et al.* Randomized, double-blind comparison of intravenous amiodarone and bretylium in the treatment of patients with recurrent, haemodynamically destabilizing ventricular tachycardia or fibrillation. Circulation 1995; 92: 3255–3263.

89. Levine JH, Massumi A, Scheiman MM *et al.* Intravenous amiodarone for recurrent sustained hypotensive ventricular tachycardias. J Amer Coll Cardiol 1996; 27: 67–75.

90. Scheinman MM, Levine JH, Cannom DS *et al*. Dose-ranging study of intravenous amiodarone in patients with life-threatening ventricular tachyarrhythmias. 1Circulation 1995; 92: 3264–3272.

91. Anastasiou-Nana MI, Nanas JN, Nans SN *et al*. Effects of amiodarone on refractory ventricular fibrillation in acute myocardial infarction: experimental study. J Am Coll Cardiol 1994; 23: 253–258.

92. Kudenchuk PJ, Cobb LA, Copass MK *et al*. Amiodarone for resuscitation after out-of-hospital cardiac arrest due to ventricular fibrillation. N Engl J Med 2000; 341: 871–878.

93. Ballew KA, Philbrick JT. Amiodarone in out-of-hospital cardiac arrest. Letter in N Engl J Med 2000; 342: 216–217.

94. Dorian P, Cass D, Schwartz B, Cooper R, Gelaznikes R, Barr A. Amiodarone as compared with lidocaine for shock-resistant ventricular fibrillation. N Engl J Med 2002; 346: 884–890.

95. Woods KI—. Possible pharmacological actions of magnesium in acute myocardial infarction. Br J Clin Pharmacol 1991; 32: 3–10.

96. Gettes LS. Electrolyte abnormalities underlying lethal ventricular arrhythmias. Circulation 1992; 85(Suppl): 170–185.

97. Woods KL, Fletcher S, Roffe C, Haider Y. Intravenous magnesium sulphate in suspected acute myocardial infarction: results of the second Leicester Intravenous Magnesium Intervention Trial (LIMIT-2). Lancet 1992; 339: 1553–1558.

98. ISIS-4 (Fourth International Study of Infract survival) Collaborative Group. ISIS-4: a randomized factorial trial assessing early oral captopril, oral mononitrate, and intravenous magnesium sulphate in 58050 patients with suspected acute myocardial infarction. Lancet 1995; 345: 669–685.

99. Thel MC, Armstrong AL, McNuity SE, Califf RM, O'Conner CM. Randomized trial of magnesium in in-hospital cardiac arrest. Lancet 1997; 350: 1272–1276.

100. Allegra J, Lavery R, Cody R *et al*. Magnesium sulphate in the treatment of refractory ventricular fibrillation in the pre-hospital setting. Resuscitation 2001; 49(3): 245–249.

101. Hassan TB, Jagger C, Barnett D13. A randomized trial to investigate the efficacy of magnesium sulphate for refractory ventricular fibrillation. Emerg Med J 2002; 19: 57–62.

102. AHA: Guidelines for cardiopulmonary resuscitation and emergency cardiac care. JAMA 1992: 268: 2171–2295.

103. AHA/ECC Guidelines 2000. Part 6: Advanced Cardiovascular Life Support. Section 6: Pharmacology ]I: Agents to optimize cardiac output and blood pressure. Circulation 2000; 102 (Suppl): 1291.

104. Bar-Joseph G. Is bicarbonate therapy during cardiopulmonary resuscitation really detrimental? Crit Care Med 2000; 28: 1693–1694. Letter.

105. Levy MM. An evidence-based evaluation of the use of sodium bicarbonate during cardiopulmonary resuscitation. Crit Care Clinics 1998; 14: 457–483.

106. Kraut JA, Kurtz L. Use of base in the treatment of severe acidaemic states. Amer J Kidney Dis 2001; 38: 703–727.

107. Bing OH, Brooks WW, Messer TV. Heart muscle viability following hypoxia: protective effects of acidosis. Science 1973; 180: 1297–1298.

108. Gazmuri RJ, von Planta M, Weil MH *et al*. Cardiac effects of carbon dioxide-generating and carbon dioxide-consuming buffers during cardiopulmonary resuscitation. J Am Coll Cardiol 1990; 15: 482–490.

109. Kette F, Weil MH, von Planta M *et al*. Buffer agents do not reverse intramyocardial acidosis during cardiac resuscitation. Circulation 1990; 81: 1660–1666.

110. Sun S, Weil MH, Tang W, Fukui M. Effects of buffer agents on post-resuscitation myocardial dysfunction. Crit Care Med 1996; 24: 2035–2041.

111. Sun S, Weil MH, Povoas HP, Mason E. Combined effects of buffer and adrenergic agents on postresuscitation myocardial dysfunction. J Pharm Experimental Therapeutics 1999; 291: 773–777.

112. Bar-Joseph G, Weinberger T, Castel T, Bar-Joseph N, Laor A, Bursztein S, Ben Haim S. Comparison of sodium bicarbonate, CarbicarbO, and THAM during cardiopulmonary resuscitation in dogs. Crit Care Med 1998; 26: 1397–1408.

113. Leong ECM, Bendall TC, Boyd AC, Einstein R. Sodium bicarbonate improves the chances of resuscitation after ten minutes of cardiac arrest in dogs. Resuscitation 2001; 51(3): 309–315.

114. Bjerneroth G. Tribonat O – A comprehensive summary of its properties. Crit Care Med 1999; 27: 1009–1013.

115. Aufderheide TP, Martin DR, Olson DW *et al*. Prehospital bicarbonate use in cardiac arrest: a three-year experience. Am J Emerg Med 1992; 10: 4–7.

116. Dybvik T, Strand T, Steen PA. Buffer therapy during out-of-hospital cardiopulmonary resuscitation. Resuscitation 1995; 29: 89–95.

117. Eisenburg MS, Bergner L, Hallstrom A. Cardiac resuscitation in the community: importance of rapid provision and implications of program planning. JAMA 1979; 241: 1905–1907.

118. Cummins RO, Eisenberg MS. Pre-hospital cardiopulmonary resuscitation: is it effective? JAMA 1985; 253: 2408–2412.

119. Waalewijn RA, de Vos R, Koster RW. Out-of-hospital cardiac arrests in Amsterdam and its surrounding areas: results from the Amsterdam resuscitation study (ARREST) in 'Utstein' style. Resuscitation 1998; 38: 157–167.

120. Holmberg M, Holmberg S, Herlitz J. The problem of out-of-hospital cardiac arrest prevalence of sudden death in Europe today. Am J Cardiol 1999; 83: 88D–90D.

121. Rea TD, Eisenberg MS, Culley LL, Becker L. Dispatcher-assisted cardiopulmonary resuscitation and survival in cardiac arrest. Circulation 2001: 104: 2513–2516.

122. Zipes DP. Saving time saves lives. Circulation 2001; 104: 2506–2508.

123. Holmberg M, Holmberg S, Herlitz for the Swedish Cardiac Arrest Registry. Factors modifying the effect of bystander cardiopulmonary resuscitation on survival in out-of-hospital cardiac arrest patients in Sweden. Eur Heart J 2001; 22: 511–519.

124. Babbs CF, Ralston SH, Geddes LA. Theoretical advantages of abdominal counterpulsation in CPR as demonstrated in a simple electrical model of the circulation. Ann Emerg Med 1984; 22: 499–506.

125. Kern KB, Paraskos JA. Co-chairs of Task Force 1: Cardiac Arrest. In 31st Bethesda Conference: Emergency Cardiac Care (1999). J Am Coll Cardiol 2000; 35(4): 833–846.

126. Sack JB, Kesselbrenner MB. Haemodynamics, survival benefits and complications of interposed abdominal compression during cardiopulmonary resuscitation. Acad Emerg Med 1994; 1: 490–497.

127. Sack JB, Kesselbrenner MB, Jarrad A. Interposed abdominal compression cardiopulmonary resuscitation and resuscitation outcome during asystole and electromechanical dissociation. Circulation 1992; 86: 1692–1700.

128. Sack JB, Kesselbrenner MB, Bregman D. Survival from in-hospital cardiac arrest with interposed abdominal counterpulsation during cardiopulmonary resuscitation. JAMA 1992; 267: 379–385.

129. Mateer JR, Stueven HA, Thompson BM, Aprahamian C, Darin JC. Prehospital IAC-CPR versus standard CPR: paramedic resuscitation of cardiac arrests. Am J Emerg Med 1985; 3: 143–146.

130. AHA/ECC Guidelines 2000. Part 6: Advanced Cardiovascular Life Support. Section 4: Devices to assist circulation. Circulation 2000; 102(Suppl): 1051.

131. Plaisance P, Lurie KG, Vicaut E *et al*. A comparison of standard cardiopulmonary resuscitation and active compression-decompression resuscitation for out-of-hospital cardiac arrest. French Active Compression-Decompression cardiopulmonary Resuscitation Group. N Engl J Med 1999; 341: 1893–1899.

132. Sikogvoll E, Wik L. Active compression-decompression cardiopulmonary resuscitation: a population-based, prospective randomized clinical trial in out-of-hospital cardiac arrest. Resuscitation 1999; 42: 163–172.

133. Stiell IG, Hebert PC, Wells GA *et al*. The Ontario trial of active compression decompression cardiopulmonary resuscitation for in-hospital and pre-hospital cardiac arrest. JAMA 1996; 275: 1417–1423.

134. Schwab TIVI, Callaham IVIL, Madsen CD, Utecht TA. A randomized clinical trial of active compression-decompression CPR vs. standard CPR in out-of-hospital cardiac arrest in two cities. JAMA 1995; 273: 1261–1268.

135. Tang W, Weil MH, Shock R *et al*. Phased chest and abdominal compression decompression: a new option for cardiopulmonary resuscitation. Circulation 1997; 95: 1335–1340.

136. Wenzel V, Lindner KH, Prengel AW *et al*. Effect of phased chest and abdominal compression-decompression cardiopulmonary resuscitation on myocardial and cerebral blood flow in pigs. Crit Care Med 2000; 28: 1107–1112.

137. Sterz F, Behringer W, Berzianovich A *et al*. Active compression-decompression of thorax and abdomen (Lifestic & CPR) in patients with cardiac arrest. Circulation 1996; 94(Suppl I): 1–9.

138. Arntz H-R, Agrawal R, Richter H *et al*. Phased chest and abdominal compression decompression versus conventional cardiopulmonary resuscitation in out-of-hospital cardiac arrest. Circulation 2001; 104: 768–772.

139. Robertson C. The value of open chest CPR for non-traumatic cardiac arrest. Resuscitation 1991; 22: 203–208.

140. Babbs CF. Hemodynamic mechanisms in CPR: theoretical rationale for resuscitative thoracotomy in non-traumatic cardiac arrest. Resuscitation 1987; 15: 37–50.

141. Kern KB, Sandersab, Badylak SF, Janas W, Carter AB, Tacker WA, Ewy GA. Long-term survival with open-chest cardiac massage after ineffective closed-chest compression in a canine preparation. Circulation 1987; 75: 498–503 [Abstract].

142. Takino M, Okada Y. The optimum timing of resuscitative thoracotomy for non-traumatic out-of-hospital cardiac arrest. Resuscitation 1993; 26: 69–74.

143. Geehr EC, Lewis FR, Auerbach PS. Failure of open-heart massage to improve survival after pre-hospital non-traumatic cardiac arrest. N Engl J Med 1986; 314: 1189–1190.

144. Cogbill TH, Moore EE, Millikan JS, Cleveland HC. Rationale for selective application of emergency department thoracotomy in trauma. J Traumal 1983; 23: 453–460.

145. Danne PD, Finelli F, Champion HR. Emergency bay thoracotomy. J Trauma 1984; 24: 796–802.

146. Eynon CA. Minimally invasive direct cardiac massage and defibrillation. Resuscitation 200; 47: 325–328.

147. Hanouz J-L, Thuaudet S, Ramakers M, Bessodes A, Charbonneau P, Gerard J-L, Bricard H. Insertion of the minimally invasive direct cardiac massage device (MIDCM): training on human cadavers. Resuscitation 2002; 52: 49–53.

148. Paiva EF, Kern KB, Hilwig RW, Scalabrini A, Ewy GA. Minimally invasive direct cardiac massage versus closed-chest cardiopulmonary resuscitation in a porcine

model of prolonged ventricular fibrillation cardiac arrest. Resuscitation 2000; 47: 287–299.

149. Lombardi G, Gallagher J, Gennis P. Outcome of out-of-hospital cardiac arrest in New York City: the Pre-Hospital Arrest Survival Evaluation (PHASE) Study. JAMA 1994; 271: 678–683.

150. Bossaert L, van Hoeyweghen RJ et al. Bystander cardiopulmonary resuscitation in out-of-hospital cardiac arrest. The Cerebral Resuscitation Study Group. Resuscitation 1989; 17(Suppl): S55–S69.

151. Becker LB, Berg RA, Pepe PE et al. A reappraisal of mouth-to-mouth ventilation during bystander-initiated cardiopulmonary resuscitation: a statement for healthcare professionals from the ventilation working group of the basic life support and pediatric life support subcommittees, American Heart Association. Circulation 1997; 96: 2102–2112.

152. Ornato JP, Hallagan LF, McMahan S13 et al. Attitudes of BLS instructors about mouth-to-mouth resuscitation during the AIDS epidemic. Ann Emerg Med 1990; 19: 151–156.

153. Brenner BE, Kaufl`man J. Reluctance of internists and medical nurse to perform mouth-to-mouth resuscitation. Arch Intern Med 1993; 153: 1763–1769.

154. Locke CJ, Berg RA, Sanders AB et al. Bystander cardiopulmonary resuscitation: Concerns about mouth-to-mouth contact. Arch Intern Med 1995; 155: 938–943.

155. Meusing BTJ, Zimmerman ANE, van Heyst ANP. Experimental evidence in favor of a reversed sequence in cardiopulmonary resuscitation. J Am Coll Cardiol 1983; 1: 610. Abstract.

156. Berg RA, Kern KB, Sanders AB, Otto CW, Hilwig RW, Ewy GA. Bystander cardiopulmonary resuscitation: Is ventilation necessary? Circulation 1993; 88: 1907–1915.

157. Berg RA, Sanders AB, Kern KB, Hilwig RW, Heidenreich JW, Porter ME, Ewy GA. Adverse haemodynamic effects of interrupting chest compressions for rescue breathing during cardiopulmonary resuscitation for ventricular fibrillation cardiac arrest. Circulation 2001; 104: 2465–2472.

158. Kern KB, Hilwig RW, Berg RA, Sanders AB, Ewy GA. Importance of continuous chest compressions during cardiopulmonary resuscitation: Improved outcome during a simulated single lay-rescuer scenario. Circulation 2002; 105: 645–649.

159. Berg RA, Hilwig RW, Kern KB et al. Simulated mouth-to-mouth ventilation and chest compressions ("bystander") CPR improves outcome in a swine model of pre-hospital pediatric asphyxial cardiac arrest. Crit Care Med 1999; 27: 1893–1899.

160. Berg RA, Hilwig RW, Kern KB et al. "Bystander" chest compressions and assisted ventilation independently improve outcome from piglet asphyxial pulseless "cardiac arrest". Circulation 2000; 101: 1743–1748.

161. Kern KB. Cardiopulmonary resuscitation without ventilation. Crit Care Med 2000; 28(Suppl): N186–N189.

162. Halistrom A, Cobb L, Johnson E, Copass M. Cardiopulmonary resuscitation by chest compression alone or with mouth-to-mouth ventilation. N Engl J Med 2000; 342: 1546–1553.

163. Turner L, Turner S, Armstrong V. Does the compression to ventilation ratio affect the quality of CPR: a simulation study. Resuscitation 2002; 52: 55–62.

164. Lurie K, Zielinski T, McKnite S, Sukhum P. Improving the efficiency of cardiopulmonary resuscitation with an inspiratory impedance threshold valve. Crit Care Med. 2000; 28(Suppl): N207–N209.

165. Lurie KG, Mulligan K, McKnite S et al. Optimizing standard cardiopulmonary resuscitation with an inspiratory threshold valve. Chest 1998; 113: 1084–1090.

166. Plaisance P, Lurie K, Payen D. Inspiratory impedance during active compression decompression cardiopulmonary resuscitation: a randomized evaluation in patients in cardiac arrest. Circulation 2000; 101: 989–994.

167. Lurie KG, Zielinski TM, McKnite SH, Aufderheide T, Voeickel W. Use of an inspiratory impedance valve impoves neurologically intact survival in a porcine model of ventricular fibrillation. Circulation 2001; 104(Suppl II): Abstract 3608.

168. Plaisance P, Lurie KG, Ducros L, Payen. Comparison of an active versus sham impedance threshold valve on survival in patients receiving active compression decompression cardiopulmonary resuscitation for out-of-hospital cardiac arrest. Circulation 2001; 104(Suppl I): Abstract 3605.

169. Eisenberg MS, Horwood BT, Cummins RG, Reynolds-Haertle R, Hearne TR. Cardiac arrest and resuscitation: a tale of 29 cities. Ann Emerg Med 1990; 19: 179–186.

170. Callaway CW. Improving neurologic outcomes after out-of-hospital cardiac arrest. Prehosp Emerg Care 1997; 1: 45–54.

171. De Vos R, De Haes HC, Koster RW, De Hann RJ. Quality of survival after cardiopulmonary resuscitation. Arch Intern Med 1999; 159: 249–254.

172. Negovsky LIA. Post-resuscitation disease. Crit Care Med 1988; 16: 942–952.

173. Leonov Y, Sterz F, Safar P et al. Mild cerebral hypothermia during and after cardiac arrest improves neurologic outcome in dogs. J Cereb Blood Flow Metab 1990; 10: 57–70.

174. Sterz F, Safar P, Tisherman S, Radovsky A, Kuboyama K, Oku K. Mild hypothermic cardiopulmonary resuscitation improves outcome after prolonged cardiac arrest in dogs. Crit Care Med 1991; 19: 379–389.

175. Safar P, Xiao F, Raddovsky A et al. Improved cerebral resuscitation from cardiac arrest in dogs with mild hypothermia plus blood flow promotion. Stroke 1996; 27: 105–113.

176. Behringer W, Pruechner S, Safar P et al. Rapid induction of mild cerebral hypothermia by cold aortic flush achieves normal recovery in a dog outcome model with 20-minute exsanguination cardiac arrest. Acad Emerg Med 2000; 7: 1341–1348.

177. Mezrow CK, Sadeghi AM, Gandsas A et al. Cerebral blood flow and metabolism in hypothermic circulatory arrest. Ann Thorac Surg 1992; 54: 609–615.

178. Kramer RS, Sanders AP, Leasage AM, Woodhall B, Seals WC. The effect of profound hypothermia on preservation of cerebral ATP content during circulatory arrest. J Thorac Cardiovasc Surg 1968; 56: 699–709.

179. Chopp M, Knight R, Tidwell CD, Helpen JA, Brown E, Welch KM. The metabolic effects of mild hypothermia on global cerebral ischaemia and recirculation in the cat: comparison to normothermia and hyperthermia. J Cereb Blood Flow Metab 1989; 9: 141–148.

180. Yanagawa Y, Ishihara S, Norio H et al. Preliminary clinical outcome study of mild resuscitative hypothermia after out-of-hospital cardiopulmonary arrest. Resuscitation 1998; 39: 61–66.

181. Zeiner A, Hoizer M, Sterz F et al. Mild resuscitative hypothermia to improve neurological outcome after cardiac arrest: a clinical feasibility trial. Stroke 2000; 31: 86–94.

182. Nagao K, Hayash N, Kanmatsise K et al. Cardiopulmonary cerebral resuscitation using emergency cardiopulmonary bypass, coronary reperfusion therapy and mild hypothermia in patients with cardiac arrest outside the hospital. J Amer Coll Cardiol 2000; 36: 776–783.

183. Felberg RA, Krieger DW, Chuang R. Hypothermia after cardiac arrest. Feasibility and safety of an external cooling protocol. Circulation 2001; 104: 1799–1803.

184. The hypothermia after Cardiac Arrest (HACA) Study Group. Mild therapeutic hypothermia to improve the neurologic outcome after cardiac arrest. N Engl J Med 2002; 346: 549–556.

185. Bernard SA, Gray TW, Buist MID, Jones BM, Silvester W, Gutteridge G, Smith K. Treatment of comatose survivors of out-of-hospital cardiac arrest with induced hypothermia. N Engl J Med 2002; 346: 557–563.

# Index